FAMILY PRACTICE REVIEW

FAMILY

PRACTICE

REVIEW

A PROBLEM ORIENTED APPROACH

SECOND EDITION

RICHARD W. SWANSON, B.S.C., M.D., C.C.F.P.

PROFESSOR OF FAMILY MEDICINE

AND

DIRECTOR, DIVISION OF CONTINUING MEDICAL EDUCATION

UNIVERSITY OF SASKATCHEWAN

SASKATOON, SASKATCHEWAN

1991

B.C. Decker Inc. · Philadelphia · Hamilton

Publisher : B.C. Decker Inc
320 Walnut Street
Suite 400
Philadelphia, Pennsylvania 19106
U.S.A.

Sales and Distribution

United States and Puerto Rico
Mosby-Year Book Inc.
11830 Westline Industrial Drive
Saint Louis, Missouri 63146

Canada
Mosby-Year Book Limited
5240 Finch Avenue E., Unit 1
Scarborough, Ontario M1S 5A2

Australia
McGraw-Hill Book Company Australia Pty. Ltd.
4 Barcoo Street
Roseville East 2069
New South Wales, Australia

Brazil
Editora McGraw-Hill do Brasil, Ltda.
rua Tabapua, 1.105, Itaim-Bibi
Sao Paulo, S.P. Brasil

Columbia
**Interamericana/McGraw-Hill de Colombia,
S.A.**
Apartado Aereo 81078
Bogota, D.E., Colombia

Europe
McGraw-Hill Book Company GmbH
Lademannbogen 136
D-2000 Hamburg 63
West Germany

France
MEDSI/McGraw-Hill
6, avenue Daniel Lesueur
75007 Paris, France

Hong Kong and China
McGraw-Hill Book Company
Suite 618, Ocean Centre
5 Canton Road
Tsimshatsui, Kowloon
Hong Kong

India
Tata McGraw-Hill Publishing Company, Ltd.
12/4 Asaf Ali Road, 3rd Floor
New Delhi 110002, India

Indonesia
Mr. Wong Fin Fah
P.O. Box 122/JAT
Jakarta, 1300 Indonesia

Italy
McGraw-Hill Libri Italia, s.r.l.
Piazza Emilia, 5
I-20129 Milano MI
Italy

Japan
Igaku-Shoin Ltd.
Tokyo International P.O. Box 5063
1-28-36 Hongo, Bunkyo-ku.
Tokyo 113, Japan

Korea
Mr. Don-Gap Choi
C.P.O. Box 10583
Seoul, Korea

Malaysia
Mr. Lim Tao Slong
No. 8 Jalan SS 7/6B
Kelana Jaya
47301 Petaling Jaya
Selangor, Malaysia

Mexico
**Interamericana/McGraw-Hill de Mexico, S.A.
de C.V.**
Cedro 512, Colonia Atlamoa
(Apartado Postal 26370)
06450 Mexico, D.F., Mexico

New Zealand
McGraw-Hill Book Co. New Zealand Ltd.
5 Joval Place, Wiri
Manukau City, New Zealand

Portugal
Editora McGraw-Hill de Portugal, Ltda.
Rua Rosa Damasceno 11A-B
1900 Lisboa, Portugal

South Africa
Libriger Book Distributors
Warehouse Number 8
"Die Ou Looiery"
Tannery Road
Hamilton, Bloemfontein 9300

Singapore and Southeast Asia
McGraw-Hill Book Co.
21 Neythal Road
Jurong, Singapore 2262

Spain
McGraw-Hill/Interamericana de Espana, S.A.
Manuel Ferrero, 13
28020 Madrid, Spain

Taiwan
Mr. George Lim
P.O. Box 87-601
Taipei, Taiwan

Thailand
Mr. Vitit Lim
632/5 Phaholyothin Road
Sapan Kwai
Bangkok 10400
Thailand

United Kingdom, Middle East and Africa
Wolfe Publishing
Brook House
2-16 Torrington Place
London WC1E 7LT

Venezuela
Editorial Interamerica de Venezuela, C.A.
2da. calle Bello Monte
Local G-2
Caracass, Venezuela

NOTICE

Authors and publisher have made every effort to ensure that the patient care recommended herein, including choice of drugs and drug dosages, is in accord with the accepted standards and practice at the time of publication. However, since research and regulation constantly change clinical standards, the reader is urged to check the product information sheet included in the package of each drug, which includes recommended doses, warnings, and contraindications. This is particularly important with new or infrequently used drugs.

Family Practice Review
A Problem Oriented Approach
Second Edition

ISBN 1-55664-319-5

Library of Congress catalog card number 90-72328

10 9 8 7 6 5 4 3

This book is dedicated to the memory of two very special men

My father, Gustav William Swanson (1900-1989)

and

My father in law, Wilmer Arnold Miller (1915-1989)

Preface

The second edition of this book, *Family Practice Review: A Problem Oriented Approach,* is written as a comprehensive review of problems commonly encountered in clinical family medicine. As in the first edition, every effort has been made to avoid esoteric, rare, or complicated management problems.

This second edition differs from the first edition in several respects. New sections on epidemiology and public health, and emergency medicine have been added. The number of problems and questions have been increased, and most of the problems have multiple cases. The number of references have been increased, and the references have been superscripted throughout the answers. A summary follows each problem.

This book is intended for senior medical students, family practice residents, other residents and interns, as well as practicing family physicians who wish to review common clinical problems as a continuing medical education exercise. This book will aid those preparing for board certifying examinations.

I hope that the physicians who read this book and work through the problem enjoy it and find it a stimulating, challenging, and useful learning experience.

Richard W. Swanson
M.D., C.C.F.P.

Acknowledgements

I wish to thank the following persons who supported and helped me during the writing of this book.

First, Mr. Walter Bailey, of B.C.Decker Inc., for his support of my problem oriented approach to learning, and for taking a chance on me with the publication of the first edition.

Second, to my reviewers, Dr. Marilyn Basinger, Dr. Randy Siemens, Dr. Gwen Siemens, Dr. Mark Cameron and Dr. Rick Spooner. A special thank you to Dr. Spooner for his many hours of work in advising on and editing all drafts of this book.

Third, to the other family medicine residents at the University of Saskatchewan in Saskatoon for their words of encouragement during the two and one-half years of preparation of this second edition.

Finally, to my wife Stella and my children, Heidi, Eric, and Jason who allowed me to pursue my obsession with this book.

Contents

Internal Medicine

Obstetrics and Gynecology

Psychiatry

Pediatrics

General Surgery and Surgical Specialities

Geriatric Medicine

Epidemiology and Public Health

Emergency Medicine

Internal Medicine

PROBLEM 1: AN OBESE 47-YEAR-OLD MALE WITH HYPERTENSION

A 47-year-old male presents to your office for a routine health assessment. He weighs 250 lb, smokes 2 packs of cigarettes/day, works 14 hours/day at the office and drinks 8 oz of hard liquor/day. His blood pressure is 180/105 mm Hg.

SELECT THE ONE BEST ANSWER TO THE FOLLOWING QUESTIONS:

1. Which of the following statements about this patient's blood pressure is FALSE?
   a) a single blood pressure reading of diastolic 105 is satisfactory for a diagnosis of hypertension
   b) this patient's alcohol intake may be a significant contributing factor to his elevated blood pressure
   c) the patient should have his blood pressure rechecked after a period of rest in the office
   d) the patient should return for reassessment of his blood pressure in 1 week
   e) the patient should not be started on antihypertensive medication at this time

2. A diagnosis of essential hypertension is established in the patient described in question 1. Therapy should be aimed at decreasing his blood pressure to a level below:
   a) 150/90 mm Hg
   b) 140/90 mm Hg
   c) 130/90 mm Hg
   d) 120/80 mm Hg
   e) 110/70 mm Hg

3. The patient described in this problem returns for two follow-up visits during the next 3 weeks. After 5 minutes of rest and two readings recorded in the supine position at each visit, his average blood pressure is 160/95 mm Hg. After appropriate laboratory evaluation you should decide to:
   a) begin treatment with hydrochlorothiazide
   b) begin treatment with a beta blocker
   c) begin treatment with a calcium-channel blocker

   d) begin treatment with an angiotensin converting enzyme inhibitor
   e) none of the above

4. If you decide to start this patient on a thiazide diuretic, what dosage should you begin with?
   a) 150 mg
   b) 100 mg
   c) 75 mg
   d) 50 mg
   e) 25 mg

5. The level of blood pressure that constitutes hypertension in the elderly has not been clearly established. Most authorities, however, would try to lower an elderly patient's blood pressure to a level of:
   a) 180/110 mm Hg
   b) 180/90 mm Hg
   c) 170/100 mm Hg
   d) 160/90 mm Hg
   e) 120/80 mm Hg

6. The benefits of drug therapy appear to outweigh any known risks to individuals with a persistently elevated diastolic blood pressure greater than:
   a) 94 mm Hg
   b) 92 mm Hg
   c) 90 mm Hg
   d) 88 mm Hg
   e) 85 mm Hg

ANSWER THE FOLLOWING QUESTIONS ACCORDING TO THE CODE:

A: 1, 2, and 3 are correct
B: 1 and 3 are correct
C: 2 and 4 are correct

D: Only 4 is correct

E: All of the above are correct

7.   Step-care therapy for hypertension has undergone considerable change in the past few years. Which of the following are now FIRST LINE agents for the management of hypertension?
1.   hydrochlorothiazide
2.   atenolol (or other beta blocker)
3.   enalapril (or other ACE inhibitor)
4.   nifedipine (or other calcium-channel blocker)

8.   The initial diagnostic work-up of a patient with hypertension should include:
1.   electrolytes/ BUN and creatinine
2.   IVP
3.   ECG
4.   24-hour urine for metanephrines

9.   A 50-year-old male is being treated for hypertension. He is currently on a low salt diet, hydrochlorothiazide 25 mg/day and propranolol 120 mg b.i.d. His blood pressure is 180/105 mm Hg. Which of the following would be reasonable choice(s) for a third line agent?
1.   atenolol
2.   nifedipine
3.   furosemide
4.   enalapril

10. Which of the following antihypertensive drug(s) are drugs of choice for patients with noninsulin-dependent diabetes mellitus?
1.   ACE inhibitors
2.   diuretics
3.   calcium-channel blockers
4.   beta blockers

11. Which of the following are characteristics of the "ideal antihypertensive" agent?
1.   effective in lowering blood pressure in at least 50% of patients as monotherapy
2.   available in a once-a-day formulation to maximize compliance
3.   minimal or no effects on electrolyte levels, serum lipid levels, and glucose metabolism
4.   minimal or no adverse effects on quality of life

12. Which of the following drugs are useful for the treatment of hypertensive emergencies and urgencies?
1.   IV labetalol
2.   oral clonidine

3.   oral or sublingual nifedipine
4.   oral propranolol

ANSWERS

1.   A. Hypertension should not be diagnosed until a sustained elevation of blood pressure has been documented. For diagnosis, at least 3 readings, averaging greater than 140 systolic or 90 diastolic, and at least 1 week apart, should be recorded.[1] If a single diastolic reading of 110 mm Hg is obtained, it is unlikely to return to normal on subsequent readings.

Alcohol abuse is a significant cause of hypertension.[1] Any patient who presents with hypertension should be questioned about alcohol intake. Studies have shown that blood pressure increases in anyone who intakes more than an average of 2 drinks/day.[1]

The patient described in this question should have his blood pressure taken again after 5 minutes of rest. If his arm circumference is greater than 33 cm the obese blood pressure cuff should be used for measurement. This will give a better idea of the baseline reading for this visit.[2] A patient whose blood pressure goes down after a period of rest has "labile hypertension." One-half of patients with "labile hypertension" will go on to develop sustained hypertension.

Home blood pressure readings are more representative of true blood pressure, and the use of home blood pressure monitoring should be considered.[3] As well, home blood pressure monitoring involves the patient more directly in the evaluation and treatment of his problem.

The patient should not be started on antihypertensive medication until it is established that his blood pressure elevation is sustained.

2.   B. The goal of antihypertensive therapy in patients under age 60 is to reduce the blood pressure to a level below 140/90 mm Hg.[1]

3.   E. The first step in the treatment of mild hypertension is nonpharmacologic therapy. In this patient this includes weight reduction, restriction of alcohol, restriction of sodium, discontinuing smoking (to reduce cardiovascular risk), and increased aerobic exercise. Only after this approach has failed should drug therapy be considered.[1]

4.   D. The ideal dose of hydrochlorothiazide appears to be approximately 25 mg/day. The efficacy of 25

mg/day appears to be equal to that of any higher dose, but the side effects including hypokalemia, hyperglycemia, hyperlipidemia, and hyperuricemia increase with increasing dosage.[4]

5. D. The level of blood pressure needed to establish the diagnosis of hypertension, and the level at which treatment should be initiated in elderly patients (>65 years) has not been established.[5] Both systolic and diastolic hypertension, however, contribute to cardiovascular and cerebrovascular mortality. Until more definitive data are available, it is reasonable to treat elderly patients with a DBP of 90 mm Hg or greater, preferably with nonpharmacologic therapy. A cautious lowering of SBP to 140–160 mm Hg also seems reasonable.[1,5]

6. A. A persistently elevated diastolic blood pressure of 94 mm Hg appears to be the level at which the benefits of drug therapy outweigh the risks in patients without other significant risk factors.[1] In patients with diabetes mellitus or hyperlipidemia, as well as patients who are cigarette smokers or who have target organ damage, the level of treatment should probably be lowered.[1]

    In patients with DBPs between 90 mm Hg and 94 mm Hg, drug therapy should be initiated with nonpharmacologic methods. Individuals with DBP's in that range who fail to respond to nonpharmacologic treatment should be assessed and treated on an individual basis.[1]

7. E. The 1984 Report of the Joint National Committee on Detection, Evaluation, and Treatment of High Blood Pressure recommended that either thiazide-type diuretics or beta blockers be used as initial therapy, unless contraindications exist.[6] Calcium antagonists and ACE inhibitors have now been included in that group.[1] Subsequent therapeutic options include increasing the dose of the first drug if it is below the recommended maximum; adding an agent from another class; or discontinuing the initial choice and substituting a drug from a different class.[1]

    Combining antihypertensive drugs with different modes of action using the step-care approach will allow smaller dosages of drugs to be used and will decrease the incidence of side effects.[1]

8. B. The basic hypertensive work-up includes a complete urinalysis, hemoglobin and hematocrit, electrolytes, BUN and creatinine, calcium, plasma cholesterol, plasma glucose and serum uric acid concentrations, CXR, and ECG.[1] Other tests including renal ultrasound, IVP, or 24-hour urines for metanephrines and VMA are only indicated in specific clinical circumstances.[1] A patient over the age of 55, for example, who has been previously normotensive and who suddenly develops hypertension should be suspected of having renal artery stenosis, and an IVP and angiography should be performed. A young person with hypertension accompanied by palpitations and sweating, on the other hand, should be suspected of having a pheochromocytoma or hyperthyroidism. In this case 24-hour urines for metanephrines and blood for thyroid function studies are indicated.

9. C. Both nifedipine and enalapril are reasonable agents to add to this patient's treatment regimen. Atenolol is a beta blocker and is not indicated as propranolol is already being prescribed.

    Furosemide is a loop diuretic and is usually only indicated in the treatment of hypertension if concomitant renal insufficiency exists.

    Other appropriate agents include the centrally acting alpha agonist clonidine and the peripheral alpha blocker prazosin.

10. B. The drugs of choice for patients with noninsulin-dependent diabetes mellitus are ACE inhibitors and the calcium-channel blockers.[7] Diuretics and beta blockers may adversely affect plasma lipids and blood sugar.[1] Diuretics are also associated with hypokalemia and hyperuricemia.

    Beta blockers also interfere with the recognition of hypoglycemia. Thus, symptoms of hypoglycemia such as palpitations, tremor, and feelings of anxiety may be blunted, and the duration of hypoglycemia may be prolonged.[1] Severe hypertension also can occur during hypoglycemia in diabetic patients treated with beta blockers.

11. E. The ideal antihypertensive agent should: (1) be effective as monotherapy, (2) be inexpensive, (3) be effective in a once-a-day dosage to increase compliance, (4) be easy to titrate, (5) have a good side-effect profile, and (6) should be safe.[8] No class of drugs meets all of these criteria. Only thiazide diuretics, beta blockers, calcium-channel blockers, and ACE inhibitors meet enough of these criteria to be considered first-line agents.

12. A. Hypertensive emergencies and urgencies are defined as follows:

1. Hypertensive emergency: a clinical situation in which blood pressure must be lowered within one hour.
   Examples are: malignant hypertension, acute myocardial ischemic syndromes, acute pulmonary edema, acute renal insufficiency, acute intracranial events, postoperative bleeding, eclampsia, and pheochromocytoma crisis.[9]

2. Hypertensive urgency: a clinical situation in which blood pressure should be lowered within 24 hours. Examples are: accelerated hypertension, marked hypertension associated with congestive cardiac failure, stable angina pectoris, transient cerebral ischemia attacks, and perioperative hypertension.[9]

A patient with a persistent diastolic blood pressure of >120 mm Hg after resting should be considered to have a hypertensive urgency until proven otherwise.

Drugs useful in treating hypertensive emergencies and urgencies include oral or sublingual nifedipine, oral clonidine, oral captopril, intravenous labetalol, and intravenous infusions of sodium nitroprusside, nitroglycerin, and diazoxide.[9]

SUMMARY OF THE DETECTION, EVALUATION AND TREATMENT OF HIGH BLOOD PRESSURE

1. **Measurement**: Three visits, with average DBP of 90 mm Hg or greater or SBP levels of 140 mm Hg or greater is required for diagnosis.

2. **Evaluation**: History, physical examination, and laboratory evaluation should include evaluation of other risk factors including family history of coronary artery disease, presence of diabetes mellitus, obesity, alcohol intake, hyperlipidemia, smoking, exercise pattern, and stress.
   Laboratory evaluation should include hemoglobin and hematocrit, complete urinalysis, measurement of serum potassium, calcium, and creatinine levels, electrocardiography, and measurement of plasma cholesterol, plasma glucose, and uric acid levels.

Treatment:
   Nonpharmacologic treatment: weight reduction, restriction of alcohol, restriction of sodium, tobacco avoidance, exercise, and modification of dietary fats are indicated.

Pharmacologic treatment:
   Step 1: diuretic, beta blocker, calcium-channel antagonist or ACE inhibitor.
   Step 2: increase dose of first drug, substitute another drug, or add a second drug of a different class.
   Step 3: substitute a second drug or add a third drug of a different class.
   Step 4: add a third or fourth drug or refer for further evaluation.

References

1. The 1988 Report of the Joint National Committee on detection, evaluation, and treatment of high blood pressure. Arch Intern Med 1988; 148: 1023–1038.

2. Frohlich ED, Grim C, Labarthe DR, Maxwell M, Perloff D, Weidman M. Report of a special task force appointed by the Steering Committee, American Heart Association. Recommendations for human blood pressure determinations by sphygmomanometer. Hypertension 1988; 11: 210A–222A.

3. MacMahon SW, Norton RN. Alcohol and hypertension: implications for prevention and treatment. Ann Intern Med 1986; 105: 124–125.

4. McVeigh G, Galloway D, Johnston D. The case for low dose diuretics in hypertension: comparison of low and conventional doses of cyclopenthiazide. Br Med J 1988; 297:95–98.

5. Amery A, Birkenhager W, Brixko P, et al. Mortality and morbidity results from the European Working Party on high blood pressure in the elderly trial. Lancet 1985; 1: 1349–1354.

6. The 1984 Joint National Committee. The 1984 report of the Joint National Committee on detection, evaluation, and treatment of high blood pressure. Arch Intern Med 1984; 144: 1045–1057.

7. Swanson R, Spooner R. Essential hypertension: when and how to initiate therapy. Can Fam Physician 1989; 35: 1821–1826.

8. Gifford R. Essential hypertension: cost-effective evaluation and treatment. Am J Med 1986(Suppl 6C):33–38.

9. Reuler J, Magarian G. Hypertensive emergencies and urgencies: definition, recognition, and management. J Gen Intern Med 1988; 3: 64–74.

Table 1 An Individualized Step-Care Approach to Hypertension

Patient	Recommended Drugs	Drugs To Avoid
Young, hyperdynamic circulation	Beta blockers	—
Elderly	Diuretics, reduced drug dosage	—
Black race	Diuretics	—
Gout	—	Diuretics
Ischemic heart disease	Beta blockers, calcium-channel blockers	—
Asthma	Calcium-channel blockers	Beta blockers
Peripheral vascular disease	Calcium-channel blockers or other vasodilators	Beta blockers
Noninsulin-dependent diabetes mellitus	ACE inhibitors, calcium-channel blockers	Diuretics
Insulin-dependent diabetes mellitus	ACE inhibitors, diuretics	Beta blockers
Hypercholesterolemia	ACE inhibitors, calcium-channel blockers, beta blockers with ISA (intrinsic sympathomimetic activity), alpha blockers	Beta blockers without ISA, diuretics without ACE inhibitors
Congestive heart failure	ACE inhibitors with diuretics	Beta blockers
Pregnancy	Beta blockers, methyldopa, hydralazine	ACE inhibitors

From Swanson, R and Spooner, R: Essential hypertension: when and how to initiate therapy, Can Fam Physician 1989, 35:1821-1826.

PROBLEM 2:   A 37-YEAR-OLD MALE WITH A HIGH CHOLESTEROL LEVEL

A 37-year-old obese male presents for a routine physical assessment. He is a 2-pack a day smoker and is hypertensive. He is currently taking hydrochlorothiazide 50 mg/day and propranolol 160 mg/day. He has no history of diabetes or hypertension. He has no family history of coronary artery disease or hyperlipidemia. Physical examination reveals a blood pressure of 150/90 mm Hg. There are no other abnormalities on physical examination. A random cholesterol determination is done and comes back at 6.3 mmol/L (244 mg%).

SELECT THE ONE BEST ANSWER TO THE FOLLOWING QUESTIONS:

13. Regarding this patient's cholesterol, which of the following statements is true?
    a) this is a normal serum cholesterol for this patient
    b) this is a borderline serum cholesterol for this patient and should be repeated in 1 year
    c) this is a high serum cholesterol for this patient and intense dietary and drug therapy should be considered
    d) although this is a high serum cholesterol, careful observation of the cholesterol is all that is required
    e) this is a high serum cholesterol; the patient should be further assessed by a fasting HDL and LDL cholesterol

14. At what level of LDL-cholesterol is treatment definitely indicated?
    a) 4.1 mmol/L (160 mg%)
    b) 3.4 mmol/L (130 mg%)
    c) 3.8 mmol/L (151 mg%)

d) 5.2 mmol/L (206 mg%)
e) 3.1 mmol/L (123 mg%)

15. The treatment of choice for hypercholesterolemia is:
a) gemfibrozil
b) colestipol
c) nicotinic acid
d) lovastatin
e) none of the above

16. The patient described in the problem is taking hydrochlorothiazide and propranolol. Which of the following statements are TRUE concerning the effect of these drugs on plasma lipoproteins?
a) hydrochlorothiazide has no effect on plasma lipoproteins
b) propranolol has no effect on plasma lipoproteins
c) neither hydrochlorothiazide nor propranolol has an effect on plasma lipoproteins
d) both hydrochlorothiazide and propranolol can adversely affect plasma lipoproteins
e) nobody worries about plasma lipoproteins any longer

ANSWER THE FOLLOWING QUESTIONS ACCORDING TO THE KEY:

A: 1, 2, and 3 are correct
B: 1 and 3 are correct
C: 2 and 4 are correct
D: Only 4 is correct
E: All of the above are correct

17. Which of the following are independent risk factors for coronary artery disease?
1) increased LDL-concentrations
2) decreased HDL-concentrations
3) increased total-cholesterol concentrations
4) increased triglyceride levels

18. The drugs of first choice for lowering plasma cholesterol levels in patients unresponsive to dietary therapy include:
1) cholestyramine
2) lovastatin
3) colestipol
4) gemfibrozil

19. Which of the following statements regarding fish oils (ω-3 fatty acids) are TRUE?

1) fish oils have been shown to lower plasma triglyceride levels
2) fish oils inhibit platelet aggregation
3) fish oils have been shown to increase HDL levels
4) fish oils may decrease blood pressure and blood viscosity

20. A 56-year-old alcoholic physician presents to your office for a complete health assessment. When you question him about his alcohol intake he replies that he simply uses alcohol to favorably affect his apolipoprotein ratio. Which of the following statements regarding alcohol and apolipoproteins are TRUE?
1) ingestion of alcohol decreases apolipoprotein A-1 levels
2) ingestion of alcohol increases apolipoprotein A-1 levels
3) ingestion of alcohol increases apolipoprotein B levels
4) ingestion of alcohol decreases apolipoprotein B levels

ANSWERS

13. E. This patient has a high serum cholesterol. Normal serum cholesterol is under 5.2 mmol/L (200 mg%). Borderline serum cholesterol is 5.2–6.2 mmol/L (240 mg%). High serum cholesterol is greater than 6.2 mmol/L.[1]

Who should be screened for hypercholesterolemia is currently being debated.[1,2] Two approaches to screening are (1) to screen all adults at periodic intervals or (2) to screen only patients who have a family history of coronary risk factors, or who have other coronary risk factors themselves.[1] The cost implications of mass screening and subsequent treatment have to be considered in making this decision.[3] The current recommendation for screening is a nonfasting sample.[1]

Patients with cholesterol levels between 5.2 mmol/L and 6.2 mmol/L require a fasting specimen to confirm the reading.[1] They should be given information on the American Heart Association Step 1 diet and rescreened in 1 year.[1]

Patients with cholesterol greater than 6.2 mmol/L require a fasting specimen to determine the HDL and the LDL cholesterol.[1] Levels of LDL above 4.1 mmol/L (160 mg%) are considered high risk; levels between 3.4 mmol/L and 4.1 mmol/L (130–159 mg%) are considered borderline.

14. A. Treatment of hypercholesterolemia is indicated if the level of LDL-cholesterol is greater than 4.1 mmol/L (160 mg%). Treatment should be initiated with diet therapy (American Heart Association Step 1 and Step 2 diets) and the goal of therapy should be an LDL-cholesterol < 3.4 mmol/L (130 mg%).[1]

15. E. The treatment of choice for hypercholesterolemia is diet therapy. The American Heart Association has produced Step 1 and Step 2 diets. Step 1 dietary therapy includes less than 30% of calories as fat, less than 10% of calories as saturated fat, and less than 300 mg/day of cholesterol. Step 2 dietary therapy includes less than 30% of calories as fat, less than 7% of calories as saturated fat, and less than 200 mg/day cholesterol.[1] Drug treatment is only indicated after dietary management has failed to achieve the desired goal.

16. D. Both hydrochlorothiazide and propranolol can adversely affect plasma lipoproteins.[4] Hydrochlorothiazide increases total cholesterol and triglyceride concentrations. In addition, very low-density lipoprotein (VLDL)-cholesterol levels and low-density lipoprotein (LDL)-cholesterol levels also increased, while the high-density lipoprotein (HDL)-cholesterol level changes are variable.[4]

    Propranolol increases plasma triglyceride levels, but does not alter total cholesterol concentrations.[4] However, propranolol does decrease HDL-cholesterol levels. LDL-cholesterol changes on propranolol are more variable.[4]

    The beta-1 selective adrenegic blockers, like the nonselective agents, increase triglyceride levels and lower HDL-cholesterol levels without altering total cholesterol concentration.[4] The adverse effects on lipoproteins tend to be less, however, than the changes observed with the nonselective agents.

    Pindolol, oxprenolol hydrochloride, and acebutolol hydrochloride are beta-adrenergic blocking agents possessing intrinsic sympathomimetic activity (ISA). The former two are nonselective, while acebutolol is beta-1 selective. Oxprenolol may increase triglyceride concentrations and lower HDL-cholesterol. Pindolol and acebutolol appear to be lipid neutral.[4]

17. A. Risk factors for coronary artery disease include increased LDL and total cholesterol concentrations, decreased HDL-concentration (below 1.0 mmol/L or 35 mg%), male sex, a family history of premature coronary artery disease, cigarette smoking, hypertension, diabetes mellitus, and severe obesity (> 30% overweight).[1]

    The relationship between plasma triglyceride levels and cardiovascular disease is controversial.[1] Although the plasma triglyceride level does not appear to be an independent risk factor, an elevated triglyceride level may reflect the presence of certain atherogenic lipoproteins.[1]

18. B. The drugs of first choice for lowering plasma cholesterol levels in patients unresponsive to dietary therapy are still the bile acid sequestrants cholestyramine and colestipol.[1] They should not, however, be used in patients with triglyceride levels above 350 mg/dL (4.0 mmol/L), as triglyceride levels may markedly increase.

    Nicotinic acid, and gemfibrozil, a fibric acid derivative, are good second-line drugs.[1,5]

    Lavostatin and other HMG-CoA reductase inhibitors are effective agents for the treatment of hyperlipidemia.[5] They are capable of lowering total cholesterol by 30–35% and LDL-cholesterol by 35–40%. At present, the indications for HMG-CoA reductase inhibitors are (1) heterozygous familial hypercholesterolemia and (2) primary severe hypercholesterolemia (total cholesterol levels 7.76–9.70 mmol/L (300–375mg%) with LDL-cholesterol levels of 5.69–7.76 mmol/L (220–300 mg%).[6] These agents are even more effective when used in combination with bile acid sequestrants.[5] Until more experience is gained with HMG Co-A inhibitors, it is probably prudent to restrict their use to the indications discussed above.

19. E. Fish and fish oil supplements may lower plasma lipid levels (especially triglycerides), inhibit platelet aggregation, and may decrease blood pressure and viscosity and increase HDL-cholesterol levels. Patients with serum triglyceride levels greater than 5.64 mmol/L and/or cholesterol levels greater than 7.75 mmol/L refractory to dietary management may benefit from a trial of fish oil supplements.[7] At this time, fish oil supplements cannot be recommended for general use.

20. C. There is an inverse relationship between low to moderate alcohol consumption and coronary artery disease.[8] This may be due to an inhibitory effect on platelet aggregation, or to increased coronary artery diameter.[8] As well, low dose al-

cohol appears to increase the cardioprotective apolipoprotein A-1 and decrease the atherogenic apolipoprotein B.[8]

Obviously, in the patient discussed, the toxic effects of alcohol outweigh any protective effect of apolipoproteins.

SUMMARY OF THE DIAGNOSIS AND MANAGEMENT OF HYPERCHOLESTEROLEMIA

1. **Screening**: Either patient-based (high-risk) or population-based (all patients). Cost-effectiveness should be considered.

2. **Cholesterol values:**
   Total Cholesterol:
    Normal: < 5.2 mmol/L (200 mg%)
    Borderline: 5.2–6.2 mmol/L (200–240 mg%)
    Elevated: >6.2 mmol/L (>240 mg%)
   LDL-Cholesterol:
    Ideal: < 3.4 mmol/L (130 mg%)
    Borderline: 3.4–4.1 mmol/L (130–159 mmol/L)
    Elevated: >4.1 mmol/L (160 mg%)

3. **Treatment:**
   Treat if LDL-cholesterol >4.1 mmol/L or >3.4 mmol/L with 2 or more risk factors.

   Dietary management is treatment of first choice. Begin with Step 1 diet and increase to Step 2 if values do not normalize. Use dietary management for at least 6 months before proceeding to drug treatment.
   Drug Treatment:
   First-line drugs:
   Bile acid sequestrants:
    Cholestyramine
    Cholestipol
   (If first-line drug ineffective, add a second-line agent.)

Second-line drugs:
1) Nicotinic acid
2) Fibrates:
    Gemfibrozil
    Clofibrate
3) HMG-CoA reductase inhibitors:
    Lovastatin
    Pravastatin
    Simvastatin

References

1. Report of the National Cholesterol Education Program Expert Panel on Detection, Evaluation, and Treatment of High Blood Cholesterol in Adults. Arch Intern Med 1988; 148(1): 36–69.

2. Canadian Consensus Conference on Cholesterol: Final Report. Can Med Assoc J 1988; 139(11) Suppl: 1–8.

3. Cummings S, Rubin S, Oster G. The cost-effectiveness of counseling smokers to quit. JAMA 1989; 261(1): 75–79.

4. Lardinois C, Neuman S. The effects of antihypertensive agents on serum lipids and lipoproteins. Arch Intern Med 1988; 148(6): 1280–1288.

5. Schaefer E. Hyperlipoproteinemia. In: Rakel R, ed. Conn's current therapy 1990. Philadelphia: WB Saunders, 1990; 516–524.

6. Grundy S. HMG-CoA reducatase inhibitors for treatment of hypercholesterolemia. N Engl J Med 1988; 319(1): 24–31.

7. Yetiv JZ. Clinical applications of fish oils. JAMA 1988; 260(5): 665–670.

8. Moore R, Smith C, Kwiterovich P, Pearson T. Effect of low-dose alcohol use versus abstention on apolipoproteins A-1 and B. Am J Med 1988; 84: 884–890.

PROBLEM 3: A 55-YEAR-OLD MALE WITH CHEST PAIN

A 55-year-old male presents to the emergency department following the acute onset of retrosternal chest pain that he describes as "severe heartburn". His chest pain came on after attending a gourmet feast. He is hypertensive and smokes 2 packs of cigarettes/day. He developed mild diaphoresis along with this chest pain.

On physical examination, the patient's blood pressure is 150/100 mm Hg. His pulse is 96 and regular. His ECG shows 1 mm of ST segment depression.

SELECT THE ONE BEST ANSWER TO THE FOLLOWING QUESTIONS:

21. Which of the following statements about this patient's chest pain is FALSE?
    a) the patient may have suffered a myocardial infarction
    b) the patient's chest pain may be due to angina pectoris
    c) the patient's chest pain may be due to esophageal spasm
    d) the administration of sublingual nitroglycerine is a very sensitive diagnostic test in distinguishing angina pectoris from esophageal spasm
    e) the patient should be admitted to the coronary care unit until the origin of the chest pain is established

22. The patient described in question 21 is admitted for observation. His pain subsides with intravenous nitroglycerin. His cardiac enzymes are reported as normal.
    Which of the following investigations is NOT INDICATED at this time?
    a) an exercise tolerance test
    b) coronary angiography
    c) an upper gastrointestinal series
    d) a plasma lipid profile
    e) a fasting blood sugar

23. The patient described in question 21 has a 2.5 mm ST segment depression on the exercise tolerance test.
    Which of the following statement(s) regarding this test result is TRUE?
    a) this probably represents angina pectoris
    b) this patient should have coronary angiography
    c) a hypotensive response with stress testing is indicative of severe ischemia
    d) a and b
    e) all of the above statements are true

24. Which of the following medications would not be indicated as a first-line drug in the treatment of the patient described in question 21?
    a) diltiazem
    b) propranolol
    c) isosorbide dinitrate
    d) prazosin
    e) nitroglycerin

ANSWER THE FOLLOWING QUESTIONS ACCORDING TO THE CODE:

A: 1, 2, and 3 are correct
B: 1 and 3 are correct
C: 2 and 4 are correct
D: Only 4 is correct
E: All of the above are correct

25. A 67-year-old male with a history of angina pectoris is brought into the emergency department by his wife. For the past 3 days, he has been having increasing chest pain, and this chest pain has been occuring at rest and has been waking him up in the middle of the night.
    On physical examination, his blood pressure is 120/70 mm Hg. His pulse is 96 and regular.
    His electrocardiogram shows ST segment depression of 1.5 mm. Flattening of the T waves is also seen.
    Which of the following statement(s) regarding this patient is(are) true?
    1) this patient has unstable angina
    2) intravenous nitroglycerin is the treatment of first choice for this condition
    3) the patient probably has complex coronary stenosis
    4) this patient should be placed on 1 aspirin/day

26. A 50-year-old female presents to the emergency department with a retrosternal chest pain that awoke her from sleep. This is the fourth episode in as many days, and she was concerned that she may be having a "heart attack." She was in to see her physician 3 weeks ago and was told that she was in "perfect health." She was told her "blood pres-

sure and cholesterol" were completely normal. She is a non-smoker and has no family history of coronary artery disease.

On physical examination, her blood pressure is 100/70 mm Hg. Her pulse is 96 and regular. The rest of the cardiovascular examination is normal.

The electrocardiogram reveals significant ST segment elevation in the anterior limb leads. Within 1 hour the ST segment has returned to normal. CPK levels done over the next 3 days are normal.

Which of the following statements regarding this patient is(are) true?
1) this patient probably has Prinzmetal's angina
2) calcium-channel blockers are the treatment of choice for this condition
3) beta blockers are contraindicated in this condition
4) ACE inhibitors are the treatment of choice for this condition.

27. Patients suitable for percutaneous transluminal angioplasty (PTCA) include:
1) patients with single-vessel disease with discrete, subtotal, noncalcified stenosis of the proximal coronary artery
2) patients with multiple vessel disease or multiple lesions in the same vessel if all or most of the stenoses are suitable for intervention
3) patients with complete occlusions that can be crossed and dilated
4) patients with left main coronary artery disease

28. Patients in whom coronary artery bypass surgery (CABG) is preferred include:
1) patients with left main stem coronary artery disease
2) patients with compromised left ventricular function
3) patients in whom an open chest is needed to allow extensive revascularization with end-arterectomy
4) all patients with myocardial ischemia not controlled by medical therapy

29. A 65-year-old male presents to your office with a history compatible with angina pectoris. He also has a long history of hypertension.

On examination, his blood pressure is 170/100 mm Hg. An exercise tolerance test is done and reveals 2.5 mm ST segment depression that strongly supports the diagnosis of angina pectoris.

Which of the following medication(s) would you consider as the agent(s) of first choice for the treatment of this patient?
1. hydrochlorothiazide
2. verapamil
3. clonidine
4. propranolol

30. Which of the following investigations should be ordered in a patient initially suspected of having angina pectoris?
1) complete blood count
2) a chest x-ray
3) a complete urinalysis
4) thyroid function tests

ANSWERS

21. D. Acute chest pain is often a diagnostic problem. Myocardial infarction must be assumed to be present until proven otherwise. This patient's 1 mm ST segment depression is not diagnostic of anything. It may or may not be due to myocardial ischemia. Pain from esophageal spasm is often confused with pain from myocardial ischemia.[1] Sublingual nitroglycerin will often relieve both pains, thus decreasing the sensitivity of its administration as a diagnostic test.

22. B. Normal cardiac enzymes essentially rule out a myocardial infarction.[2] However, the origin of the patient's chest pain is still unclear. Myocardial ischemia, esophageal spasm, and musculoskeletal chest wall pain are the main diagnostic considerations. Because he is a high-risk candidate for coronary artery disease, his other potential risk factors, including plasma lipid profile and plasma glucose, should be checked. Because the patient has a significant pretest probability of coronary artery disease, a treadmill stress test will further delineate his risk of coronary artery disease. An upper gastrointestinal series may determine any contribution from reflux esophagitis. An invasive test such as coronary angiography should not be done unless the patient has a positive stress test.[1,3]

23. E. This patient probably has angina pectoris. An exercise tolerance test is considered positive if there is 1 mm horizontal or downsloping ST segment depression (beyond baseline) measured 80 ms after the J point.[1] If this interpretation is applied, 60–80% of patients with anatomically significant coronary artery disease will have a

positive test, but 10–20% of those without significant disease will also have a positive test.[1] The false-positive rate is decreased significantly by increasing the ST segment depression criterion from 1 mm to 2 mm.[1] Severe ischemia is suggested if there is (1) an early ischemic response (<3 min of testing or when heart rate is <120 to 130 /min, (2) ST segment depression > 2.5 mm, (3) there is significant hypotension with stress, (4) a prolonged recovery period (> 8 min) before ECG changes or symptoms become normal, or (5) there are prolonged complex ventricular arrhythmias.[3]

24. D. Angina pectoris has traditionally been managed with sublingual nitroglycerin being the drug of choice for acute episodes, and long acting nitrates such as isosorbide dinitrate being the agents of first choice for prophylaxis. Beta-adrenergic receptor blockers such as propranolol were considered as the agents of second choice.[1,3]

Calcium-channel blockers such as nifidepine, diltiazem, and verapamil have changed the pharmacologic management of angina.[3] Any one of the three classes of drugs mentioned above is now acceptable first line therapy. Caution should be used in combining these agents.[1,3] Prazosin is an alpha-adrenergic blocker that acts peripherally and is used in the treatment of hypertension. It is not indicated in the treatment of angina pectoris.

Nitroglycerin for the treatment of an acute attack may now be conveniently administered in the form of a spray. This has the advantage of having a significantly longer shelf life than the sublingual tablets.

25. E. This patient has unstable angina. Unstable angina is the term used to describe accelerating or "crescendo" angina in a patient who has previously had stable angina. Unstable angina can be diagnosed when the angina occurs with less exertion or at rest, lasts longer, and is less responsive to medication.

Many patients with unstable angina have complex coronary stenosis consisting of plaque ulceration, hemorrhage, or thrombosis. This unstable situation may progress to complete occlusion and infarction or may heal, with reendothelialization and a return to a stable though probably more severe pattern of ischemia.[4]

Nitrates are first-line therapy for unstable angina. Nonparenteral therapy with sublingual or oral nitrates or nitroglycerin ointment is usually sufficient. If pain persists despite the addition of other agents, intravenous nitroglycerin should be started.[4] Intravenous beta blockers are an alternative to intravenous nitrates to control acute pain. Once the acute episode is controlled, therapy can be initiated or changed using a combination of nitrates, beta blockers, and calcium-channel blockers.

Heparin and thrombolytic therapy should also be considered during the acute phase.[5] As well, a single aspirin/day should be used in patients with unstable angina.

26. A. Prinzmetal's angina (coronary artery vasospasm) is angina that occurs in the absence of precipitating factors. It is most common in the early morning, often awakening the patient from sleep. It is usually associated with ST segment elevation rather than ST depression.[1] Coronary angiography should be performed to rule out coexisting fixed stenotic lesions.

Calcium-channel blockers are probably the drugs of choice for Prinzmetal's angina. Nitrates are also effective.[1,5]

Beta blockers are contraindicated in patients who have vasospasm without fixed, stenotic lesions.

ACE inhibitors are not indicated in the treatment of Prinzmetal's angina.

27. A. The initial indications for PTCA were quite limited. They included patients who had (1) angina pectoris or substantial myocardial ischemia, (2) lesions suitable for surgical revascularization, (3) well preserved left ventricular function, and (4) single vessel disease with discrete, subtotal, noncalcified stenosis of the proximal coronary artery.[6] The expanded list of indications now includes patients with (1) multivessel disease or multiple lesions in the same vessel if all or most of the stenoses are suitable for intervention, (2) complete occlusions that can be crossed and dilated, (3) less optimal left ventricular function, and (4) other risk factors such as controlled diabetes or hypertension.[6]

Left main coronary artery disease is still considered by most authorities to be a contraindication to PTCA.

28. A. Coronary artery bypass grafting is preferred when (1) left main coronary artery disease is present, (2) poor left ventricular function is demonstrated, and (3) when open chest technique is needed to allow extensive revascularization with

endarterectomy.[6] Many cardiovascular surgeons are now using the internal mammary artery much more extensively than previously. A graft using this artery is thought to have a longer patency life than a saphenous vein graft.

29. C. A patient who initially presents with angina pectoris and hypertension should be treated with either a calcium-channel blocker or a beta blocker as the agent of first choice.[7] Thus, verapamil or propranolol are the drugs of choice in this patient. Extreme caution should be used when combining these agents because of their additive negative inotropic and chronotropic effects. Hydrochlorothiazide and clonidine will treat the hypertension but not the angina. Thus, an agent that treats both is probably preferable. If the blood pressure is not well controlled, hydrochlorothiazide, clonidine, or a number of other agents could be added to the treatment regimen.

30. E. Patients suspected of having angina pectoris should have a complete blood count, a complete urinalysis, a chest x-ray, electrocardiogram, and thyroid function tests.[4] In addition, renal function, electrolytes, blood glucose, and a lipid profile should be obtained.[4] If the patient appears to have significant chronic lung disease, arterial blood gas studies may be helpful.

SUMMARY OF THE DIAGNOSIS AND MANAGEMENT OF ANGINA PECTORIS

1. **Definition**: An imbalance between myocardial requirements for oxygen and the amount delivered through the coronary arteries resulting from either increased demand or diminished coronary flow or both.

2. **Symptoms**: Chest discomfort or "tightness," "burning," "pressing," "choking," "aching," "gas," or "indigestion" typically located in the retrosternal area or the left chest. Usual radiation to the left shoulder, left arm, or jaw. Typical angina is aggravated by exercise and relieved by rest.

3. **Signs**: Physical examination is often normal although hypertension is sometimes present.

4. **Initial laboratory evaluation**: CBC, urinalysis, electrolytes, blood glucose, blood lipids, thyroid function tests, CXR, ECG.

5. **Additional investigations once angina is suspected**:
Exercise tolerance testing with or without thallium-201 scintigraphy or radionuclide angiography. This is often followed by coronary angiography.

6. **Treatment**:
Acute attacks:
Sublingual nitroglycerin or nitroglycerin spray
Prophylaxis:
Long acting nitroglycerin, beta blockers, and calcium-channel blockers alone or in combination
Intervention/Surgery:
Percutaneous transluminal angioplasty
Coronary artery bypass surgery

7. **Angina variants**:
Prinzmetal's angina: coronary artery spasm with or without fixed stenotic lesions. Usually seen in women. ST segment elevation rather than ST segment depression is characteristic. Calcium-channel blockers are the treatment of choice.

Unstable angina: an accelerating or "crescendo" pattern of angina. May represent intermittant incomplete occlusion of coronary arteries. Acute treatment includes intravenous nitroglycerin or an intravenous beta blocker. Prophylaxis is with a combination of drugs previously discussed and with antiplatelet therapy (1 aspirin/day).

References

1. Sokolow M, Massie B. Angina pectoris. In: Schroeder S, Krupp M, Tierney L, McPhee S, eds. Current medical diagnosis and treatment. Norwalk: Appleton and Lange, 1989: 222–229.

2. Sokolow M, Massie B. Myocardial infarction. In: Schroeder S, Krupp M, Tierney L, McPhee S, eds. Current medical diagnosis and treatment. Norwalk: Appleton and Lange, 1989: 229–236.

3. Wilson D, Vacek J. Angina and coronary artery disease: manifestations and management. Postgrad Med 1988; 84(7): 77–86.

4. Selwyn A, Braunwald E. Ischemic heart disease. In: Braunwald E, Isselbacher K, Petersdorf R, Wilson J, Martin J, Fauci A, eds. Harrison's principles of internal medicine. 11th Ed. New York: McGraw-Hill, 1987: 975–982.

5. Klopf F, Ridner M. Ischemic heart disease. In: Dunagan W, Ridner M, eds. Manual of medical therapeutics. 26th Ed. Boston: Little, Brown, 1989: 90–95.

6. Wehrmacher W. Angioplasty versus bypass surgery: where do we stand today. Postgrad Med 1988; 84(7): 62–68.

7. Swanson R, Spooner R. Essential hypertension: when and how to initiate treatment. Can Fam Physician 1989; 35: 1821–1826.

PROBLEM 4:   A 62-YEAR-OLD MALE WITH ACUTE CHEST PAIN

A 62-year-old farmer is brought into the emergency department of his local rural hospital by his wife. Apparently, he developed a "twinge of chest pain" while shoveling grain 3 hours ago. He wanted to stay home and rest, but his wife insisted that he come into emergency. He states that the pain is "almost gone." He is obese, smokes two packs of cigarettes/day, drinks "a goodly amount of beer," and has been told that his cholesterol level is very high.

On examination, he is sweating and diaphoretic. He has vomited twice since the pain began. His blood pressure is 160/100 mm Hg. His pulse is 120 and regular.

His electrocardiogram reveals a Q wave in V1–V4 with significant ST segment elevation in the same leads.

SELECT THE ONE BEST ANSWER TO THE FOLLOWING QUESTIONS:

31. The most likely diagnosis in this patient is:
    a) acute inferior wall myocardial infarction
    b) acute anterior wall myocardial infarction
    c) acute myocardial ischemia
    d) acute pericarditis
    e) chest wall pain

32. Given the history and physical examination presented, your first priority would be to:
    a) call the ambulance for immediate transport
    b) admit the patient for observation
    c) administer streptokinase intravenously
    d) administer heparin intravenously
    d) none of the above

ANSWER THE FOLLOWING QUESTIONS ACCORDING TO THE CODE:

A: 1, 2, and 3 are correct
B: 1 and 3 are correct
C: 2 and 4 are correct
D: Only 4 is correct
E: All of the above are correct

33. Which of the following criteria should be met before a patient is given thrombolytic therapy following a myocardial infarction?
    1) patient age preferable less than 70 years
    2) typical chest pain of myocardial infarction
    3) ECG changes confirming myocardial infarction
    4) absence of other disease that would explain the symptoms

34. Which of the following is (are) contraindications to the use of thrombolytic therapy in patients with acute myocardial infarction?
    1) active gastrointestinal bleeding
    2) recent (within 2 weeks) trauma or surgery
    3) history of cerebrovascular accident
    4) atrial fibrillation or mitral stenosis

35. Which of the following statements regarding the use of heparin in patients with acute myocardial infarction is(are) true?
    1) heparin therapy is used routinely with or without thrombolytic therapy during acute myocardial infarction
    2) full-dose anticoagulation is recommended whenever there is echocardiographic evidence of left ventricular thrombi
    3) heparin therapy should be administered (unless contraindicated) to all patients with acute anterior wall myocardial infarction
    4) heparin is not contraindicated in patients with uncontrolled hypertension

36. Which of the following agents is(are) useful in the management of acute myocardial infarction?
    1) intravenous lidocaine
    2) intravenous beta blocker therapy
    3) intravenous nitrate therapy
    4) intravenous morphine

37. Which of the following statements regarding patients admitted to the coronary care unit following myocardial infarction is(are) true?
    1) patients should have a determination of left ventricular ejection fraction by radionuclide ventriculography or echocardiography within the early hours of admission to the coronary care unit
    2) patients without complications should have submaximal exercise stress testing with thallium-201 imaging performed on the fourth or fifth hospital day
    3) patients with negative submaximal stress tests should have a maximal exercise stress test performed after 4 to 6 weeks
    4) patients with positive submaximal stress tests should have coronary angiography performed to determine the need for PTCA and/or coronary artery bypass grafting

38. In which of the following circumstances is the risk of reinfarction and/or mortality following myocardial infarction significantly increased?
    1) postinfarction angina
    2) left ventricular ejection fraction <40%
    3) exercise-induced ischemia
    4) non Q-wave infarction

39. Which of the following medications have been shown to be of benefit in some postmyocardial infarction patients?
    1) beta blockers
    2) calcium-channel blockers
    3) aspirin
    4) antiarrhythmics

40. Which of the following statements regarding rehabilitation of the patient following a myocardial infarction is(are) true?
    1) sexual intercourse should be prohibited for at least 4 months
    2) an exercise program can be safely initiated by 3–4 weeks post-MI
    3) patients who have suffered a myocardial infarction should stay off work for at least 4 months
    4) the involvement of the spouse or significant other is a key element in post-MI rehabilitation.

ANSWERS

31. B. This patient has most likely suffered an anterior wall MI.[1] His history suggests that he is at high risk for an infarct and the Q waves and ST segment elevation in the anterior limb leads confirm the diagnosis.

    An inferior wall MI would present with ST segment elevation and possibly Q waves in leads II, III, and AVF.

    Acute pericarditis would present with elevation of the ST segment in all leads.

    Chest wall pain does not produce abnormalities in the electrocardiogram as seen in this patient.

32. C. In a patient with a documented myocardial infarction whose pain began less than 6 hours ago, your first priority should be to administer streptokinase.[2] The streptokinase can be administered as 1.5 million units IV over 1 hour.[2]

    Thrombolytic therapy reduces the mortality rate and limits infarct size in many patients when started within 3–6 hours after the onset of infarction.[3] It may also be effective (to a lesser extent) if given within 24 hours. The benefits of thrombolytic therapy are clear in those patients with anterior wall infarcts; the benefit in those patients with inferior wall infarcts has yet to be proved.[3] The recanalization rate utilizing intracoronary streptokinase is somewhat greater than using intravenous streptokinase. This procedure, however, can only be done in specialized centers.

    Urokinase and recombinant tissue plasminogen activator[2] can also be used as thrombolytic agents.

    Heparin therapy will be discussed in a subsequent question.

    The sooner the thrombolytic agent is administered, the better the prognosis.[4]

33. E. A number of criteria should be met before a patient is given thrombolytic therapy.[2-4] These include:
    a) age: although there is no specific cut-off age for thrombolytic therapy, elderly patients are at greater risk for complications.
    b) absence of other life-threatening or terminal illnesses.
    c) typical chest pain: the patient should have typical anginal chest pain that lasts at least 20 minutes.
    d) ECG changes compatible with myocardial injury: Q waves in the anterior limb leads, ST

segment elevation in the same leads, and poor R wave progression suggest anterior wall myocardial infarction.

e) there should be no evidence of another cause for the chest pain

34. E. The contraindications to thrombolytic therapy include (a) active gastrointestinal bleeding; (b) aortic dissection; (c) recent (within 2 weeks) trauma or surgery; (d) uncontrolled hypertension (blood pressure > 180/100 mm Hg); (e) history of cerebrovascular accident, cardiopulmonary resuscitation, head trauma, or intracranial neoplasm; (f) known bleeding diathesis or current use of anticoagulants; (g) atrial fibrillation or mitral stenosis; (h) increased likelihood of left ventricular embolization; (i) significant liver dysfunction; (j) diabetic retinopathy and/or other hemorrhagic ophthalmic conditions; (k) pregnancy; and (l) age > 75.[4]

35. A. Heparin therapy is used in patients with acute myocardial infarction who have left ventricular thrombi, deep venous thrombosis, or anterior wall MI. If inferior wall MI is accompanied by atrial arrhythmias, congestive cardiac failure, or ventricular wall motion abnormalities, it is also recommended.[4]

Contraindications include age greater than 75 years, uncontrolled hypertension, hemorrhagic diathesis, malignancy, peptic ulcer, acute bleeding, and active liver disease.[4]

36. E. Prophylaxis with intravenous lidocaine is favored after reperfusion therapy, although its routine use remains controversial.[5]

The use of intravenous beta blockers and intravenous nitrates appear to reduce mortality rates in acute myocardial infarction.[5]

Intravenous morphine is the drug of choice for treating the acute chest pain of myocardial infarction.[2] An intravenous dose of 3–5 mg usually provides substantial relief.

37. E. The length of time spent in the coronary care unit after acute infarction is decreasing.[5] Intermediate care can usually begin in 48–72 hours.

Patients admitted to the coronary care unit should probably have their ejection fraction determined by either radionuclide ventriculography or echocardiography within the early hours after the patient is admitted to the unit.[5]

Patients without complications can undergo submaximal exercise stress testing (thallium-201) on the fourth or fifth day. If this test is negative, a maximal exercise tolerance test can be performed after 4 to 6 weeks. Patients with a positive submaximal test require coronary angiography performed early to determine the feasibility of PTCA or coronary artery bypass grafting.[5]

Patients with complications (pulmonary edema, congestive heart failure, dysrhythmias, heart block, or postinfarction angina) require a more prolonged stay since congestion, dysrhythmias, heart block, or postinfarction angina require intensive evaluation and therapy.[5]

38. E. Risk of subsequent infarction and/or mortality following discharge from hospital is increased in patients with (1) postinfarction angina, (2) non Q wave infarction, (3) congestive cardiac failure, (4) left ventricular ejection fraction less than 40%, (5) exercise-induced ischemia diagnosed by electrocardiography or scintigraphy, and (6) ventricular ectopy (> 10 VPBs/h).[6]

39. A. Beta blockers, aspirin, and calcium-channel blockers have been shown to improve prognosis in some patients following myocardial infarction.[4]

Beta blockers appear to reduce the risk of sudden death in patients who are at increased risk (see critique of question 38).

Antiplatelet agents, particularly aspirin (325 mg/day), have been shown to be of benefit in patients who have had a myocardial infarction.[4]

Calcium-channel blockers (particulary diltiazem) has been shown to decrease the risk of reinfarction after a non Q wave infarction.[4]

Anticoagulants have not been shown to improve prognosis, although they do reduce peripheral embolization in the early discharge phase.

Antiarrhythmics other than beta blockers have not been shown to be effective as prophylactic therapy.

40. C. The patient who has suffered an MI should be able to resume sexual activity by 4 to 6 weeks post-MI. If a patient is able to climb two flights of stairs, sexual activity is unlikely to be hazardous. In other words, if the patient can make it up the stairs to the bedroom the rest is probably safe also.

Most patients who have suffered an uncomplicated MI may return to work by 8 weeks postinfarction.

Patients who have suffered an uncomplicated MI may be safely started in an activity program at 3 to 4 weeks post MI. By that time, most patients should be able to enjoy a light workout and still have enough energy left to get through the rest of the day.

In many patients, the psychological impact of myocardial infarction outweighs the physical impact. In many cases, the spouse is affected more than the patient himself. The commonest error in cardiac rehabilitation is to fail to involve the spouse at every stage of the program.[7]

SUMMARY OF THE DIAGNOSIS AND MANAGEMENT OF MYOCARDIAL INFARCTION

1. **Symptoms and signs:** The pain of myocardial infarction, unlike angina pectoris, usually occurs at rest. The pain is similar to angina in location and radiation but is more severe, and it builds up rapidly. Other symptoms include diaphoresis, weakness, nausea, vomiting, and abdominal discomfort (especially in inferior wall MI).

2. **ECG changes:** The classical evolution of changes is from peaked (hyperacute) T waves, to ST segment elevation, to Q wave development, to T wave inversion. This may occur over a few hours to several days.

3. **Other diagnostic procedures:** Other diagnostic procedures that may be helpful in making the diagnosis of acute myocardial infarction include echocardiography, scintigraphic studies (technetium-99 and thallium-201), and radionuclide angiography.

4. **Treatment of myocardial infarction:**
   Acute:
   > Pain: nitroglycerin or morphine sulfate
   > Thrombolytic therapy: streptokinase (1,500,000 units IV over 1 hour)
   > Anticoagulation: heparin 1000 units/hour adjusted to keep PTT at 1.5 times control, asprin 325 mg daily

   > Other agents: intravenous nitrates and intravenous beta blockers have been shown to decrease acute mortality
   > Lidocaine prophylaxis is indicated after thrombolytic therapy
   > PTCA and CABG may be indicated in acute situation

   Postdischarge:
   > Beta blockers
   > Aspirin (1/day)

5. **Cardiac rehabilitation:**
   > Exercise program within 3–4 weeks
   > Return to work within 8 weeks
   > Sexual intercourse within 4–6 weeks
   > Involvement of spouse is critical

References

1. Pasternak R, Braunwald E, Alpert J. Acute myocardial infarction. In: Braunwald E, Isselbacher K, Petersdorf R, Wilson J, Martin J, Fauci A, eds. Harrison's principles of internal medicine. 11th Ed. New York: McGraw-Hill, 1987: 982–992.

2. Klopf F, Ridner M. Ischemic heart disease. In: Dunagan W, Ridner M, eds. Manual of medical therapeutics. 26th Ed. Boston: Little, Brown, 1989: 96–114.

3. Sokolow M, Massie B. Heart and great vessels. In: Schroeder S, Krupp M, Tierney L, McPhee S, eds. Current medical diagnosis and treatment. Norwalk: Appleton and Lange, 1989: 229–236.

4. Leya F. Acute myocardial infarction. Postgrad Med 1989; 85(2): 131–142.

5. Pitt B. Acute myocardial infarction. Treatment in the coronary care unit. Postgrad Med 1989; 85(2): 145–152.

6. Del Core M, Sketch M. Acute myocardial infarction: management after discharge from the coronary care unit. Postgrad Med 1989; 85(2): 157–166.

7. Wenger N. Rehabilitation of the patient with coronary artery disease. Postgrad Med 1989; 85(5): 369–380.

PROBLEM 5:   AN 80-YEAR-OLD FEMALE WITH DYSPNEA AND FATIGUE

An 80-year-old woman presents with a 3-week history of fatigue and shortness of breath, especially on exertion. She mentions having to get up at night because of acute shortness of breath to "open the window to get some air." She denies edema, weight gain, or other symptoms. Physical examination reveals rales in both lung bases.

SELECT THE ONE BEST ANSWER TO THE FOLLOWING QUESTIONS:

41. Based on this history and these physical findings the most likely diagnosis is:
    a) left ventricular heart failure
    b) right ventricular heart failure
    c) biventricular heart failure
    d) cor pulmonale
    e) asthma

42. The patient described in question 41 is treated with bed rest and appropriate medication. She returns 1 month later complaining of dyspnea and fatigue as before, but now has developed dependent edema. She has gained 10 pounds in weight since her last visit. On examination, her jugular venous pressure is elevated. At this time, the most likely diagnosis is:
    a) left ventricular heart failure
    b) right ventricular heart failure
    c) biventricular heart failure
    d) cor pulmonale
    e) asthma

ANSWER THE FOLLOWING QUESTIONS ACCORDING TO THE CODE:

A: 1, 2, and 3 are correct
B: 1 and 3 are correct
C: 2 and 4 are correct
D: Only 4 is correct
E: All of the above are correct

43. Which of the following statements regarding the nonpharmacologic management of congestive cardiac failure is (are) true:
    1) dietary salt restriction should be part of the management
    2) weight loss may be of benefit
    3) cessation of cigarette smoking is even more important than in the general population
    4) bed rest is an important part of management

44. The patient described in question 41 is begun on medical therapy. Which of the following drug(s) is/are indicated as first-line therapy?

1) digoxin
2) prazosin
3) nifedipine
4) furosemide

45. Which of the following drugs is/are potassium-sparing diuretics?
   1) chlorothalidone
   2) spironolactone
   3) ethacrynic acid
   4) triamterene

46. Which of the following are useful vasodilator drugs in the treatment of congestive cardiac failure?
   1) prazosin
   2) hydralazine/isosorbide dinitrate
   3) nifedipine
   4) enalapril

47. The place of digitalis in congestive cardiac failure is controversial. In which instances is digitalis definitely indicated in the treatment of congestive cardiac failure?
   1) congestive heart failure with atrial fibrillation
   2) congestive heart failure with left ventricular dysfunction
   3) congestive heart failure with tachycardia
   4) congestive heart failure with normal sinus rhythm

ANSWERS

41. A. This patient has left ventricular heart failure. Dyspnea is the most common symptom of congestive cardiac failure.[1] Initially, the dyspnea is present only with moderate amounts of exertion, but as the severity of the heart failure increases, the shortness of breath may occur with only minimal exertion or even at rest. Other common complaints are fatigue and lethargy. With left-sided heart failure, lying flat is often followed by increasing shortness of breath. Paroxysms of nocturnal dyspnea (PND) are the hallmark of severe left ventricular failure.[1] These bouts are characterized by marked breathlessness, often described as a "suffocating" feeling, and are often accompanied

by severe anxiety. The patient has to sit upright or even stand to breathe and may have the urge to rush to an open window to relieve his breathlessness. Many patients find that sleeping on extra pillows will reduce the number and severity of attacks, and some patients resort to sleeping in reclining chairs. In severe cases, any type of semirecumbent position is intolerable. In such cases, pulmonary edema is usually severe and the shortness of breath is accompanied by cough, sometimes productive of frothy, blood-tinged secretions, and wheezing.[1] Occasionally, an isolated nocturnal cough may be the first sign of heart failure.

In this patient signs of right-sided heart failure have not yet developed. Asthma is not associated with the PND picture described in this question although left ventricular failure is sometimes referred to as "cardiac asthma."

42. C. At this time, the patient has developed signs of right ventricular heart failure as well. Chronic left ventricular failure usually leads to right ventricular failure. Right ventricular failure is manifested more by signs than by symptoms, although the pitting edema and weight gain may produce discomfort. In addition, enlargement of the liver and elevated jugular venous pressure occur.[1] If right atrial pressure is markedly elevated, splanchnic engorgement may accompany ascites, resulting in anorexia, nausea, vomiting and, eventually cachexia.[1]

43. A. Symptoms of heart failure are mostly due to sodium retention and circulatory congestion. The classic signs of congestive heart failure, including peripheral edema, jugular venous distention, and pulmonary rales, are directly related to the volume overload associated with a reduced natriuretic capacity of the kidney.[2] Therefore, dietary salt restriction (2–3 g Na/day) is an important part of therapy.[2]

Other nonpharmacologic treatments including weight loss, cessation of cigarette smoking, and alcohol reduction are even more important in patients with congestive cardiac failure than in the general population.[2] Weight loss will reduce afterload and discontinuing cigarette smoking will reduce vasoconstriction secondary to nicotine. The excess consumption of alcohol, a known cardiotoxin, should be avoided.

Bed rest was once considered a cornerstone of therapy for congestive cardiac failure. Bed rest, however, reduces exercise tolerance. Exercise

conditioning, on the other hand, increases exercise tolerance.[2] Thus, a carefully tailored moderate exercise program to the point of symptoms may be recommended for the patient in congestive cardiac failure.

44. D. Peripheral edema or pulmonary congestion are the most frequent presenting symptoms in patients with congestive cardiac failure. A diuretic is therefore the drug of first choice.[2] In mild cases of heart failure, a thiazide diuretic may be sufficient. In more severe cases, a loop diuretic such as furosemide or ethacrynic acid will be required.[2] A potassium-sparing diuretic, or the addition of an angiotensin-converting enzyme inhibitor will prevent the hypokalemia that often accompanies diuretic therapy. It is not difficult to overdiurese a patient in congestive heart failure and produce volume depletion. The intermittent use of diuretics, combined with careful regular assessment of the patient should guard against this complication. Prazosin (a peripheral alpha-receptor antagonist) and nifedipine (a calcium-channel blocker) have limited usefulness in the management of congestive cardiac failure.[3] Digitalis is not a first-line drug, but is useful in some patients (see question 47).

45. C. Hypokalemia occurs with both thiazide and loop diuretics. Hypokalemia is sometimes associated with life-threatening ventricular dysrhythmias.[3] Hypokalemia can usually be prevented (or if not effectively treated) by using potassium supplements, potassium-sparing diuretics such as spironolactone or triamterene, or by adding an angiotensin-converting enzyme inhibitor to the treatment regime.

46. C. Vasodilator therapy is the most important recent advance in the management of congestive cardiac failure.[2] Two regimens, one a combination of hydralazine and isosorbide dinitrate, and the second an ACE inhibitor such as captopril or enalapril, have emerged as front-line therapy in the treatment of congestive cardiac failure. Some authors are suggesting that vasodilator therapy be used even before diuretic therapy.[2] Evidence suggests that these regimens will prolong life in patients with congestive cardiac failure.

47. A. Digitalis, once a first-line drug in all patients with congestive heart failure, is now most commonly used in patients with atrial fibrillation and

a moderately fast ventricular response, in patients with other tachycardias, and in patients with left ventricular dysfunction, either clinical or radiologic.[3] It may actually provoke dysrhythmias and thus is not usually recommended for CHF patients in sinus rhthym.

SUMMARY OF TREATMENT OF CONGESTIVE CARDIAC FAILURE

1. **Nonpharmacologic:**
    Limitation of salt intake
    Weight reduction
    Discontinuation of cigarette smoking
    Avoidance of excessive alcohol intake
    Exercise conditioning

2. **Pharmacologic:**
    First-line drugs:
    Diuretics: Thiazides for mild failure
    Loop diuretics for moderate to severe failure
    Combination therapy often indicated (e.g., Dyazide and Lasix)
    Vasodilators: Angiotension-converting enzyme inhibitors (e.g., enalapril, captopril)
    Hydralazine/isosorbide dinitrate
    Second-line drug: digitalis (atrial fibrillation, tachycardia, left ventricular dysfunction)

3. **Cardiac transplantation**

References

1. Braunwald E. Heart failure. In: Braunwald E, Isselbacher K, Petersdorf R, Wilson J, Martin J, and Fauci A, eds. Harrison's principles of internal medicine. 11th Ed. New York: McGraw-Hill, 1987: 905–916.

2. Cohn J. Current therapy for heart failure. Am J Med 1988; 84(Supp 3B): 51–55.

3. Kopitsky R, Genton R. Myocardial and valvular heart failure. In: Dunagan W, Ridner M, eds. Manual of medical therapeutics. 26th Ed. Boston: Little, Brown, 1989: 114–124.

PROBLEM 6: A 65-YEAR-OLD FEMALE WITH CYANOSIS, SHORTNESS OF BREATH, AND SUBSTERNAL CHEST PAIN

A 65-year-old female is admitted to the emergency department with a 3-hour history of cyanosis, shortness of breath, and substernal chest pain. She was discharged from hospital 5 days earlier following a total hip replacement for osteoarthritis. Her surgery and postoperative course had been uneventful.

On examination, the patient is in acute distress. Her respiratory rate is 50/minute and her breathing is labored. Her blood pressure is 100/70 mm Hg. She is cyanotic. There are rhonci heard in both lung fields.

SELECT THE ONE BEST ANSWER TO THE FOLLOWING QUESTIONS:

48. Based on the information provided, the most likely diagnosis in this patient is:
    a) late onset gram-negative nosocomial pneumonia with septic shock
    b) acute myocardial infarction
    c) dissecting aortic aneurysm
    d) pulmonary embolism
    e) late onset status asthmaticus

49. Which of the following scintigraphic findings is most sensitive for the detection of the condition described above?
    a) no perfusion defects
    b) two or more medium to large perfusion defects with no ventilation-perfusion mismatch
    c) two or more medium to large perfusion defects with ventilation-perfusion mismatch
    d) a single medium or large perfusion defect with ventilation-perfusion mismatch
    e) none of the above

ANSWER THE FOLLOWING QUESTIONS ACCORDING TO THE CODE:

A: 1, 2, and 3 are correct
B: 1 and 3 are correct
C: 2 and 4 are correct
D: Only 4 is correct
E: All of the above are correct

50. Which of the following laboratory abnormalities would you expect to find in the patient described above?
    1) decreased PO_2
    2) increased PCO_2
    3) increased LDH
    4) increased CK (MB fraction)

51. Which of the following is, or may be, appropriate treatment for the condition described above?
    1) heparin
    2) streptokinase
    3) warfarin
    4) isosorbide dinitrate

52. Which of the following is(are) risk factors for deep venous thrombosis?
    1) post-traumatic immobility
    2) pregnancy
    3) previous episodes of deep venous thrombosis
    4) nephrotic syndrome

53. Which of the following statements regarding deep venous thrombosis is(are) true?
    1) deep venous thrombosis is usually readily detectable on clinical examination
    2) the most specific test for the detection of deep venous thrombosis is ascending venography
    3) calf-vein thrombi are just as likely to lead to pulmonary embolism as are iliofemoral thrombi
    4) impedance plethysmography (IPG) and Doppler ultrasonography are highly sensitive tests for detecting proximal deep venous thrombi

54. Which of the following is(are) recommended as specific preventive therapy for venous thromboembolism?
    1) patients at moderate risk for any reason should receive low-dose heparin or intermittent pneumatic compression
    2) patients undergoing neurosurgical procedures should be treated with intermittent pneumatic compression
    3) patients undergoing urological procedures should be treated with intermittent pneumatic compression
    4) patients undergoing surgery for hip fracture should receive prophylactic therapy with moderate-dose warfarin to prolong the prothrombin time to 1.2–1.5 times the control value

ANSWERS

48. D. This patient has a pulmonary embolus. Hip surgery is a common predisposing factor for pulmonary embolism.

Symptoms of pulmonary embolism are often not as revealing as those described above, especially in elderly patients. It is often impossible to distinguish pulmonary embolism from myocardial infarction on the basis of symptoms alone. Chest pain, dyspnea, anxiety, hyperventilation, and syncope are common to both conditions.[1] Other symptoms of pulmonary embolism include adventitious breath sounds, fever, and cyanosis.

Pulmonary embolism is suggested by the triad of cough, hemoptysis, and pleuritic chest pain.[1]

Pulmonary embolism can produce acute cor pulmonale. When this complication arises signs include neck vein distention, tachycardia, an accentuated and split pulmonic heart sound, Kussmaul's sign (distention of the jugular veins on inspiration), and pulsus paradoxus (exaggerated fall in blood pressure on inspiration).[1] Systemic hypotension and shock suggests massive pulmonary embolism.

49. C. If two or more medium or large perfusion defects with ventilation-perfusion mismatch are present, there is a 90% probability of pulmonary embolus.[2] Although a negative ventilation/perfusion scan virtually excludes a pulmonary embolism (high sensitivity), a positive scan does not confirm the diagnosis (low specificity). If only a single medium or large defect with mismatch is present, the probability of pulmonary embolism drops to under 50%. Small perfusion defects with ventilation-perfusion mismatch confer a low probability of pulmonary embolism.

50. B. Pulmonary embolism is typically accompanied by a low PO_2 (<80 mm Hg) and a low PCO_2 (<40 mm Hg). The low PCO_2 is produced by hyperventilation. Pulmonary embolism, the arterial PO_2 is usually under 80 mm Hg and the PCO_2 below 40 mm Hg.[1]

The chest x-ray may or may not be abnormal. Abnormalities that may be seen include infiltrates, effusions, decreased pulmonary vascular markings, and radiographic evidence of acute cor pulmonale.[1]

Except for sinus tachycardia, the electrocardiogram is often normal. The pattern of a deep S1, a prominent Q III, and an inverted TIII is usually only found in patients with acute cor pulmonale.[1] The ECG will, however, rule out a myocardial infarction as a cause of the patient's symptoms.

An increase in LDH isoenzyme 3 is found in most cases of pulmonary embolus. Liver enzymes and CK-MB (cardiac isoenzyme) levels are usually normal.

51. C. The medical treatment of deep venous thrombosis and pulmonary embolism is heparin, thrombolytic therapy, or both.

Heparin may be given at 1000 units/hour following a 5000 unit bolus. The heparin dose should be adjusted according to the level of the activated thromboplastin time (ATT). Heparin should be continued for 7–10 days, after which warfarin should be substituted.[1,3]

Thrombolytic therapy with streptokinase or urokinase may be the treatment of choice for patients with massive pulmonary embolism, submassive pulmonary embolism with shock, and severe deep venous thrombosis.[1] The details of this therapy are beyond the scope of this book.

Warfarin therapy, if begun within 3 days of initial hospitalization, may shorten hospital stay.[1] Warfarin, (adjusted to prothrombin time of 1.2–1.5 × control) should be continued for at least 3 months.[3]

Isosorbide nitrate is, of course, not indicated in the treatment of deep venous thrombosis and pulmonary embolism.

52. E. Deep venous thrombosis and pulmonary embolism are among the most common causes of morbidity and mortality in hospitalized patients. Risk factors include immobility (both post-traumatic and postoperative), history of DVT, oral contraceptive or estrogen use, pregnancy, cerebrovascular accidents, obesity, malignancy, autoimmune diseases, nephrotic syndrome, polycythemia, inflammatory bowel disease, and congestive cardiac failure.[1]

53. C. A well performed clinical examination is only 50% sensitive in detecting deep venous thrombosis.

The most reliable test for diagnosing deep venous thrombosis is ascending venography.[1] A normal venogram essentially rules out the diagnosis of deep vein thrombosis.[1]

Calf-vein thrombi, unlike iliofemoral thrombi, rarely result in clinically significant pulmonary emboli.[1]

Impedance plethysmography (IPG) and Doppler ultrasonography are highly sensitive for detecting proximal deep vein thrombi but not for detecting thrombi in the calves.[1] Radionuclide scanning is a sensitive test for detecting thrombi in the calves but not in the thighs.

54. E. In 1986, a national conference on antithrombotic therapy was held.[4] The recommendations of this conference were:
1) patients at moderate risk of venous thromboembolism for any reason should receive preventive therapy with low-dose heparin (5000 units q12h) or with intermittent pneumatic compression.
2) patients undergoing neurosurgical procedures, urologic procedures, and major knee surgery should be treated with intermittent pneumatic compression
3) patients undergoing elective hip surgery should receive prophylaxis with adjusted-dose heparin therapy or moderate-dose warfarin therapy.
4) patients who are undergoing repair of a hip fracture should receive prophylactic therapy with moderate-dose warfarin therapy.

SUMMARY OF THE DIAGNOSIS AND TREATMENT OF VENOUS THROMBOEMBOLISM

1. **Diagnosis:** Most patients who develop DVT and subsequent pulmonary embolism have one of the risk factors discussed in question 52. DVT is often clinically silent. Pulmonary embolism, however, is often heralded by the abrupt onset of dyspnea, chest pain, apprehension, hemoptysis, or syncope. When massive pulmonary embolism is present, the signs of acute cor pulmonale are evident. With pulmonary embolism, rhonchi are frequently heard in the chest.

2. **Laboratory evaluation:**
Low PO_2 and low PCO_2 are characteristic
LDH is often elevated
Chest x-ray is nonspecific
ECG is most useful in distinguishing pulmonary embolism from acute myocardial infarction

3. **Radiologic confirmation:**
Deep venous thrombosis:
    Most reliable test in ascending venography.

Impedance plethysmography (IPG) and Doppler ultrasonography are highly sensitive for detecting proximal deep vein thrombi but not for detecting thrombi in the calves.

Radionuclide scanning is sensitive for detecting thrombi in the calves.

Pulmonary embolism:

Ventilation-perfusion scanning is procedure of choice. Two or more medium or large perfusion defects with ventilation-perfusion mismatch produce a 90% probability of pulmonary embolism.

Pulmonary angiography remains the gold standard.

4. **Treatment:**

Deep venous thrombosis: heparin followed by warfarin therapy. Warfarin therapy should be continued for at least 3 months.

Pulmonary embolism: heparin or thrombolytic therapy (streptokinase or urokinase) followed by warfarin therapy. Pulmonary embolectomy may be life-saving in moribund patients. Warfarin should be continued for at least 3 months.

5. **Prevention:** Follow standards set out by the National Conference on Antithrombotic Therapy to prevent venous thromboembolism in patients at risk (see question 54).

References

1. Rubenstein E. Thromboembolism. In: Rubenstein E, Federman D, eds. Scientific American medicine. New York: Scientific American Medicine Inc, 1989: 1(XVIII), 1–14.

2. Hull RD, Hirsh J, Carter CJ, et al. Pulmonary angiography, ventilation lung scanning, and venography for clinically suspected pulmonary embolism with abnormal perfusion lung scan. Ann Intern Med 1983; 98: 891.

3. Shapiro S, Campbell E. Pulmonary embolism. In: Dunagan W, Ridner M, eds. Manual of medical therapeutics. 26th Ed. Boston: Little, Brown, 1989: 209–213.

4. American College of Chest Physicians and the National Heart, Blood, and Lung Institute national conference on antithrombotic therapy. Chest 1986; 89 (Suppl): 1S.

PROBLEM 7:   A 78-YEAR-OLD MALE WITH SUDDEN ONSET HEMIPLEGIA

A 78-year-old male presents with the acute onset of a left-sided paralysis. The paralysis seemed to evolve over several hours in the middle of the night. His past medical history is significant for hypertension, which has been well controlled on hydrochlorothiazide and captopril.

On examination, the patient's blood pressure is 170/100 mm Hg. His pulse is 96 and regular. His neurological examination reveals left-sided hemiplegia along with hemianesthesia. There is also a left homonymous hemianopsia. His head and eyes are deviated to the right side.

SELECT THE ONE BEST ANSWER TO THE FOLLOWING QUESTIONS:

55. The most likely artery involved with the symptoms described above is the:
    a) anterior cerebral artery
    b) right middle cerebral artery
    c) vertebral artery
    d) posterior cerebral artery
    e) left middle cerebral artery

56. The diagnostic procedure of choice for the patient described in question 55 is:
    a) digital subtraction angiography
    b) carotid arteriography
    c) CT scanning
    d) lumbar puncture
    e) NMR scanning

57. The diagnostic procedure of choice for the patient described in question 55 is performed. It reveals an ischemic infarction. The neurologic deficits appear to be worsening. The drug of choice for the treatment of this patient in the acute phase is:
    a) warfarin
    b) aspirin
    c) dipyridamole
    d) heparin
    e) mannitol

58. The single most important risk factor for stroke is:
    a) hypertension

b) age
c) diabetes mellitus
d) coronary artery disease
e) cigarette smoking

59. The single most common cause of stroke is:
a) embolism from a cardiac source
b) intracranial hemorrhage secondary to hypertension
c) thrombosis secondary to atherosclerosis of the carotid system
d) subarachnoid hemorrhage
e) thrombosis secondary to atherosclerosis of the vertebral system

60. Which of the following statements about transient ischemic attacks (TIAs) is FALSE?
a) transient ischemic attacks refer to episodes of neurologic dysfunction that last less than 24 hours
b) almost all patients that experience TIAs go on to develop completed strokes
c) the peak age for the development of TIAs is in the seventh decade
d) transient ischemic attacks result largely from thromboembolism
e) transient ischemia of the retina results in amaurosis fugax

61. A patient presents with a left-sided neurological deficit including weakness and decreased sensation in both the left arm and left leg. The symptoms evolved over 3 hours and lasted 10 days. The symptoms then cleared completely. The phenomenon is called:
a) a transient ischemic attack (TIA)
b) a reversible ischemic neurological disability (RIND)
c) a partial nonprogressing stroke (PNS)
d) a completed stroke
e) a progressing stroke or stroke-in-evolution

ANSWER THE FOLLOWING QUESTIONS ACCORDING TO THE CODE:

A: 1, 2, and 3 are correct
B: 1 and 3 are correct
C: 2 and 4 are correct
D: Only 4 is correct
E: All of the above are correct

62. The drug(s)of choice for the prevention of transient ischemic attacks is(are):

1) warfarin
2) dipyridamole
3) vitamin E
4) aspirin

63. Which of the following statements regarding carotid endarterectomy is(are) true?
1) carotid endarterectomy is indicated in the presence of a completed stroke
2) carotid endarterectomy is indicated in the presence of a complete arterial occlusion
3) randomized, controlled trials have established the benefit of carotid endarterectomy over standard medical therapy for the treatment of carotid artery stenosis
4) carotid endarterectomy may be superior to medical therapy when operative morbidity and mortality are low, but relative benefits of endarterectomy and aspirin are unknown.

SELECT THE ONE BEST ANSWER TO THE FOLLOWING QUESTION:

64. A 25-year-old female is admitted to the emergency department with the sudden onset of a severe headache. She describes this headache as "the worst headache she has ever had." She has no previous history of other significant medical illness, including migraine headache.

On examination, the patient has a stiff neck. Her blood pressure is 150/95 mm Hg. The headache persists despite an injection of 100 mg of intramuscular meperidine.

The most likely diagnosis in this patient is:
a) subarachnoid hemorrhage
b) intracerebral hemorrhage
c) cerebrovascular malformation
d) acute migraine headache
e) none of the above

ANSWERS

55. B. The patient described in question 55 has the classical presentation of a middle cerebral artery thrombosis. The middle cerebral artery is the most frequent site of intracranial vascular thrombosis.[1] Symptoms of middle cerebral artery thrombosis include hemiplegia, hemianesthesia, homonymous hemianopsia, and a deviation of the head and eyes toward the side on which the lesion is located.[1] Smaller lesions will produce less profound symptoms.

Thrombosis of the anterior cerebral artery is less common than thrombosis of the middle cerebral artery. With involvement of this artery, there is usually greater involvement of the leg than the arm.[1]

Thrombosis in the vertebrobasilar system tends to produce cranial nerve lesions, ataxia, vertigo, dysarthria, weakness or sensory disturbances in some or all of the limbs, and sometimes intranuclear ophthalmoplegia.

56. C. Computerized cranial tomography will differentiate an ischemic stroke from a hemorrhagic stroke.[2] This is of critical importance in deciding whether or not to use anticoagulants in the acute phase.

Digital subtraction angiography is not helpful in the diagnosis of acute stroke. Carotid arteriography is contraindicated in the acute phase of stroke and lumbar puncture for the detection of subarachnoid hemorrhage has been replaced by CT scanning.

Magnetic resonance imaging, although valuable in the detection of cerebellar and cerebral pathology, has not yet replaced CT scanning as the diagnostic procedure of choice in acute stroke.

57. D. Anticoagulation with heparin should probably be used when the neurologic deficits are found to worsen progressively (stroke-in-evolution), unless there is CT evidence of cerebral hemorrhage.[3] Prophylactic anticoagulation is also indicated in patients who have suffered a cerebral embolism as a result of rheumatic heart disease or atrial fibrillation.[3] The use of vasodilators and antiedema agents such as mannitol have not gained widespread acceptance.

Aspirin is recommended in the chronic phase of stroke and for the prevention of TIAs.[3] Aspirin and dipyridamole are recommended for the prevention of cerebral embolism following insertion of an artificial heart valve. Warfarin is sometimes used in the treatment of TIAs if they are relatively recent in onset (within months).

58. A. Stroke remains the third leading cause of death in North America. The single most important risk factor for stroke is hypertension.[2] The decrease in the incidence of stroke is most likely due, for the most part, to the effective treatment of hypertension.

Other factors that are important are age, coronary artery disease, cigarette smoking, diabetes mellitus, complicated migraine headaches, and use of the oral contraceptive pill.

59. C. The single most common cause of stroke is thrombosis secondary to atherosclerosis.[2] The thrombus originates from the carotid artery system twice as often as from the vertebral artery system.

Cerebral embolism accounts for up to 20% of strokes. The embolism most commonly arises from a cardiac source.

Subarachnoid hemorrhage accounts for 10% of the total number of strokes. This usually occurs secondary to a rupture of a congenital berry aneurysm around the area of the circle of Willis.

Intracerebral hemorrhage accounts for 5% of strokes, with most of this total being due to hypertensive intracerebral hemorrhage.

60. B. Cerebral transient ischemic attacks (TIAs) are episodes of neurologic dysfunction that develop suddenly and clear completely within 24 hours.[2] The peak age for the development of TIAs is in the seventh decade. Although the incidence is not precisely known, the majority of patients with TIAs do not go on to develop completed strokes.

TIAs result mainly from thromboembolism. Aggregated platelets or debris from ulcerated atheromatous plaques in the extracranial carotid system are the most common type of emboli.[2]

Transient ischemia of the retina, which results from microembolization in the ophthalmic branch of the internal carotid artery, causes transient blackness of vision (amaurosis fugax). Patients often feel as though a shade has been pulled down over one eye.

Cerebral hemisphere ischemia produces the sudden onset of such symptoms as contralateral monoparesis or hemiparesis, localized tingling or numbness, hemianopic visual loss, or aphasia.[1,2] Vertebrobasilar ischemia produces visual symptoms such as dim, grey, blurred vision, transient disturbance of conjugate gaze, or even total blindness. Brainstem symptoms include dysarthria, dysphagia, perioral numbness, and weakness or paraethesias of all four limbs. Drop attacks, in which there is a sudden loss of postural tone in the legs, are also characteristic of basilar insufficiency.[1,2]

61. B. This patient has a reversible ischemic neurologic deficit (RIND). This is defined as an ischemic neurologic deficit that lasts longer than 24 hours but resolves within 3 weeks.[4]

An ischemic event leaving persistent disability but short of a calamitous stroke is defined as a partial nonprogressing stroke (PNS).[4] More severe ischemia producing major permanent neurologic disability is termed a completed stroke. A stroke-in-evolution is a gradual worsening of neurological symptoms over hours or weeks.[4]

62. D. The drug of choice for the prevention of TIAs is aspirin.[3] No benefit has yet been demonstrated for the other known platelet antiaggregants, sulfinpyrazone and dipyridamole.

Some authorities recommend the use of anticoagulants for recently developed TIAs in carotid and vertebrobasilar territory,[3] recommending them for 2 to 3 months if a cluster of TIAs occurs that is not relieved by platelet antiaggregant therapy. Vitamin E has no place to play in the treatment of TIAs.

63. D. Carotid endarterectomy may be superior to medical therapy when operative morbidity and mortality are low, but relative benefits of endarterectomy and aspirin are not known.[3] Patients who may be considered for carotid endarterectomy include patients with TIA, RIND, or a minimal persistent deficit.[3]

Carotid endarterectomy is not indicated in the presence of a completed stroke or in the presence of a complete arterial occlusion appropriate to the symptoms.

64. A. This patient has most likely had a subarachnoid hemorrhage. The most likely etiology is a cerebral aneurysm in or near the circle of Willis.[1,2]

The symptoms of subarachnoid hemorrhage include a sudden violent headache (the worst ever experienced), confusion, agitation, collapse, and coma. Nuchal rigidity and other signs of meningeal irritation are usually present. Grossly bloody CSF on lumbar puncture confirms the diagnosis.[1,2,4]

Cerebral hemorrhage will usually present with a hemiplegia.

A cerebrovascular malformation could cause the symptoms described, but a subarachnoid hemorrhage would be much more likely.

Acute onset migraine headache is not a diagnostic consideration.

SUMMARY OF THE DIAGNOSIS AND TREATMENT OF CEREBROVASCULAR ACCIDENTS

1. **Diagnosis:**
Middle cerebral artery thrombosis or embolism (most common syndrome): hemiplegia, hemianesthesia, homonymous hemianopsia, and a deviation of the head and eyes toward the side on which the lesion is located. Thrombosis of artery branches produces less severe neurological deficit; motor and sensory impairment will be greater in the face and arm than in the leg.

Anterior cerebral artery thrombosis or embolism: less common than middle cerebral artery thrombosis. A thrombosis in this area usually produces a more profound degree of impairment in the leg than in the face and arm.

Vertebrobasilar artery thrombosis or embolism: cranial nerve lesions, ataxia, nystagmus, dysarthria, vertigo, motor or sensory disturbance in some or all of the limbs, intranuclear ophthalmoplegia.

Lacunar syndromes: small areas of infarction (lacunes), resulting from atheromatous occlusion of deep penetrating branches of the major cerebral arteries.

Cerebral hemorrhage:
Deep in cerebral hemisphere: flaccid hemiplegia, dense hemianesthesia, and hemianopsia

Pontine hemorrhage: paralysis of conjugate gaze, marked pupillary miosis, and flaccid-quadriplegia.

Cerebellar hemorrhage: headache, vomiting, unsteadiness of gait, and collapse. Nuchal rigidity, ipsilateral paresis of conjugate gaze, dysarthria, reduced corneal reflex, and peripheral facial weakness.

Subarachnoid hemorrhage: Sudden onset of "the most severe headache". Sudden violent headache followed rapidly by confusion, agitation, collapse, and coma. Nuchal rigidity present.
Classification of stroke syndromes: Transient ischemic attack (TIA): neurologic deficit resolving within 24 hours

Reversible ischemic neurologic disability (RIND): neurologic deficit persisting more than 24 hours but resolving within 3 weeks

Partial nonprogressing stroke (PNS): an ischemic event leaving persistent disability short of a calamitous stroke

Completed stroke: a stroke that results in permanent neurologic disability

Progressing stroke or stroke-in-evolution: neurological deficits worsening gradually or stepwise over hours to weeks

2. **Evaluation:**

A CT scan will differentiate an ischemic stroke from a hemorrhagic stroke.

Carotid ultrasound is useful in the evaluation of TIA's

3. **Treatment:**

Anticoagulants (heparin and warfarin) are used in the management of acute ischemic stroke.

Aspirin is the drug of choice for the treatment of TIAs.

Aneurysm clipping should be performed if subarachnoid hemorrhage is due to cerebral aneurysm (confirmed by angiography)

Careful lowering of blood pressure if the patient is hypertensive is necessary in the treatment of acute stroke.

Long-term physical therapy for rehabilitation, and attention to the needs of the patient and his(her) family are most important. Depression is common in both the patient and family following a sudden stroke; this may require therapy with tricyclic antidepressants.

References

1. Cutler R. Cerebrovascular diseases. In: Rubenstein E, Federman D, eds. Scientific American Medicine. New York: Scientific American Inc, 1987: 11(X) 1–9.

2. Kistler P, Ropper A, Martin J. Cerebrovascular diseases. In: Braunwald E, Isselbacher K, Petersdorf R, Wilson J, Martin J, Fauci A, eds. Harrison's textbook of internal medicine. 11th Ed. New York: McGraw-Hill, 1987: 1930–1959.

3. Applegate C, Fox P. Cerebrovascular disease. In: Dunagan M, Ridner M, eds. Manual of medical therapeutics. 26th Ed. Boston: Little, Brown, 1989: 468–473.

4. Barnett H. Cerebral ischemia and infarction. In: Wyngaarden J, Smith L, eds. Cecil textbook of medicine. 18th Ed. Philadelphia: WB Saunders, 1988: 2163–2173.

PROBLEM 8: A 55-YEAR-OLD MALE WITH A CHRONIC COUGH

A 55-year-old male presents to your office for assessment of a chronic cough. He states that he has "been coughing for the last 10 years," but the cough is becoming more bothersome lately. The cough is productive of sputum that is usually mucoid; occasionally it becomes purulent.

His significant past history is a 35-year history of smoking 2 packs of cigarettes/day.

On examination, he is obese (280 pounds). He wheezes while he talks. On auscultation, adventitious breath sounds are heard in all lobes.

His chest x-ray reveals increased markings at the lung bases.

SELECT THE ONE BEST ANSWER TO THE FOLLOWING QUESTIONS:

65. The most likely diagnosis in this patient is:
    a) smoker's cough
    b) subacute bronchitis
    c) emphysema
    d) chronic bronchitis
    e) allergic bronchitis

ANSWER THE FOLLOWING QUESTIONS ACCORDING TO THE CODE:

A: 1, 2, and 3 are correct
B: 1 and 3 are correct
C: 2 and 4 are correct
D: Only 4 is correct
E: All of the above are correct

66. Which of the following statements regarding the condition described in question 65 is(are) true?

1) the disease develops in 10–15% of cigarette smokers
2) cigarette smokers in whom this disease develops usually report the onset of cough with expectoration 10–12 years after they begin smoking
3) dyspnea is noted initially only on extreme exertion, but as the condition progresses, it becomes more severe and occurs with mild activity
4) pneumonia, pulmonary hypertension, cor pulmonale, and chronic respiratory failure characterize the late stage of the disease

67. Which of the following statements regarding the patient discussed in question 65 is(are) true?
   1) this patient is a "pink puffer"
   2) this patient will probably have a decreased PCO_2.
   3) this patient will probably demonstrate hyperinflation on the chest x-ray
   4) this patient will probably demonstrate an increased inspiratory resistance

68. Which of the following abnormalities in pulmonary function testing are commonly seen in patients with the disease described above?
   1) reduced FEV_1
   2) reduced FEV_1/FVC
   3) reduced FEF_{25-75}
   4) decreased residual volume

69. Which of the following statements regarding the use of bronchodilators in the condition described above is(are) true?
   1) bronchodilators have been shown to alter the course of COPD and improve life expectancy
   2) bronchodilators may provide symptomatic relief of dyspnea and improve exercise tolerance
   3) inhaled anticholinergics appear to be less effective than inhaled beta agonists.
   4) when inhaled anticholinergics are combined with inhaled beta agonists, the effect is additive

70. Which of the following statements regarding the use of corticosteroids in the condition described above is(are) true?
   1) steroids should be used in patients with uncomplicated COPD
   2) corticosteroids are effective in some patients with asthmatic bronchitis
   3) when a corticosteroid trial is given to a patient with the condition described, it may be reasonable to continue it even if there is lack of objective evidence of improvement
   4) corticosteroids should be used in the smallest effective dosage in the condition described

71. Which of the following statements regarding the use of long-term oxygen in the treatment of the condition described above is(are) true?
   1) chronic hypoxemia causes secondary erythrocytosis and contributes to exercise limitation; this may be reversed by long-term oxygen therapy
   2) chronic hypoxemia causes pulmonary hypertension and right heart failure; this may be ameliorated and improved by long-term oxygen therapy
   3) patients with the condition described above should receive long-term oxygen therapy if the resting PO_2 level is 55 mm Hg or less
   4) long-term oxygen therapy improves the quality and the quantity of life in patients with the condition described above

72. Which of the following treatment modalities is(are) often useful in the treatment of the condition described above?
   1) antibiotics
   2) physiotherapy
   3) smoking cessation
   4) digoxin

ANSWERS

65. D. This patient has chronic bronchitis. Chronic bronchitis is defined as cough and sputum production on most days for at least 3 months of the year of a minimum of 2 years in succession.[1] Chronic bronchitis is most often caused by cigarette smoking.

Acute bronchitis is an inflammation of the bronchi caused by an infectious agent or acute exposure to a nonspecific irritant.[2] Acute bronchitis is most often caused by a viral infection. Acute bronchitis may occur as a complication of chronic bronchitis.

Emphysema is a destructive process involving the lung parenchyma. It is defined as abnormal permanent enlargement of air spaces distal to the terminal bronchiole accompanied by destruction of alveoloar walls.[1]

Subacute bronchitis is a nondiagnosis.

Allergic bronchitis refers to reversible airflow obstruction that is caused by exposure to an environmental agent.

Chronic bronchitis and emphysema are responsible for the majority of chronic obstructive pulmonary disease (COPD).

66. E. All of the statements are true. Chronic bronchitis usually develops in cigarette smokers, 10–12 years after they began smoking. Patients with chronic bronchitis have an increased susceptibility to recurrent respiratory infections.

Obstructive lung disease develops in 10–15% of patients who are cigarette smokers, and in these patients, airflow obstruction worsens over time if cigarette smoking is continued.[1]

Dyspnea is initially noted only on extreme exertion, but as the condition progresses, it becomes more severe and occurs with mild activity. In severe disease, dyspnea occurs at rest.

Complications of COPD include pneumonia, pulmonary hypertension, cor pulmonale, and chronic respiratory failure.[1]

67. D. There are two types of COPD patients: Type A or "pink puffers" and Type B or "blue bloaters."[3] The patient described in the question is a classic "blue bloater." Pink puffers are: (1) usually thin, (2) usually present with dyspnea, (3) have hyperinflated lungs on chest x-ray, and (4) have a slightly decreased PO_2 and a normal or slightly decreased PCO_2. Blue bloaters are: (1) often stocky or obese, (2) usually present with cough and sputum production, (3) have normal or increased lung markings, (4) usually have a markedly reduced PO_2 and elevated PCO_2, and (5) often develop pulmonary hypertension and cor pulmonale.

68. A. COPD is characterized by several abnormalities on pulmonary function testing. Abnormalities include an increased residual volume (RV) and a normal to increased functional residual capacity. There is a decrease in the forced vital capacity in 1 second (FEV_1) and the ratio of FEV_1/FVC. Also, there is a decrease in the FEF_{25-75}.[3]

69. C. Chronic bronchitis and emphysema are generally considered to be diseases manifested by fixed airflow obstruction. Most patients have some degree of reversible airflow obstruction. Patients with dyspnea should be given a trial of bronchodilators even if pulmonary function testing does not demonstrate signficiant bronchodilation.[1] Patients may respond with decreased dyspnea and improved exercise tolerance.

At present, there is no evidence that bronchodilators affect the course of the disease or improve life expectancy.

In COPD, inhaled anticholinergics may be equally or more effective than inhaled beta agonists. When these two agents are combined, they are synergistic. They may be used regularly by metered-dose inhaler or as needed depending on the symptomatic response.[4]

70. C. Corticosteroids should not be used in patients with uncomplicated COPD. Only those patients with a reversible airflow component, or asthma, should be treated with corticosteroids.[1,4] There may be a significant therapeutic effect of corticosteroids in suppressing the inflammation associated with asthmatic bronchitis.

Corticosteroids should only be continued in those patients in whom objective improvement can be demonstrated. If improvement occurs, the oral corticosteroid should be tapered to the lowest effective maintenance level and an attempt should be made to substitute an inhaled corticosteroid. In patients who do not respond to prednisone, there is no rationale to continue either oral or inhaled corticosteroids.

71. E. The single most important treatment modality in patients with COPD is the use of long-term supplementary oxygen therapy.[4]

Chronic hypoxemia causes secondary erythrocytosis, limits exercise capabilities, and causes pulmonary hypertension, right-sided heart failure, and impaired mental functioning. All of these consequences of COPD can be improved by the administration of oxygen at levels that are sufficient to maintain the arterial oxygen saturation at values exceeding 90%. This value (corresponding to a PO_2 of 60–80 mm Hg) can usually be achieved with oxygen supplementation delivered at a rate of 2 L/min via nasal cannula.

Survival is significantly improved when supplemental oxygen is given 24 hours/day. Shorter periods of daily therapy do, however, improve symptoms.

Patients with COPD who should receive home oxygen include those with resting PO_2 levels less than 55 mm Hg or those with PO_2 levels of less than 59 mm Hg if one or more of the following conditions are present: peripheral edema (a sign of cor pulmonale), a hematocrit of 55% or greater, or evidence of P pulmonale on the electrocardiogram.[3]

72.   A. If infection supervenes in chronic bronchitis, antibiotics should be administered for a 10-day course. Infection is suspected when there is a change in sputum color (to purulent) or a change in sputum volume. Secondary infection in COPD is usually caused by either *Hemophilus influenzae* or *Streptococcus pneumoniae*. Regular antibiotic administration may, in some patients, be reasonable.[1,3]

Smoking cessation should be advocated in all patients with chronic bronchitis.[3] Cough and sputum production will often be significantly reduced or completely disappear over a period of 4–6 months following cessation of cigarette smoking.

Active physiotherapy including chest percussion and vibration may be extremely helpful in patients who have sputum that is difficult to mobilize.[1]

Digoxin is contraindicated in the right-sided heart failure of cor pulmonale with the exception of supraventricular tachydysrhythmias.

SUMMARY OF THE DIAGNOSIS AND TREATMENT OF COPD

1.   **Definitions:**
Chronic bronchitis: the presence of cough and sputum production on most days for at least 3 months of the year and for a minimum of 2 years in succession
Emphysema: permanent and abnormal enlargement of the acinus (primary lobule of the lung), with destruction of alveolar walls

2.   **Etiology:** in almost all cases cigarette smoking

3.   **Differentiation of subtypes of COPD:**
Type A: The "pink puffer": emphysema
Type B: The "blue bloater": chronic bronchitis

4.   **Pulmonary function test abnormalities:**
a)   decreased FEV_1
b)   decreased ratio of FEV_1/FVC
c)   decreased FEF_{25-75}
d)   increased residual volume
e)   normal to increased functional residual capacity

5.   **Treatment:**
a)   continuous home oxygen: the only therapy that has been shown to improve survival in patients with COPD
b)   bronchodilators: beta agonists and anticholinergics may improve dyspnea and exercise tolerance. They are synergistic.
c)   corticosteroids: reduce inflammation in patients with a reversible component. They should only be used if there is objective evidence of improvement, tapered, and switched from oral to inhaled as soon as possible
d)   antibiotics
e)   physiotherapy
f)   diuretics (with caution)
g)   smoking cessation
h)   counseling/support groups

References

1.   Stauffer J. Pulmonary diseases. In: Krupp M, Schroeder S, Tierney L, McPhee S, eds. Current medical diagnosis and treatment. Norwalk: Appleton and Lange, 1989: 141–145.

2.   Rodnick J, Gude J. The respiratory system. In: Taylor R, ed. Family medicine: principles and practice. 3rd Ed. New York: Springer-Verlag, 1988: 210–214.

3.   Fanta C, Ingram R. Chronic obstructive diseases of the lung. In: Federman D, Rubensteins E, eds. Scientific American medicine. New York: Scientific American Medicine Inc, 1988; 14(III): 1–22.

4.   Tullis E, Grossman R. Outpatient management of patients with chronic obstructive lung disease. Can Fam Physician 1989; 35: 1527–1531.

PROBLEM 9:   A 75-YEAR-OLD MALE WITH METASTATIC BONE PAIN
SECONDARY TO PROSTATE CANCER

A 75-year-old male was discovered to have Stage IV cancer of the prostate. As he was not symptomatic at the time of diagnosis, therapy was postponed. Six months after diagnosis he developed mild pain in the lumbar region.

On examination, there is tenderness over the L2–L5 vertebrae. No other abnormalities are found on physical examination.

A bone scan is performed and reveals increased uptake of radionuclide in the L2–L5 area, compatible with metastatic disease.

SELECT THE ONE BEST ANSWER TO THE FOLLOWING QUESTIONS:

73. The initial treatment of choice for his patient's mild bone pain is:
    a) morphine sulfate
    b) palliative radiotherapy
    c) a nonsteroidal anti-inflammatory drug
    d) Brompton's cocktail
    e) acetaminophen

74. You begin the patient described above on a treatment regimen. His pain is well controlled for 6 weeks. However, at that time, he once again develops severe pain in his lumbar spine and pain in the area of the right ischium. You suspect progression of the metastatic disease. At this time, you would add which of the following drugs to the patient's treatment regimen.
    a) pentazocine
    b) meperidine
    c) morphine sulfate
    d) a nonsteroidal anti-inflammatory drug
    e) acetaminophen

75. You make the appropriate change to the patient's treatment regimen. With increasing dosage of the analgesic you selected, he remains pain free for 6 months. However, as the dosage continues to be increased, he begins to become nauseated. You institute appropriate antinauseant therapy, but he fails to respond. Which of the following narcotic agents would you now consider as the agent of choice to switch to for the management of this patient's cancer pain?
    a) methadone
    b) pentazocine
    c) heroin
    d) hydromorphone
    e) meperidine

76. The average starting dosage of morphine sulfate in a patient with terminal cancer is:

    a) 1–2 mg every 4 hours
    b) 5–10 mg every 4 hours
    c) 10–20 mg every 4 hours
    d) 5–10 mg every 6 hours
    e) 20–30 mg every 6 hours

77. The most common type of pain in patients with terminal cancer is:
    a) visceral pain
    b) bone pain
    c) soft-tissue inflammatory pain
    d) nerve root compression pain
    e) pain due to secondary infection

ANSWER THE FOLLOWING QUESTIONS ACCORDING TO THE CODE:

A: 1, 2, and 3 are correct
B: 1 and 3 are correct
C: 2 and 4 are correct
D: Only 4 is correct
E: All of the above are correct

78. Which of the following statements regarding the use of morphine in the treatment of cancer pain is(are) false?
    1) morphine produces rapid tolerance
    2) morphine produces euphoria
    3) morphine produces addiction
    4) morphine produces respiratory depression

79. Which of the following agents are effective co-analgesic(s) in the management of cancer pain?
    1) dexamethasone
    2) Tegretol
    3) amitriptyline
    4) diazepam

80. Which of the following statements regarding the use of antinauseants and antiemetics in the treatment of cancer pain is(are) true?
    1) antinauseants should be initiated when a narcotic analgesic is begun

2) antinauseants are sometimes more effective in combination than as single agents

3) antinauseants may be discontinued in many cancer patients after the effective dosage of narcotic analgesic is established

4) antinauseants usually produce signficant side effects in cancer patients

81. Which of the following statements regarding the prevention of constipation in patients who are being treated with narcotic analgesics is(are) true?

1) stool softeners and peristaltic stimulants should be started when a patient is begun on an oral narcotic

2) a combination of docusate and a standarized senna concentrate is a good prophylactic regimen to prevent constipation

3) the dosage of stool softener and peristaltic stimulant may have to be increased as the dose of oral narcotic is increased

4) psyllium hydrophilic mucilloid is a good choice for the prevention of constipation in a patient on an oral narcotic analgesic

82. Which of the following is(are) aims of pain management in palliative care?

1) to identify the cause of the pain

2) to prevent the pain from occurring

3) to maintain a clear sensorium

4) to maintain a normal effect

83. Which of the following factors modify the pain threshold in patients with cancer pain?

1) insomnia

2) fear

3) anxiety

4) sadness

84. Which of the following statements concerning the use of narcotic analgesics in the treatment of cancer pain is(are) true?

1) most patients with cancer pain can be effectively treated with oral narcotics

2) intramuscular narcotic administration on a regular basis is not recommended for terminally ill patients

3) narcotic analgesics may be effectively administered by the rectal route

4) the subcutaneous infusion of fluids, narcotic analgesics and other medications is preferred to intravenous therapy in terminally ill patients

ANSWERS

73. C. The treatment of first choice for mild bone pain due to secondary cancer is a nonsteroidal anti-inflammatory drug.[1] Tumors in bone, and possibly elsewhere, liberate prostaglandins, which sensitize nerve endings to painful stimuli. Anti-inflammatory drugs such as diclofenac, aspirin, ibuprofen, and naproxen inhibit prostaglandin synthesis and are therefore effective at the site of the pain. In contradistinction, narcotic analgesics act centrally.[2]

Many cancer patients with metastatic disease can be controlled on nonsteroidal anti-inflammatory drugs. When the drug becomes ineffective, a narcotic analgesic should be added.[1] Nonsteroidal anti-inflammatory agents and narcotic analgesics work by two different mechanisms; therefore, their effects, especially with bony metastatic disease, are additive.[1]

Palliative radiotherapy[1] could be used as a treatment option following the failure of a nonsteroidal agent. However, it may be better to try a narcotic analgesic first and keep palliative radiotherapy as a future consideration.

The drug of second choice, in the opinion of Tywcross and others[2] is a combination of aspirin-codeine or acetaminophin-codeine. However, because of the highly constipating effect of codeine, you may wish to go straight to a morphine preparation. Acetaminophen may be effective in the treatment of some patients with mild cancer pain; however, it is inferior to the nonsteroidal anti-inflammatory agents in bony metastatic disease.[2]

Brompton's cocktail is a mixture of cocaine, alcohol, a phenothiazine, and morphine or heroin. It has been replaced by more effective agents in the treatment of cancer pain.[2]

74. C. At this time, you should add a narcotic analgesic to the patient's treatment regimen. Morphine sulfate would be a good choice. Morphine sulfate can be begun in oral liquid or tablet form. The initial dose is 10–20 mg every 4 hours.[1] The dose is rapidly increased as needed. It is appropriate to write a dosage range to give the nurses added flexibility in controlling the patient's cancer pain. As well, morphine and other narcotic analgesics should never be given on a PRN basis in the treatment of terminal cancer pain. Additional morphine should always be available for breakthrough pain, but the patient must be given the analgesic on a regular basis.

Once the total daily dosage is established, the patient can be switched to a long-acting morphine preparation.[3] The total daily dose is given in two or three equal doses. This allows both patient and family to have a restful night, and eliminates the fear of waking up in pain. When a patient is switched to a long-acting preparation, the shorter-acting preparation should still be available for breakthrough pain. If a patient is getting significant breakthrough pain, the dosage of the longer acting preparation should be increased. As well, a short-acting preparation can be extremely useful in patients with bony metastatic disease before they are turned in bed. Ten or 15 mg of morphine given 20 minutes before turning the patient will significantly alleviate discomfort associated with movement.

An alternative to beginning morphine at this time would be to begin an aspirin-codeine preparation.[1] Because the pain is severe, however, this may not be appropriate.

Pentazocine (Talwin) and meperidine (Demerol) should never be used in the treatment of cancer pain. Pentazocine is an agonist-antagonist, and its use in chronic pain is therefore totally illogical.[1] Meperidine is a narcotic analgesic with a very short half-life. It is not, therefore, suitable for use in chronic cancer pain. In addition, oral meperidine is a poor analgesic, and repeated intramusuclar injections of meperidine in an emaciated cancer patient are both ineffective and uncomfortable.

Acetaminophen and other nonsteroidal anti-inflammatory agents are first-line, not second-line analgesics.

75. D. The agent of choice in this situation is hydromorphone (Dilaudid). Dilaudid is four times as potent on a milligram/milligram basis as morphine and is a good choice when side effects limit the use of morphine.[3] The dosage of morphine should be divided by four to arrive at the correct Dilaudid dose. Dilaudid must be given every 4 hours to produce complete pain control, and this may sometimes present a problem.[3]

Levorphanol and methadone[1] have both been successfully used in the management of cancer pain. In this situation, levorphanol would be a good alternative to hydromorphone. Methadone should only be used when other oral analgesics have failed.

Heroin, although an effective analgesic, is converted in the body to morphine. Thus, it seems to offer no real advantage over the analgesics that we presently have.[3]

As discussed previously, neither meperidine nor pentazocine has any place in the management of cancer pain.

76. C. The average starting dosage of morphine sulfate for a patient with terminal cancer is 10–20 mg every 4 hours.[1,4] Morphine (except sustained release) must be given every 4 hours. The nursing staff should be given some flexibility in dosing, and thus an order of 10–20 mg is a good starting dose. The dose can be increased by 5–10 mg every 4 hours until complete pain control is obtained. The patient can then be switched to a long-acting preparation and the total daily dosage given in two equal doses (occasionally three doses are required). The short acting preparation, however, should be maintained for breakthrough pain.

77. B. The most common type of cancer pain is metastatic bone pain. Nerve root compression pain is the second most common type of pain. Visceral pain and pain caused by tumor infiltration of soft tissue also occur frequently.

Many cancer patients have multiple cancer pains occurring at the same time.[2] Therapy for these pains may be different. Thus, it is important to try and determine which pain(s) are occurring at a given time in your patient.

78. E. All of the statements are false. These statements are known as the "morphine myths," and do not apply to patients who are in the terminal phase of illness.[2]

There is no maximum morphine or other analgesic equivalent dosage. Each patient requires his(her) dosage to be individualized. This should be done by starting at lower doses and increasing the dose until you have achieved total pain control.

79. E. All of the above are effective co-analgesics. Co-analgesics (drugs that act synergistically with analgesics to increase the pain threshold) include corticosteroids, dilantin, tricyclic antidepressants, and benzodiazepines.[1]

80. E. Antinauseants should be begun when a patient is begun on an oral narcotic agent.[1] Metoclopramide (Maxeran, Reglan), dimenhydrinate (Gravol), prochlorperazine (Stemetil), or chlorpromazine (Largactil) are the most commonly used agents.

In many cases, you can discontinue the antinauseant 1–2 weeks after beginning the oral narcotic. As the dosage is increased you may have to reinstitute the antinauseants.[2]

In cases of resistant nausea, either narcotic-analgesic induced or due to progression of disease, a combination of agents such as metoclopramide and Gravol may be more effective than either agent used alone.

Antinauseants usually do not produce significant side effects in terminally ill patients.

81. A. Stool softeners and peristaltic stimulants should be started when a patient is placed on an oral narcotic agent. This prevents constipation that is inevitably associated with the use of narcotic agents.[1,2]

A good treatment regimen is a combination of a stool softener such as docusate (Colace) and a peristaltic stimulant such as a concentrated senna preparation (Senokot). An alternative is a lactulose preparation.

Psyllium hydrophilic mucilloid (Metamucil) is not recommended as a prophylactic agent. It usually aggravates rather than relieves the problem.

Unlike the antinausents, this prophylactic bowel regimen usually cannot be discontinued.[2] The dosage of the agents used may have to be increased as the narcotic requirements are increased.

82. E. The aims of pain management in palliative care are to identify the cause of the pain, prevent the pain from occurring again, erase the memory of the pain, and at the same time maintain a clear sensorium and a normal effect.[2] With careful drug selection and titration, this can usually be done.

83. E. Cancer pain is a complex entity that requires treatment of not only the somatic source(s), but also the other aspects including depression, anxiety, anger, and isolation. Pain threshold is raised by relief of symptoms, sleep, rest, empathy, understanding, diversion, elevation of mood, effective analgesic, anxiolytics, and antidepressants. Pain threshold is lowered by discomfort, insomnia, fatigue, anxiety, fear, anger, sadness, depression, mental isolation, introversion, and past painful experiences.[2]

84. E. Most patients with terminal cancer pain can be effectively and completely treated with the regular administration of oral narcotic analgesics.[1,4] In the patients who cannot keep down an oral medication, the rectal suppository route will usually provide effective control.

In patients whose cancer pain is not effectively controlled by either the oral or the rectal route, a subcutaneous infusion of narcotic analgesic, along with antiemetics and other medications, may be established. This procedure requires the enzyme hyaluronidase to permit dispersion of the medication and to prevent buildup of fluid subcutaneously. This is known as hypodermoclysis,[5] and is preferable to intravenous administration because of friable, difficult-to-catheterize veins in terminally ill patients. Hypodermoclysis also allows complete mobilization. Subcutaneous infusion pumps are also available.

The regular use of intramuscular injections for the terminally ill cancer patient is not recommended. This is uncomfortable for a patient who is cachectic and emaciated, and the half-life of medications delivered by the intramuscular route is generally shorter than those delivered by the oral route.

SUMMARY OF THE TREATMENT OF CANCER PAIN

1. Cancer pain must be treated with attention to the physical, psychological, social, and spiritual manifestations of pain.

2. **Treatment of cancer pain:**
   A. First-line agents: NSAIDs, acetaminophen
   B. Optional second line agent: aspirin-codeine, acetaminophen-codeine
   C. Second line agent: morphine sulfate. Once total daily dosage is established switch to a sustained-release preparation. If side effects limit use, switch to hydromorphone. Other useful agents are levorphanol and anileridine. Begin morphine sulfate at 10–20 mg q4h. Increase or decrease at 5–10 mg q4h.
   D. The oral route will provide complete control in most cases. If patient is unable to keep down oral medication, consider rectal suppositories or hypodermoclysis.
   E. Consider the use of co-analgesics when appropriate.
   F. Consider palliative radiotherapy for metastatic bone pain.

3. **Bowel regimen:** All patients who are on oral narcotics should be on a bowel regimen to prevent

constipation. Docusate sodium and senna preparation or lactulose may be used. This should be continued for as long as the patient is on the oral narcotic and may have to be increased as the analgesic requirements change.

4. **Antiemetics**: Nausea and vomiting may be a side effect of narcotic analgesic use or may be due to the progression of the disease itself. All patients who are begun on narcotic analgesics should be started on an antiemetic for the first week or two. After that time, the drug dosage may be decreased or the drug stopped if there is no nausea or vomiting.

5. **Analgesic equivalency chart:**[3]

	Oral	*Subcutaneous*
Morphine	30 mg	15 mg
Hydromorphone	7.5 mg	3.75 mg
Levorphanol	4 mg	2 mg

6. **The Ten Commandments**[4,6]

1. *Thou shalt not assume that the patient's pain is due to the malignant process.* Always begin with steps aimed at making a specific diagnosis.
2. *Thou shalt consider the patient's feelings.* Pain threshold varies with mood and morale. Given the opportunity to express fears, the patient's pain may improve.
3. *Thou shalt not use the abbreviation "PRN."* Achieving balanced pain control means avoiding the return of pain because of gaps in medication administration. Less medication will be required if given round the clock as opposed to PRN dosing.
4. *Thou shalt prescribe adequate amounts of medication.* The right dose of medication is not dictated by a recommendation from a book, but rather by the patient's level of pain. Use what it takes to relieve the pain, titrating for effect.
5. *Thou shalt always try nonnarcotic medications first.* Mild to moderate pain is relieved in most instances by acetaminophen or non-

steroidal anti-inflammatory drugs. Nonsteroidal anti-inflammatory drugs are particularly useful for bony metastases.
6. *Thou shalt not be afraid of narcotic analgesics.* When nonnarcotic agents fail, move to a narcotic agent quickly.
7. *Thou shalt not limit thyself to using only drug therapies.* Nondrug therapies such as distraction, self-hypnosis, imagery techniques, talking, reading, and listening to music should be added. Some patients will benefit from radiation, nerve blocks, or immobilization.
8. *Thou shalt not be reluctant to seek a colleague's advice.* When you have exhausted your skills or run out of ideas, ask someone else to evaluate your patient.
9. *Thou shalt provide support for the entire family.* Treatment of the anticipatory grief experienced by the family will help to prevent isolation and loneliness. Be able to intervene quickly when a crisis occurs.
10. *Thou shalt maintain an air of quiet confidence and cautious optimism.* Aim for "graded relief," choosing small goals that can be accomplished to build the patient's trust and hope. Exhibit a determination to succeed.

References

1. Driscoll C. Pain management. Prim Care 1987; 14(2): 337–352.

2. Twycross R, Lack S. Symptom control in far advanced cancer. London: Pitman, 1983: 117–291.

3. Billings JA. Outpatient management of advanced cancer. Philadelphia: JB Lippincott, 1985: 27.

4. Silverman H, Crocker N. Pain management in terminally ill patients. Postgrad Med 1988; 83(8): 181–188.

5. Hays H. Hypodermoclysis for symptom control in terminal care. Can Fam Physician 1985; 31:1253–1256.

6. Twycross R. Principles and practice of pain relief in terminal cancer. In: Corr C, Corr D, eds. Hospice care—principles and practice. New York: Springer, 1983: 55–72.

PROBLEM 10: A 51-YEAR-OLD FEMALE WITH SEVERE NAUSEA AND VOMITING AND ADVANCED OVARIAN CARCINOMA

You are called to the home of a 51-year-old female with advanced ovarian carcinoma. She began vomiting 3 days ago (twice/day) and has had severe nausea and associated anorexia. In addition, she describes a sore mouth and difficulty breathing.

On examination, the patient's breathing is slightly labored. Her respiratory rate is 24/minute. She has numerous white patches in her mouth. She is cachectic. She has a large abdominal mass with ascites present.

SELECT THE ONE BEST ANSWER TO THE FOLLOWING QUESTIONS:

85. With respect to this patient's anorexia, which of the following treatments may be beneficial?
    a) prednisone 5 mg t.i.d.
    b) alcohol 1 oz prior to meals
    c) cyproheptadine 4 mg t.i.d.
    d) maltevol 12 multivitamin preparation
    e) all of the above may be of benefit

86. The nausea and vomiting that this patient has developed may be treated with various measures or drugs. Which of the following WOULD NOT be recommended as a treatment for this patient's nausea at this time?
    a) prochlorperazine 5–10 mg q4h
    b) dimenhydrinate 75 mg b.i.d.
    c) chlorpromazine 10–25 mg q4h
    d) metoclopramide 10 mg t.i.d.
    e) intravenous fluids

87. The patient described in the question has had a sore mouth for the past 6 days. You suspect a thrush infection. Your examination confirms your suspicions. Which of the following may be helpful in the treatment of this problem?
    a) nystatin oral suspension 100,000 units q4h
    b) anetholetrithion (Sialor) 25 mg t.i.d.
    c) hydrogen peroxide 1/4 strength
    d) a and c
    e) all of the above

88. The patient described in the question above undergoes palliative radiotherapy for severe bone pain that develops 1 month after the problems described above. Following this, she develops bloody diarrhea. Which of the following treatments may be helpful in the treatment of this problem?
    a) diphenoxylate HCl 2.5 mg t.i.d. to a maximum of 20 mg/day
    b) loperamide HCl 2 mg after each unformed stool to a maximum of 16 mg/day
    c) codeine phosphate 30–60 mg t.i.d.

d) a and b
e) all of the above

ANSWER THE FOLLOWING QUESTIONS ACCORDING TO THE CODE:

A: 1, 2, and 3 are correct
B: 1 and 3 are correct
C: 2 and 4 are correct
D: Only 4 is correct
E: All of the above are correct

89. The patient described in the question becomes increasingly short of breath. You suspect a pleural effusion.

    On examination there is dullness to percussion over the area of the left lung. A chest x-ray confirms the diagnosis of left pleural effusion.

    Which of the following treatments may be useful in alleviating this symptom?
    1) palliative radiotherapy
    2) prednisone 10–15 mg t.i.d.
    3) morphine sulfate 5–10 mg q4h
    4) dexamethasone 8–12 mg daily

90. You treat the patient's pleural effusion effectively. One week later she develops increasing abdominal distention, nausea, and vomiting. You suspect a bowel obstruction.

    On examination, there are increased bowel sounds. A plain film of the abdomen confirms a partial bowel obstruction. Which of the following may be indicated in the treatment of this patient at this time?
    1) decreased fluid intake
    2) metoclopramide
    3) chlorpromazine
    4) nasogastric suction

91. A 53-year-old male presents to the emergency department with the sudden onset of left-sided weakness. He has been previously well, apart from mild chronic obstructive pulmonary disease due to cigarette smoking.

On examination, the patient has a left-sided hemiplegia. A chest x-ray shows a left-sided mass lesion and prominent hilar lymphadenopathy. You suspect a bronchogenic carcinoma.

Which of the following statements regarding this patient is(are) true?

1) there is likely no relationship between the hemiplegia and the chest x-ray findings
2) recovery from the hemiplegia is unlikely
3) the cause of the hemiplegia is likely a cerebral embolus
4) dexamethasone may be used both as a diagnostic test and a therapeutic maneuver in this patient

92. You are called to the home of a 42-year-old female with disseminated breast cancer. She has a fungating breast carcinoma that is giving off a very offensive odor. Her friends have stopped coming to see her because of the odor. The patient and her family have tried numerous remedies without success.

    Which of the following may be useful in the treatment of the odor associated with this fungating growth?

    1) frequent cleansings with Dakin's solution
    2) application of yogurt dressings
    3) application of buttermilk dressings
    4) charcoal briquets strategically placed throughout the house

93. You are called to the home of a 51-year-old patient with terminal colon cancer. He has become increasingly depressed and agitated and now is unable to get to sleep at night.

    As you talk to the patient you realize that he has a significant agitated depression.

    Which of the following may be indicated in the treatment of this patient's condition?

    1) a tricyclic antidepressant in the evening
    2) an anxiolytic agent given on a PRN basis
    3) supportive psychotherapy
    4) attention to other symptoms, including pain

ANSWERS

85. E. Anorexia is a very common and distressing symptom occurring in all types of cancer. Mouth discomfort, changes in sense of taste, dehydration, malnutrition, some drugs, and chemotherapy may all contribute to it.

    Small food helpings on small plates with patients' preferred foods attractively prepared will make meals more appealing. Prednisone 5 mg t.i.d. may improve appetite.[1] Maltevol 12 or cyproheptadine 4 mg t.i.d.[1] before meals may be used. Alcohol, such as 1 oz of brandy, may also be beneficial. It is important to reassure the patient and family members that large feeds are unnecessary.

    Certain foods seem to appeal to patients who are terminally ill. Contrary to common belief, terminally ill patients do not appreciate foods that have been pulverized in a blender. Rather, spicy foods such as fried chicken, fast food hamburgers, and pizza in small helpings often offer much greater appeal to these patients.

86. E. Nausea and vomiting may result from stimulation of the emetic center in the brain stem by impulses from the gut, vestibular apparatus, cerebral cortex, or the chemoreceptor trigger zone.[2] There are multiple causes including the following:

    a) drugs—digoxin, morphine, and estrogens
    b) biochemical changes—uremia, hypercalcemia, liver failure, and ketosis
    c) bowel obstruction
    d) psychological causes

    If nausea and vomiting are caused by an oral narcotic, a phenothiazine should be given concurrently. These work on the chemoreceptor trigger zone in the medulla and have a tranquilizing action. The most widely used are:

    a) metoclopramide 10 mg q.i.d.
    b) chlorpromazine 10–25 mg q4h
    c) dimenhydrinate 75 mg b.i.d .
    d) prochlorperazine 5–10 mg q4h

    In addition to working on the central chemoreceptor zone, metoclopramide also works on the upper gut to increase gastric peristalsis, and relax the pyloric antrum.

    Often, if one antiemetic is not effective, a combination of two agents may be more effective. A common combination that is utilized is dimenhydrinate 75 mg b.i.d. and metoclopramide 40–60 mg/day in three or four divided doses.

    Although rehydration may be indicated, subcutaneous infusions are preferable to intravenous fluid administration.[3] Terminally ill patients are often cachectic, and have friable veins that make intravenous therapy difficult.

87. E. Although a sore mouth in terminally ill patients can be caused by ill-fitting dentures, aphthous ulcerations, vitamin deficiency, and blood dys-

crasias, the most common cause of sore mouth is thrush. Monilial infection is treated with nystatin oral suspension 100,000 units (1 ml) q4h until 48 hours after clinical cure.[2] Dentures must be treated with the same solution.

Good mouth care is essential in terminally ill patients. Hydrogen peroxide 1/4 strength, used as a rinse, will help prevent monilia infection.[2]

The other major mouth complaint is dry mouth. This can be treated with ice chips, lemon candies, frozen pineapple chunks, and tart juice mixtures such as cranberry cocktail/carbonated beverage. Sialor 25 mg t.i.d. (artificial saliva) is also useful in increasing salivation and preventing dry mouth.[2]

88. D. The diarrhea in this case is likely due to the effect of the radiotherapy on the bowel. In this case, any of diphenoxylate, loperamide, or codeine phosphate are good treatment choices.[1] In most patients, the diarrhea will settle down 1–2 weeks after completion of the course of radiotherapy.

89. E. Dyspnea and pleural effusion in terminally ill patients should be treated with reassurance and a number of symptomatic measures. As well, a number of medications are useful in the treatment of these symptoms. Having the patient's window open and the patient in a semi-Fowler's position gives the patient significant relief.

Although thoracentesis and the installation of chemotherapeutic agents may be used initially, repeated thoracentesis is uncomfortable, and other treatment options should be sought.

Bronchodilators such as theophylline may be helpful in relieving air hunger.[4]

Palliative radiotherapy may have an important role to play in some patients.

Steroids such as prednisone 10–15 mg t.i.d. or dexamethasone 8–12 mg/day may help to mobilize the pleural effusion and will decrease the subjective sensation of dyspnea.[2]

Morphine sulfate 5–10 mg q4h, and antianxiety agents such as sublingual lorazepam are also helpful in the symptomatic relief of dyspnea.[2] Thiazide and/or loop diuretics may be useful in treating a pleural effusion in a terminally ill patient.

90. A. A partial bowel obstruction in a patient who is terminally ill should be treated symptomatically with decreased fluid intake, antinauseants, narcotic analgesics, and perhaps prednisone.[5]

A decreased fluid intake (to 25–50 cc/hr) will decrease the number of episodes of emesis/day. Antinauseants including metoclopramide, prochlorperazine, chlorpromazine, and dimenhydrinate are useful singly or in combination (metoclopramide/dimenhydrinate).[5] Prednisone in a dosage of 5 mg t.i.d. may help mobilize fluid from the small bowel.

Nasogastric tubes are uncomfortable, and as all care should be directed to making the patient more comfortable, this intervention is not reasonable.

91. D. This patient has cerebral edema secondary to brain metastases from a primary bronchogenic carcinoma. In this case, dexamethasone can be used both as a diagnostic test and as therapy for the cerebral edema. Dexamethasone in a dosage of 16–100 mg/day should significantly improve cerebral edema secondary to brain metastases.[1] Recovery of hemiplegia caused by cerebral edema should occur rapidly. Cimetidine or another H_2 receptor antagonist should be used along with the dexamethasone to ensure that iatrogenic peptic ulcer does not develop.

92. E. Fungating growths (especially breast cancers) can produce very offensive odors that isolate the patient and her family.

Scrupulous cleanliness, frequent dressing changes, frequent washing with dilute hydrogen peroxide, and the application of unpasteurized yogurt or buttermilk dressings to the lesion can eliminate the odor associated with fungating tumors.[2] As well, the strategic placement of charcoal briquets throughout the house will significantly improve the general odor of the house and will allow visitors to visit with the patient in comfort.

93. E. Depression and anxiety are common symptoms in terminally ill patients. Before instituting specific drug therapy for depression and anxiety, the health care team should address all aspects of physical and mental stress that the patient is currently undergoing. Other symptoms, including pain, may be manifested by depression and anxiety, and indeed, the overall perception of pain involves physical, psychological, social, and spiritual aspects. Supportive psychotherapy may be effective in some cases.

Drug therapy for depression may be initiated with a tricyclic antidepressant such as amitriptyline, best given a couple of hours before bed. Anxiolytic therapy with sublingual lorazepam or another benzodiazepine may be effective in relieving the anxiety component of a terminal illness.[1]

Depression and anxiety in terminal illness are usually due to fear. The two biggest fears that terminally ill cancer patients describe are the fear of pain and the fear of dying alone. Terminally ill patients need permission to talk about these fears; this in itself is very therapeutic.

SUMMARY OF SYMPTOM MANAGEMENT IN TERMINALLY ILL PATIENTS

1. **Nausea and Vomiting:**
   Small frequent meals
   Antiemetics: metoclopramide, prochlorperazine, chlorpromazine, and dimenhydrinate.

2. **Constipation:**
   Docusate sodium, senna concentrate, lactulose

3. **Anorexia:**
   Small frequent meals
   Prednisone
   Alcohol
   Avoid blended, pulverized foods

4. **Dry mouth:**
   Good mouth care imperative; treat thrush with nystatin
   Hydrogen peroxide 1/4 strength, lemon drops, pineapple chunks, tart juices

5. **Dehydration:**
   Usually not symptomatic; do not treat with subcutaneous or intravenous fluids unless you feel that the dehydration is causing the patient discomfort

6. **Diarrhea:**
   Diphenoxylate, loperamide, or codeine

7. **Dyspnea and pleural effusion:**
   Open windows, fresh air, semi-Fowler's position, bronchodilators, prednisone, narcotic analgesics, anxiolytics, diuretics, palliative radiotherapy, repeated thoracocentesis will likely cause more discomfort than give relief

8. **Bowel obstruction:**
   Restrict fluids
   Antiemetics (emesis × 3/day is acceptable)
   Prednisone
   Narcotic analgesics
   Avoid use of nasogastric tubes

9. **Cerebral edema:**
   Dexamethasone

10. **Fungating growths:**
    Frequent dressing changes; Dakin's solution or hydrogen peroxide
    Yogurt or buttermilk dressings
    Charcoal briquets around the house

11. **Depression and anxiety:**
    Address all aspects of pain; physical, psychological, social, and spiritual
    Psychotherapy/support: "be there, be sensitive, be silent"
    Tricyclic antidepressants/anxiolytics

References

1. Driscoll C. Symptom control in terminal illness. Prim Care, 1987: 14(2): 353–363.

2. Billings J. Outpatient management of advanced cancer. Philadephia, JB Lippincott, 1985: 40–138.

3. Hays H. Hypodermoclysis for symptom control in terminal care. Can Fam Physician 1985; 31: 1253–1256.

4. Norton W, Lack S. In: Twycross R, Ventafridda V, eds. The continuing care of terminal cancer patients. Oxford: Pergamon Press, 1979: 44–45.

5. Ajemian I. General principles of symptomatic management. In: Ajemian I, Mount B, eds. The R.V.H. manual on palliative/hospice care. Salem: The Ayer Company, 1982: 184–198.

PROBLEM 11:   A 17-YEAR-OLD FEMALE WITH WEIGHT LOSS, POLYURIA AND POLYDYPSIA

A 17-year-old female comes into your office with a 6-month history of weight loss in spite of increased appetite, along with polyuria and polydypsia. She has had no other significant illnesses.

On physical examination, the patient looks unwell. Her blood pressure is 110/60 mm Hg. Her pulse is 72 and regular. There are no other abnormalities found on examination.

A spot blood sugar is performed and reveals a venous plasma glucose of 13.2 mmol/L (237 mg%). You suspect diabetes mellitus.

SELECT THE ONE BEST ANSWER TO THE FOLLOWING QUESTIONS:

94. Which of the following statements regarding this patient is false?
    a) the diagnosis of diabetes should be confirmed with a glucose tolerance test
    b) a diabetic diet will be an essential part of treatment
    c) this illness may have been precipitated by a viral infection
    d) insulin will be required to control her disease
    e) hospital inpatient stabilization is not necessary to begin treatment

95. Which of the following statements regarding the diagnosis of diabetes mellitus is(are) true?
    a) diabetes mellitus is confirmed if the fasting venous plasma glucose is $\geq$ 7.8 mmol/L (140 mg%) on one occasion
    b) diabetes mellitus is confirmed if the venous plasma glucose exceeds 11.1 mmol/L (200 mg%) on one occasion in the presence of symptoms
    c) if the fasting venous plasma glucose is normal, the diagnosis of diabetes can be confirmed if, following a 75-gram glucose load, the plasma glucose equals or exceeds 11.1 mmol/L (200 mg%) twice within a 2-hour period
    d) all of the above statements are true
    e) b and c are true

96. The patient in question 94 begins treatment for diabetes mellitus. Long-term control of her disease will probably best be accomplished by:
    a) a single daily injection of intermediate acting insulin
    b) twice daily injections of intermediate acting insulin
    c) twice daily injections of intermediate acting and regular insulin
    d) twice daily injections of short acting insulin
    e) oral glyburide 5–10 mg/day

97. The patient described in question 94 is started on insulin therapy. The initial daily dose of insulin that the patient should receive is approximately:
    a) 1–2 units
    b) 4–8 units
    c) 15–20 units
    d) 30–50 units
    e) 60–75 units

98. Which one of the following statements regarding diet and diabetes is false?
    a) diet is basic in the treatment of all diabetics
    b) new evidence suggests that diabetics do not have to avoid sweets and foods that contain simple carbohydrates
    c) the diabetic on insulin therapy must have three meals at fixed times each day
    d) the diabetic on insulin therapy should have frequent snacks
    e) the diabetic on insulin therapy should have a fixed caloric distribution

99. Which of the following statements regarding morning hyperglycemia in an insulin-dependent diabetic is false?
    a) morning hyperglycemia can be due to the Somogyi effect
    b) morning hyperglycemia can be due to the "dawn phenomenon"
    c) the "dawn phenomenon" can be distinguished from the Somogyi effect by determination of the 3 AM sugar
    d) none of the above statements are false

100. A 17-year-old female is brought into your office with a 3 day history of nausea, vomiting, generalized abdominal pain, and lethargy. She appears acutely sick.

    On examination, the patient's blood pressure is 170/70 mm Hg, and her pulse 140 and regular. Her respirations are 45/minute and regular.

    She has no history of significant disease.

    Her chemstrip is 40 mmol/L (718 mg%). Her urine has +4 sugar and +4 ketones.

    Which of the following statements regarding this patient is(are) true?
    a) this patient is at risk for going into hyperosmolar diabetic coma
    b) this patient can safely be treated as an outpatient

Family Practice Review

c) this patient should be treated with intravenous fluids, intravenous insulin, and intravenous potassium
d) a and c
e) b and c

101. A 65-year-old asymptomatic obese female has a routine fasting sugar drawn at the time of her annual physical examination. The level comes back at 240 mg/dl (13.4 mmol/L). Her urine is negative for ketones. The test is repeated the following day and comes back at the same level. Which of the following statements about this patient is INCORRECT?
a) the patient has noninsulin-dependent diabetes mellitus (NIDDM)
b) insulin is the agent of first choice in the management of this condition
c) a diabetic diet forms the cornerstone of therapy
d) insulin and oral hypoglycemics may be used together in the treatment of this condition
e) monitoring of this condition is best done by home glucose monitoring

ANSWER THE FOLLOWING QUESTIONS ACCORDING TO THE CODE:

A: 1, 2, and 3 are correct
B: 1 and 3 are correct
C: 2 and 4 are correct
D: Only 4 is correct
E: All of the above are correct

102. Which of the following drugs may increase the blood glucose level and lead to diabetes mellitus?
1. thiazide diuretics
2. indomethacin
3. propranolol
4. diazepam

103. Which of the following statements regarding the complications of diabetes mellitus is(are) true?
1) complications of diabetes mellitus are much less frequent with NIDDM than with IDDM
2) patients with NIDDM have a 30% decrease in life expectancy secondary to complications of diabetes
3) retinopathy is an unusual complication of NIDDM
4) atherosclerosis is a common complication of NIDDM

ANSWERS

94. A. The patient described in question 94 has insulin-dependent diabetes mellitus (IDDM). Although IDDM may originate at any age, the onset is usually before 40 years of age. The classic symptoms of hyperglycemia include polyuria, polydypsia, and polyphagia. Weight loss often occurs despite an increased intake of food.[1]

In IDDM, an absolute insulin deficiency exists. Insulin is necessary to prevent ketoacidosis and to sustain life. The inability of the pancreas to produce insulin may be due to direct damage of the islet cells or to autoimmune destruction of the beta cells in genetically susceptible individuals.[1] The direct damage or the autoimmune destruction may be caused by a viral infection.[1]

Therapy is comprised of insulin and a diabetic diet. In the diabetic diet, 55–60% of calories should come from carbohydrate sources, 12–20% from protein sources, and less than 30% from fat sources. In addition, total cholesterol should be less than 300 calories/day, and 40 g of fiber should be eaten per day.[2,3]

A single glucose level in excess of 11 mmol/L (200 mg/dl) in the presence of the classic symptoms of diabetes is diagnostic, and therefore the glucose tolerance test is unnecessary (see critique of question 95).

Most new cases of diabetes mellitus (in the absence of ketosis) can be initially managed in an outpatient setting.

95. E. Although there is no clear distinction between normal and abnormal glucose levels, especially when age is considered, National Diabetes Study Group standards are as follows:[4]
1. If the fasting venous plasma glucose is greater than 7.8 mmol/L (140 mg%) *on more than one occasion* the diagnosis is confirmed.
2. A single glucose level of 11.1 mmol/L (200 mg%) in the presence of classic symptoms of diabetes is diagnostic.
3. If the fasting venous plasma glucose is normal, the presence of diabetes mellitus can be established if, following a 75-g glucose load, the serum glucose levels equals or exceeds 11.1 mmol/L (200 mg%) twice within a two-hour period. (1/2 hour, 1 hour, 1 1/2 and 2 hour samples are checked).
4. If the fasting plasma glucose is normal, and the patient has only one value exceeding 11.1

mmol/L in the glucose tolerance test, the patient has impaired glucose tolerance.

96. C. Most patients with IDDM can be controlled on two daily injections of a combination of intermediate acting insulin (Humulin-N or NPH) and regular insulin (Humulin-R or Toronto). Twice daily injections are usually required for optimum control because the peak activity of intermediate acting insulin occurs in 6–14 hours and declines thereafter.

Human insulin (Humulin), which is synthesized artificially from DNA recombinant techniques, is the insulin of choice because of lack of antigenicity and antibody formation. For patients who are already on pork or beef insulin and who are not having any problems it is reasonable to continue them on the same regimen.

Intensive insulin therapy, which refers to multiple injections (at least 4) of short acting (Humulin-R, Toronto) insulin, combined with an ultralong acting preparation (Humulin-U), or a continuous insulin pump, is not necessary for good control in most cases.

A usual treatment regimen involves 2/3 of the total insulin dose in the morning and 1/3 in the evening; with 2/3 of each dose being an intermediate acting insulin and 1/3 of the total dose being a short acting insulin. Although the regimen discussed above will usually be required for excellent control, some authorities still begin with a single daily injection of an intermediate acting insulin (15–20 units for a nonobese patient and 25–30 units for an obese patient).[1,3] Patients who can be controlled on a single injection probably have some residual pancreatic function.

In some patients, intensive insulin therapy with a daily injection of ultralente and preprandial boluses of regular insulin is required.[3]

Oral hypoglycemic agents like glyburide are not indicated for the treatment of IDDM.

97. C. The usual starting dose of insulin is 15–20 units per day. The obese individual may need 25–30 units per day.[1] The dose, however, must be individualized; some persons require much more and some persons require much less.

98. B. Diet is an essential component of treatment in all patients with diabetes. It is, however, especially important for the insulin-dependent diabetic. In the diabetic on insulin the rate at which insulin enters the blood from an injection site is fixed, and therefore the diabetic must match meals to the pattern of insulin absorption. The diabetic's diet should be the same as the diet suggested for nondiabetics of the same age.[2,3]

During the past several years, the avoidance of sweets and foods that contain simple carbohydrates has been challenged, but until further information is forthcoming, it still seems reasonable to instruct diabetics to avoid beverages with sucrose and desserts that are highly sweetened.[2]

The diabetic on insulin therapy must have three meals at fixed times each day, with a fixed distribution of calories. Also, frequent snacks, also with a fixed distribution of calories, are recommended.[2,3]

If a diabetic patient is overweight, a weight-reducing program should be initiated. This may be facilitated by substituting complex carbohydrates with high residue for simple sugars. As well, saturated animal fats should be replaced with polyunsaturated vegetable fats. One fifth of the daily caloric intake should be consumed at breakfast and about two-fifths each at lunch and supper. The caloric intake at lunch and supper may be reduced slightly to allow for a small snack, such as crackers or fruit, in midafternoon or at bedtime.[2,3]

99. D. Morning hyperglycemia in a diabetic on insulin may be due to relative insulin deficiency (the "dawn phenomenon") or to rebound hyperglycemia (the "Somogyi effect").[1] Because the treatment is different, these conditions must be distinguished.

The "dawn phenomenon," which is a relative insulin deficiency due to a waning of insulin action in the early morning hours, and likely mediated by an increased nocturnal output of growth hormone (which has anti-insulin activity) is treated by increasing the dosage of evening insulin.[1]

The Somogyi effect, which is rebound hyperglycemia following a hypoglycemic reaction, is treated by decreasing, not increasing, the dosage of evening insulin.[1]

The "dawn phenomenon" can be distinguished from the Somogyi effect by determination of the 3:00 AM glucose. Therefore, all diabetic patients should periodically measure their 3:00 AM blood sugar, in addition to regularly measuring their blood sugars four times per day.[1]

100. D. This patient is in diabetic ketoacidosis. Diabetic ketoacidosis is often the initial presentation of diabetes mellitus in children, adolescents, and young adults.

Patients in diabetic ketoacidosis usually present with nausea, vomiting, abdominal pain, and lethargy. Tachycardia, hyperventilation, and hypothermia are often present. Diabetic ketoacidosis is a complication in diabetes in younger patients; hyperglycemic hyperosmolar coma usually occurs in elderly patients. Hyperventilation is unusual in hyperosmolar coma, as is a low HCO_3 level. Obtundation is common.[1]

Diabetic ketoacidosis is treated by large volumes of fluid; initially normal or hypotonic saline (first liter), followed by 5% dextrose in water when the blood sugar falls below 14 mmol/L (250 mg%). Following a loading dose of 0.2 units/kg, insulin should be given by constant infusion at 0.1 units/kg/hour.[1,5] Potassium, initially in a dosage of 40 mEq/L, is almost always required. In patients with severe acidosis (pH <7.1), sodium bicarbonate may be considered.[1,5]

Once the acute condition has been treated, the patient should be put on a combination of regular and intermediate acting insulin.

101. **B.** This patient has noninsulin-dependent diabetes mellitus (NIDDM). NIDDM account for 90–95% of all diabetes. NIDDM is characterized by both an impairment of beta-cell function and a decreased tissue sensitivity to insulin.[1,6]

NIDDM is often discovered in asymptomatic patients by the finding of an elevated blood sugar.[1] It may also present with nonspecific symptoms including fatigue, weakness, blurred vision, vaginal and perineal pruritus, impotence, or paresthesias. Weight loss is uncommon in the patients. The majority of patients with NIDDM are obese; many have a strong family history of obesity and diabetes.[1]

A diabetic diet is the therapy of first choice. If diet is not sufficient, an oral hypoglycemic agent should be tried first.

All oral hypoglycemic agents currently available are sulfonylurea agents. The first generation agents include tolbutamide, chlorpropamide, acetohexamide, and tolazamide. The second generation agents include glyburide and glipizide. At this time, there is no conclusive evidence that the second generation agents are more effective, have fewer side effects, or produce fewer interactions with other drugs.[6,7]

Oral hypoglycemic therapy should begin with the lowest effective dose, which can then be increased every several days to achieve maximal control.[6] Self-monitoring of blood glucose is the key to evaluation of efficacy in this type of treatment program.

About 25–30% of NIDDM patients fail to respond to sulfonylurea drugs. These patients are called primary failures. In addition, about 5% of patients per year who initially responded to these drugs will lose their responsiveness. These patients are termed secondary failures.[6] Sometimes, a combination of an oral hypoglycemic (given in the morning) and an intermediate acting-insulin (given at night) can be beneficial in lowering blood sugar to normal.[8]

Home glucose monitoring is the method of choice for monitoring blood sugars in diabetic patients. It is recommended that blood sugars be initially checked four times per day until control is achieved. When the blood sugar falls towards normal, the frequency of monitoring can be decreased to two or three times weekly (3–4 times per day).[3] Also, the 3 AM sugar should be occasionally checked.

102. **A.** Many drugs are known to raise the blood glucose level and lead in some cases to diabetes mellitus. These include thiazide diuretics, furosemide, corticosteroids, propranolol (and some other beta blockers), indomethacin (and some other nonsteroidal anti-inflammatory drugs), isoniazid, lithium, oral contraceptives and other estrogens, clonidine, diphenylhydantoin, tricyclic antidepressants, and nicotinic acid.[9–11] Diazepam does not raise the plasma glucose level.

103. **C.** NIDDM is not a benign disease. Both microvascular and macrovascular complications resulting from long-term NIDDM result in signficant morbidity and mortality.[1,12]

Complications of diabetes mellitus (both IDDM and NIDDM) include the macrovascular complications of atherosclerosis; the microvascular complications of microangiopathy including retinopathy and nephropathy; and other complications neuropathy and gastroparesis.[1,12]

SUMMARY OF THE DIAGNOSIS AND MANAGEMENT OF DIABETES MELLITUS

1. **Diagnosis:** Two fasting levels of > 7.8 mmol/L (140 mg%); a single level greater than 11.1 mmol/L (200 mg%) in the presence of symptoms; two or more values of > 11.1 mmol/L in a 2 hour period following a 75 g glucose tolerance test. If the venous plasma glucose level is < 7.8 mmol/L

fasting; greater than 11.1 mmol/L at either 1/2 hour, 1 hour or 1 1/2 hours; and greater than 11.1 mmol/L at 2 hours the diagnosis is impaired glucose tolerance (IGT)

2. **Treatment:**
IDDM:
a) diet
b) insulin: usually a split daily dose with 2/3 of the total daily dose being given in the morning and 1/3 in the evening; and with 2/3 of each dose being intermediate-acting and 1/3 being short-acting is the treatment regimen of choice. Humulin insulin should be used whenever a newly-diagnosed diabetic is started on insulin.
c) monitoring: Home glucose monitoring is essential for monitoring short-term control; hemoglobin A1C should be used for monitoring long-term control.

NIDDM:
a) diet
b) oral hypoglycemics: tolbutamide, chloropropamide, glyburide, and glipizide
c) insulin: insulin should be used after primary or secondary failure with oral hypoglycemics
d) insulin may be used alone or used in combination with the oral hypoglycemics
e) monitoring: as with IDDM, home glucose monitoring is essential

3. **Complications:**
Acute: diabetic ketoacidosis, hyperosmolar coma
Long-term complications: atherosclerosis, retinopathy, nephropathy, neuropathy (both IDDM and NIDDM)

References

1. Foster D. Diabetes Mellitus. In: Braunwald E, Isselbacher K, Petersdorf R, Wilson J, Martin J, Fauci A, eds. Harrison's principles of internal medicine. 11th Ed. New York: McGraw-Hill, 1987: 1778–1796.

2. Anderson J, Geil P. New perspectives in nutrition management of diabetes mellitus. Am J Med 1988; 85(5A):159–165.

3. Nathan D. Modern management of insulin-dependent diabetes mellitus. Med Clin North Am 1988; 72(6): 1365–1378.

4. National Diabetes Data Group: Classification and diagnosis of diabetes mellitus and other categories of glucose intolerance. Diabetes 1979; 28(12): 1039–1057.

5. Kitabchi A, Murphy M. Diabetic ketoacidosis and hyperosmolar hyperglycemic nonketotic coma. Med Clin North Am 1988; 72(6): 1545–1563.

6. Lebovitz H. Oral hypoglycemia agents. Prim Care 1988; 15(2): 353–369.

7. Ferner R. Oral hypoglycemic agents. Med Clin North Am 1988; 72(6): 1323–1335.

8. Firth R. Insulin: either alone or combined with oral hypoglycemic agents. Prim Care 1988; 15(3): 665–679.

9. Dunn F. Treatment of lipid disorders in diabetes mellitus. Med Clin North Am 1988; 72(6): 1379–1398.

10. Sowers J, Levy J, Zemel M. Hypertension and diabetes. Med Clin North Am 1988; 72(6): 1399–1414.

11. Hatcher R, Guest F, Stewart F, Stewart G, Trussell J, Bowen S, Cates W. Drug interactions. In: Breedlove B, Judy B, Martin N, eds. Contraceptive technology 1988–1989. New York: Irvington Publishers, 1988: 436.

12. Flint M, Clements R. Prevention of the complications of diabetes. Prim Care 1988; 15(2): 277–284.

PROBLEM 12: A 45-YEAR-OLD MALE WEIGHING 320 POUNDS AND COMPLAINING OF FATIGUE

A 320-pound, 45-year-old male presents to your office complaining of fatigue. You decide that his fatigue is mainly due to his morbid obesity and send him for dietary counseling. The dietician puts him on a 1300 Kcal/day diet and calculates his ideal weight at 170 lbs.

SELECT THE ONE BEST ANSWER TO THE FOLLOWING QUESTIONS:

104. Assuming that his activity level does not change, that his total energy expenditure is 2300 Kcal/day, and that he sticks to his diet, how long will it take him to reach his ideal weight?
    a) 125 days
    b) 225 days
    c) 325 days
    d) 425 days
    e) 525 days

105. Obesity is generally defined as:
    a) an increase in the ponderal index of 20% above normal
    b) a decrease in the ponderal index of 30% below normal
    c) an increase in the body mass index of 20% above normal
    d) an increase in the body mass index of 30% above normal
    e) none of the above

106. The overall prevalence of obesity in North Americans is:
    a) 1%
    b) 5%
    c) 10%
    d) 20%
    e) 50%

107. Which of the following conditions is MOST CONSISTENTLY associated with obesity?
    a) alveolar hypoventilation syndrome
    b) hypertension
    c) hyperlipidemia
    d) diabetes mellitus
    e) angina pectoris

108. The use of severe calorie restricted diets (<800 Kcal/ day) has been responsible for many deaths. The most common cause of death in these cases has been:
    a) sudden cardiac death
    b) congestive cardiac failure secondary to anemia
    c) hepatic failure
    d) renal failure
    e) septicemia

ANSWER THE FOLLOWING QUESTIONS ACCORDING TO THE CODE:

A: 1, 2, and 3 are correct
B: 1 and 3 are correct
C: 2 and 4 are correct
D: Only 4 is correct
E: All of the above are correct

109. Which of the following statements regarding the use of anorectic drugs is(are) true?
    1) short-term studies demonstrate that weight loss is greater with these agents at 1 month than with placebo
    2) hypertension is a documented side effect
    3) renal failure is a documented side effect
    4) long-term studies suggest that these agents are not beneficial as part of a weight loss program

110. Which of the following is(are) advocated as part of a weight loss program?
    1) a nutritionally balanced diet
    2) behavior modification techniques
    3) an exercise program
    4) caloric restriction to 1000 cal/day or less

111. The practical management of weight loss by the family physician should involve:
    1) multiple office visits over 8–12 weeks
    2) changes to the act of eating
    3) the patient keeping a food diary
    4) the patient keeping a daily weight chart

ANSWERS

104. E. One pound of fat is equal to 3500 Kcal. Therefore, if his total energy expenditure is 2300 Kcal/day and he is only taking in 1300 Kcal/day, his energy deficit is 1000 Kcal/day. His excess weight above ideal weight of 150 lb corresponds to 525,000 Kcal. Therefore, it will take him 525 days to lose the 150 extra pounds if he sticks to his diet.

105. C. Obesity is defined as an increase in relative weight for height (body mass index) of greater than 20% above desirable weight.[1] Less than 20% above ideal body weight is simply defined as being "overweight." Ponderal index is a measure of height/weight.

106. D. The overall prevalence of obesity in North Americans is approximately 20% of the popula-

tion.[2,3] In certain groups the incidence is as high as 40–50%. The highest incidence appears in those individuals in the lowest socioeconomic groups with some improvement as socioeconomic level increases.

107. B. Obesity is associated with many chronic diseases. These include cardiomyopathy, alveolar hypoventilation syndrome, angina pectoris and sudden cardiac death, hyperlipidemia, diabetes mellitus, degenerative joint disease, cholelithiasis, gout, varicose veins, thromboembolic disease, and endometrial carcinoma. The disease most consistently correlated with obesity, however, is hypertension.[4]

108. A. The most common cause of death recorded in patients on severe calorie restricted diets has been sudden cardiac death.[3] This is most likely due to hypokalemia-induced dysrhythmias (particularly ventricular fibrillation). The other causes listed have not been frequently documented as causes of death.

109. E. The drugs that are currently used to treat obesity are central nervous system stimulants. Although these agents demonstrate significantly greater efficacy in producing weight loss at 1 month, there is no documentation of their efficacy in long-term studies.[5] There is some evidence, in fact, that their use may impair long-term weight loss. Complications of anoretic agents include hypertension, psychosis, seizures, renal failure, cardiac arrhythmias, and myocardial infarction.[5]

110. A. A structured program is essential for successful weight loss. A program that offers a nutritionally balanced diet, behavioral techniques, and exercise at the least expense is the treatment of choice.[6] A nutritionally balanced diet with a caloric intake approximately 500 Kcal/day less than maintenance is recommended.

111. A. The practical management of the obese patient in the family physician's office includes multiple office visits over 8–12 weeks, changes to the act of eating (most importantly slowing the act), keeping of a food diary, and keeping of a daily weight chart, and increasing exercise activity.[7] The weight loss goal is 1–2 pounds/week.

The purpose of office visits[7] is outlined below:

1st visit:
a) orientation to the weight loss program
b) examination of current eating patterns (food diary)
c) A complete history and physical examination. The history should include age of onset of obesity, number and success of previous weight loss attempts, and present motivation. The patient should be weighed at this time.

2nd visit:
a) review of weight
b) review of food diary (including what, where, and with whom food eaten)
c) the prescription of a nutritionally sound diet including nutrition facts

3rd visit:
a) review of food diary
b) review of weight (positive reinforcement if weight loss attained, explanation as to why if not attained

4th and subsequent visits:
a) review of food diary
b) review of weight
c) exercise prescription and review

Once weight loss has begun, the frequency of visits can be decreased. Patients should be followed for 6–12 months to ensure continued adherence to the program.

SUMMARY OF THE MANAGEMENT OF OBESITY

1. Set nutritionally sound diet at 500 Kcal below maintenance level (1–2 pounds/week)

2. Use behavior modification techniques in multiple office visits

3. Have patient keep an accurate food diary that is reviewed at every office visit

4. Encourage exercise program to burn extra calories and compensate for lowered basal metabolic rate

5. Use positive reinforcement to help patient continue program

6. Continue to see patient at regular intervals once weight loss pattern is established or goal weight is attained

References

1. Simopoulos AP, Van Itallie TB. Body weight, health, and longevity. Ann Intern Med 1984; 100: 285–295.

2. Van Italie TB. Health implications of overweight and obesity in the United States. Ann Intern Med 1985; 103: 983–988.

3. Steffie W. The medical syndrome of obesity. Prim Care 1982; 9(3): 581–593.

4. NIH. Health implications of obesity. National Institutes of Health consensus development conference statement. Ann Intern Med 1985; 103: 147–151.

5. Elliot D, Goldberg L, Girard D. Obesity: pathophysiology and practical management. J Gen Intern Med 1987; 2: 188–198.

6. Weinsier RL, Wadden TA, Ritenbaugh C, et al. Recommended therapeutic guidelines for professional weight loss programs. Am J Clin Nutr 1984; 40: 865–872.

7. Smith S. Management of obesity: an office strategy. Can Fam Physician 1988;34: 1793–1796.

PROBLEM 13: AN 80-YEAR-OLD FEMALE WITH PAINFUL FINGER JOINTS

An 80-year-old female presents with a 6-month history of stiffness in her hands bilaterally. This stiffness is worse in the morning, and quickly subsides as the patient begins her daily activities. She has no other significant medical problems.

On examination, the patient has bony swelling at the margins of the distal interphalangeal joints on the second to the fifth digits on both hands. No other abnormalities are found on physical examination.

SELECT THE ONE BEST ANSWER TO THE FOLLOWING QUESTIONS:

112. Which of the following statements regarding this patient's condition is true?
    a) these swellings may represent Heberden's nodes
    b) these swellings may represent Bouchard's nodes
    c) this patient will most likely demonstrate an elevated ESR and positive rheumatoid factor
    d) synovial fluid analysis will probably demonstrate low viscosity and normal mucin clotting
    e) the total leukocyte count in the synovial fluid will probably be greater than 1000 cells/mm.

113. Which of the following statements regarding the symptomatology of the condition described above is false?
    a) pain is the chief symptom of osteoarthritis and is usually deep and aching in character
    b) stiffness of the involved joint is common but of relatively brief duration
    c) the pain of osteoarthritis does not originate from the degenerating cartilage
    d) the major physical finding in osteoarthritis is bony crepitus
    e) the presence of osteophytes is sufficient for the diagnosis of osteoarthritis

114. Which of the following statements regarding the condition described above is false?
    a) this condition is the most common form of joint disease in the population
    b) 80% of the population have radiographic features of this condition in weight-bearing joints by the age of 65 years
    c) this condition has both primary and secondary forms
    d) narrowing of the joint space is unusual
    e) pathologically, the articular cartilage is first roughened and finally worn away

115. A 65-year-old female with moderately severe osteoarthritis of her left hip comes into your office requesting an exercise prescription. She wishes to "get into shape."
    Which of the following would you recommend to this patient at this time?
    a) exercise is not good for osteoarthritis; rest is much more appropriate
    b) a graded exercise program that consists of brisk walking gradually increasing the distance to 3–4 miles/day will probably not cause pain and will be good for her
    c) a passive isotonic exercise program is preferable to an active exercise isometric one
    d) any exercise program will probably hasten her need for total hip replacements

e) swimming is the best exercise prescription you can give her as it promotes cardiovascular fitness and at the same time keeps pressure off the weight-bearing joints

ANSWER THE FOLLOWING QUESTIONS ACCORDING TO THE CODE

A: 1, 2, and 3 are correct
B: 1 and 3 are correct
C: 2 and 4 are correct
D: Only 4 is correct
E: All of the above are correct

116. Which of the following radiographic changes are seen in the condition described above?
    1. narrowing of the joint space
    2. bony sclerosis
    3. osteophyte formation
    4. subchondral cysts

117. Which of the following is(are) useful treatment modalities in the condition described above?
    1. weight loss in obese patients
    2. canes, crutches, and walkers
    3. the application of heat to involved joints
    4. nonsteroidal anti-inflammatory agents

ANSWERS

112. A. The patient described in this question has osteoarthritis. Heberden's nodes (bony swellings of the distal interphalangeal joints) are pathognomonic for osteoarthritis.[1] Bouchard's nodes are bony swellings of the proximal interphalangeal joints. A significantly elevated ESR is seldom seen with osteoarthritis. The rheumatoid factor will be negative. Synovial fluid analysis will probably demonstrate high viscosity and normal mucin clotting. The total leukocyte count in the synovial fluid will probably be less than 1000 cells/mm.[1]

113. E. The most common symptom of osteoarthritis is pain. It is usually described as deep and aching.[2] The pain is usually aggravated by joint use and relieved by rest.[2] Joint stiffness in weight-bearing joints, usually lasting only a short period of time, is common after prolonged rest. Osteoarthritic pain is due to movement against joint surface irregularities, subchondral bone microfractures, irritation of periosteal nerve endings, ligamentous stress, muscular strain, and soft tissue inflamma-

tion such as bursitis and tendinitis. It is not due to degenerating cartilage.[2]

Bony crepitus is the most common physical finding in osteoarthritis.[2] Osteophytes are a common radiologic finding, especially with advancing age. The diagnosis of osteoarthritis is clinical, the mere presence of osteophytes on an x-ray is insufficient for diagnosis.[2]

114. D. Osteoarthritis is the most common joint disease. By age 65, over 80% of the population have radiographic features compatible with osteoarthritis. As aging progresses, symptomatology increases.[2]

Osteoarthritis can be either primary or secondary. Primary osteoarthritis usually most affects the terminal interphalangeal joints, the metacarpophalangeal and carpometacarpal joints of the thumb, the hip, the knee, the metatarsophalangeal joint of the great toe, and the cervical and lumbar spine.[1] Secondary osteoarthritis[2] may occur after articular injury resulting from either intra-articular (including rheumatoid arthritis) or extra-articular causes. The most common extra-articular cause of osteoarthritis is obesity. Other causes include fractures, bad posture, joint overuse, or metabolic diseases such as hyperparathyroidism.

In the pathogenesis of osteoarthritis, articular cartilage is first roughened, and finally worn away. Spur formation and lipping at the joint surface occur.

115. E. Muscle spasm and muscle atrophy can be prevented by a graded exercise program. Active exercises are preferred to passive exercises; isometric exercises are preferred to isotonic exercises.[3] With minimal involvement of weight-bearing joints swimming can be recommended as an ideal exercise. A graded exercise program that includes walking 3–4 miles/day will result in trauma to the joints and should not be advised. It may very well hasten the need for total hip replacement. When walking it is best to advise the patient to keep pressure off the involved joint; patients should be encouraged to use canes and other devices to accomplish that goal.

116. E. Radiographic changes in osteoarthritis include narrowing of the joint space due to loss of articular cartilage, bony sclerosis due to thickening of subchondral bone, subchondral bone cysts, and osteophytes (bone spurs).[2]

117. E. The treatment of osteoarthritis includes rest, avoidance of overuse of the affected joint; walking aids such as canes, crutches, and walkers; weight loss; the application of heat and other physiotherapy techniques; nonsteroidal anti-inflammatory drugs; local steroid injections; and sometimes orthopedic surgery (specifically hip joint and knee joint replacement).[3]

SUMMARY OF THE DIAGNOSIS AND TREATMENT OF OSTEOARTHRITIS

1. **Essentials of diagnosis:**
   a) a degenerative disorder without any systemic organ effects. May be primary or secondary.
   b) most commonly affects the joints of the hand, the hip, the knee, and the cervical and lumbar spine
   c) pain is aggravated by activity and relieved by rest. Morning stiffness is brief.
   4) radiologic findings include narrowed joint spaces, subchondral bone cysts, osteophyte formation, and bony sclerosis

2. **Treatment:**
   a) General measures: rest, weight loss, walking aids, local heat
   b) Specific measures: nonsteroidal anti-inflammatories, corticosteroid injections, and orthopedic surgery

References

1. Gilliland B. Degenerative joint disease. In: Braunwald E, Isselbacher K, Petersdorf R, Wilson J, Martin J, Fauci A, eds. Harrison's principles of internal medicine. 11th Ed. New York: McGraw-Hill, 1987: 1456–1458.

2. Eyanson S, Brandt K. Osteoarthritis. Prim Care 1984; 11(2): 259–269.

3. Shearn M. Arthritis and musculoskeletal disorders. In: Krupp J, Schroeder S, Tierney L, eds. Current Medical Diagnosis and Treatment. Norwalk: Appleton and Lange, 1987: 508–509.

PROBLEM 14: A 35-YEAR-OLD FEMALE WITH MALAISE, WEIGHT LOSS, VASOMOTOR DISTURBANCE, AND VAGUE PERIARTICULAR PAIN AND STIFFNESS

A 35-year-old female presents with a 6-month history of malaise, a 10 lb weight loss, paraesthesias in both hands, and vague pain in both wrists. Approximately 1 month ago, the patient began to notice morning stiffness in both hands and swelling in the metacarpophalangeal joints of both hands.

On examination, there is swelling in the 2nd and 3rd metacarpophalangeal joints of both hands. There is pain on motion of the affected joints. No other abnormalities are noted on physical examination.

SELECT THE ONE BEST ANSWER TO THE FOLLOWING QUESTIONS:

118. The most likely diagnosis in this patient is:
    a) nonarticular rheumatism
    b) synovitis
    c) gonococcal arthritis
    d) rheumatoid arthritis
    e) systemic lupus erythematosus

119. Which of the following statements regarding the condition described in the patient in question 118 is false?
    a) this is a disease that chiefly affects synovial membranes of multiple joints
    b) this disease is more common in females than in males
    c) serum protein abnormalities are often present in this condition
    d) the knees are uncommonly involved in this condition
    e) entrapment syndromes are not unusual

120. Instability of the cervical spine is a major problem in patients with rheumatoid arthritis. This instability usually develops between:
    a) C5 and C6
    b) C4 and C5
    c) C3 and C4
    d) C2 and C3

e) C1 and C2

121. The drug of first choice for suppressing inflammation in patients with rheumatoid arthritis is:
    a) aspirin
    b) gold
    c) D-penicillamine
    d) naproxen
    e) indomethacin

122. The drug of first choice for the induction of remission in rheumatoid arthritis is:
    a) aspirin
    b) gold
    c) D-penicillamine
    d) naproxen
    e) indomethacin

123. The treatment of choice for the prevention of joint deformity in a single joint or multiple small joints in a patient with rheumatoid arthritis who is already on remission-inducing therapy is:
    a) systemic corticosteroids
    b) intra-articular corticosteroids
    c) D-penicillamine
    d) gold
    e) aspirin

ANSWER THE FOLLOWING QUESTIONS ACCORDING TO THE CODE:

A: 1, 2, and 3 are correct
B: 1 and 3 are correct
C: 2 and 4 are correct
D: Only 4 is correct
E: All of the above are correct

124. Which of the following is(are) classical radiologic features of rheumatoid arthritis?
    1) loss of juxta-articular bone mass
    2) narrowing of the joint space
    3) bony erosions
    4) subarticular sclerosis

125. Which of the following is(are) extra-articular manifestations of rheumatoid arthritis?
    1) episcleritis/scleritis
    2) pleuritis with pleural effusion
    3) pericarditis
    4) hypochromic, microcytic anemia

126. Which of the following statements regarding the use of oral corticosteroids in rheumatoid arthritis is(are) true?
    1) oral corticosteroids alter the natural progression of the disease
    2) symptoms frequently reappear once corticosteroids are discontinued
    3) corticosteroids often do not produce immediate and dramatic anti-inflammatory effects in the disease
    4) the least amount of steroid that will achieve the desired clinical effect should be given

ANSWERS

118. D. The patient presented in this question has rheumatoid arthritis by the criteria of the American Rheumatologic Society.[1] The criteria (based on a duration of at least 6 weeks) are:
    1) morning stiffness
    2) pain on motion or tenderness in at least one joint
    3) swelling (soft-tissue thickening of fluid, not bony overgrowth alone) in at least one joint
    4) swelling of at least one other joint
    5) symmetrical joint swelling with simultaneous involvement of the same joint on both sides of the body; terminal phalangeal joint involvement will not satisfy this criteria
    6) subcutaneous nodules over bony prominences, on extensor surfaces, or in juxta-articular regions
    7) roentgenographic changes typical of rheumatoid arthritis (which must include at least bony decalcification localized to or greatest around the involved joints and not just degenerative changes
    8) positive agglutination (anti-gammaglobulin) test
    9) poor mucin precipitate from synovial fluid
    10) characteristic histologic changes in synovial membrane
    11) characteristic histologic changes in nodules

Rheumatoid arthritis often presents with prodromal symptoms of malaise, weight loss, vasomotor symptoms (paresthesias, Raynaud's phenomenon), and vague periarticular pain or stiffness. These symptoms usually progress to more definite symptomatology.

With the joint involvement described nonarticular rheumatism is by definition not a consideration. Synovitis is a pathologic diagnosis and not a disease. Gonococcal arthritis does not present with these signs and symptoms. None of the other organ manifestations that would make systemic lupus erythematosus a consideration are present.

119. D. Rheumatoid arthritis affects synovial membranes of multiple joints. There is considerable variability in articular and extra-articular manifestations.

    The prevalence is 1–2%, with a 3/1 female/male ratio. The pathologic findings in the joint include chronic synovitis with pannus formation. The pannus erodes cartilage, bone, ligaments, and tendons. In acute rheumatoid arthritis, effusion and other manifestations of inflammation are common. As the disease progresses, organization may result in fibrous ankylosis. In both acute and chronic phases, inflammation of soft tissues around the joints may be prominent and is a significant factor in joint damage.[2]

    Serum protein abnormalities are frequently seen. A number of serologic techniques may be used to detect rheumatoid factor, an IgM antibody directed against other globulins. One of these, the latex fixation test, is positive in 75% of cases. During both the acute and chronic phases, the erythrocyte sedimentation rate and the gamma globulins (IgM and IgG) are frequently elevated. An anemia, usually hypochromic normocytic, is often seen. The white blood cell count may be normal or slightly elevated.[2]

    Entrapment syndromes, especially the carpal tunnel syndrome, are common.

    The most commonly affected joints in rheumatoid arthritis are the proximal interphalangeal joints and metacarpophalangeal joints of the fingers, the wrists, the knees, the ankles, and the toes. Any joint, however, may be affected. Monarticular disease is occasionally seen early.[2]

120. E. Instability of the cervical spine is a life-threatening complication of rheumatoid arthritis. The instability results from a cervical ligament synovitis in the region of the first two cervical vertebrae.[3] This complication may occur in 30–40% of patients who develop rheumatoid arthritis. Five percent of RA patients eventually develop a myelopathy or cord injury as a result of this instability.

121. A. Aspirin is the drug of first choice in treating rheumatoid arthritis.[3] Aspirin is usually increased to the maximally tolerated dosage and then cut back slightly. Enteric coated aspirin or nonacetylated salicylates[5] may be preferable as they are easier to take and cause fewer side effects.

    Gold and D-penicillamine may be used to induce remission if spontaneous natural remission does not occur. Naproxen and indomethacin are nonsteroidal anti-inflammatory agents that can be used in place of aspirin if intolerance, side effects, or other reasons limit its use.

122. B. The drug of first choice for the induction of remission in rheumatoid arthritis is gold.[3] Gold may retard the bone erosions in rheumatoid arthritis.[4] About 60% of patients may be expected to benefit from gold therapy, although complete remissions are uncommon. The exact method of action is unknown. Gold can be given either intramuscularly or orally.[3,5]

    D-penicillamine is the second-line agent but has considerably more toxicity than gold. Aspirin, naproxen, and indomethacin are nonsteroidal anti-inflammatory agents and have no effect on inducing remission of the disease.

    Hydroxychloroquinine, glucocorticoids, and other immunosuppressive agents may be used in patients with crippling disease that do not respond to other therapies.[5]

123. B. Joint deformities are a major complication of rheumatoid arthritis. Sometimes, even after inflammation has been suppressed with aspirin or other nonsteroidal anti-inflammatory agents and remission has been induced, one or more joints will flare up. The removal of accumulated intrasynovial fluid and the injection of an intra-articular steroid may provide dramatic relief.[3,5] Oral corticosteroids can also be used but have many more side effects (especially a tendency to osteoporosis).

124. A. In early rheumatoid arthritis, few radiologic findings are seen. Soft-tissue changes in synovial fluid or capsular thickening may occasionally be seen on the radiograph, but are more readily detected by physical examination. Loss of juxta-articular bone mass (osteoporosis) is most often detected near the finger joints and may be seen early in the disease. Narrowing of the joint space, which is due to thinning of the articular cartilage, is usually seen late in the disease. Bony erosions are usually best seen at the margins of the joint. Subarticular sclerosis is a feature of osteoarthritis but not of rheumatoid arthritis.[3]

125. E. Rheumatoid arthritis may involve many extra-articular systems.

Sjogren's syndrome is usually present if ocular involvement occurs. Sjogren's syndrome usually presents with decreased tear formation and a sensation of grittiness. Common ocular problems associated with rheumatoid arthritis include episcleritis and scleritis.[3]

Pulmonary abnormalities are commonly associated with rheumatoid arthritis. The most common form of lung involvement is pleuritis with effusions. This may present with gradual onset of pain and dyspnea.

Other pulmonary manifestations include rheumatoid nodules; progressive, symptomatic, interstitial pulmonary fibrosis, and obliterative bronchiolitis.[3]

Cardiac abnormalities in rheumatoid arthritis are common. Pericarditis, the most significant of the rheumatoid cardiac lesions, is most prominent in patients who have severe seropositive disease. Rheumatoid nodules in the valves and conduction system may occur.[3]

The most common hematologic abnormality is a hypochromic, normocytic anemia.[3] Iron deficiency anemia may occur from gastrointestinal blood loss secondary to aspirin or nonsteroidal anti-inflammatory drugs.

Neuromuscular involvement and vasculitis are other complications of rheumatoid arthritis.

126. C. Oral corticosteroids usually produce an immediate and dramatic anti-inflammatory effect in rheumatoid arthritis; they do not, however, alter its natural progression. The anti-inflammatory effect appears to be limited only to as long as the drug is being used; clinical symptomatology commonly reappears when the steroids are discontinued. The long term use of corticosteroids is recommended only when the patient does not respond to conservative management and when they are contraindications to other remittive agents.[4]

The smallest amount of corticosteroid that will control the inflammation is the right dose.

Localized symptoms can also be treated with corticosteroid injections.

SUMMARY OF THE DIAGNOSIS AND TREATMENT OF RHEUMATOID ARTHRITIS

1. Make diagnosis according to criteria of the American Rheumatologic Society (see question 118)

2. Recognize that rheumatoid arthritis is a systemic disease with extra-articular manifestations including pulmonary changes (effusions, fibrosis), pericarditis and valvular lesions, vasculitis, atrophy of muscles, and subcutaneous nodules

3. Recognize radiologic features of rheumatoid arthritis: juxta-articular osteoporosis, joint erosions, and narrowing of the joint spaces

4. **Treatment:**
   A. Conservative Management:
      i) systemic rest
      ii) articular rest
      iii) physical therapy including active-assistive exercises
      iv) heat and cold
      v) nonsteroidal anti-inflammatory drugs: aspirin remains the drug of choice; other NSAIDs also valuable
   B. Remittive Agents:
      i) gold salts (either oral auranofin or intramuscular gold) are the drugs of choice
      ii) if gold is contraindicated or produces signficant side effects penicillamine, hydroxychloroquine, or methotrexate may be used
   C. Corticosteroid therapy:
      i) intra-articular steroids are indicated when one or two joints are the chief source of pain and symptoms
      ii) although oral corticosteroids are potent anti-inflammatory agents, they do not produce disease remission. They should be used in the smallest possible dose and for the shortest period of time

References

1. Ropes MW, Bennett GA, Cobb S, et al. 1958 Revision of the diagnostic criteria for rheumatoid arthritis by a committee of the American Rheumatism Association. Arthritis Rheum 1959; 2: 16.

2. Lipsky P. Rheumatoid arthritis. In: Braunwald E, Isselbacher K, Petersdorf R, Wilson J, Martin J, Fauci A, eds. Harrison's principles of internal medicine. 11th Ed. New York: McGraw-Hill, 1988: 1423–1428.

3. Krane S. Rheumatoid arthritis. In: Rubenstein E, Federman D, eds. Scientific American medicine. New York: Scientific American Medicine Inc, 1986: 15(II), 1–20.

4. Drugs for rheumatoid arthritis. Med Lett 1989; 31(Issue 795), June 30.

5. Klearman M, Pereira M. Arthritis and rheumatologic diseases. In: Dunagan W, Ridner M, eds. Manual of medical therapeutics. 26th Ed. Boston: Little, Brown, 1989: 436–445.

PROBLEM 15: A 26-YEAR-OLD MALE WITH ACNE VULGARIS

A 26-year-old male presents to your office with multiple facial acne scars. The scars are broad-based. The disease is quiescent at the present time. He is depressed and wishes to have the scars removed.

SELECT THE ONE BEST ANSWER TO THE FOLLOWING QUESTIONS:

127. You should tell the patient described in the question that:
    a) there is no hope for removing existing acne scars
    b) the treatment of choice is collagen implant
    c) the treatment of choice is dermabrasion
    d) a prolonged course of isotretinoin should significantly improve his complexion
    e) cryotherapy is the treatment of choice

128. Which of the following statements regarding acne and diet is(are) TRUE?
    a) chocolate may aggravate acne
    b) shellfish and iodized salt may aggravate acne
    c) nuts may aggravate acne
    d) all of the above are correct
    e) none of the above are correct

ANSWER THE FOLLOWING QUESTIONS ACCORDING TO THE CODE:

A: 1, 2, and 3 are correct
B: 1 and 3 are correct
C: 2 and 4 are correct
D: Only 4 is correct
E: All of the above are correct

129. Which of the following statements regarding skin care and acne is(are) correct?
    1) vigorous washing will unblock pores and resolve the lesions
    2) manual manipulation of acne lesions may result in more inflammation and scarring
    3) patients who use cosmetics should use oil-based products as opposed to water-based products
    4) if moisturizers are used, an oil-free moisturizer should be used

130. Which of the following statements is(are) TRUE regarding the use of benzoyl peroxide in the treatment of acne?
    1) it normalizes keratinization
    2) it is often used as a drying and desquamating agent
    3) it is generally applied three times per day
    4) the gel form is usually more effective than the lotion

131. Which of the following antibiotic(s) is(are) effective when used in topical form for the treatment of acne vulgaris?
    1) erythromycin
    2) tetracycline
    3) clindamycin
    4) gentamicin

132. The antibiotic(s) of choice for the systemic therapy of acne vulgaris is(are):
    1) clindamycin
    2) tetracycline
    3) chloramphenicol
    4) erythromycin

133. Which of the following statements about the use of oral isotretinoin (Accutane) is(are) TRUE?
    1) it is the only drug that works against all components of acne genesis
    2) isotretinoin is a teratogen
    3) isotretinoin prevents scarring and improves existing scars
    4) isotretinoin often causes significant elevation of serum triglycerides

ANSWERS

127. C. The treatment of choice for the removal of sharp-bordered, deep acne scars is dermabrasion.[1] Dermabrasion evens out the skin contour by means of a high-speed wire brush. The results of der-

mabrasion are somewhat unpredictable, with 30–75% of patients achieving improvement.[2] The patient most likely to benefit from dermabrasion is the one with broad-based scars and quiescent disease.[1] Complications of dermabrasion include infection, hypertrophic scarring, hyperpigmentation, and hypopigmentation.

Collagen implants are most effective for soft, pliable scars with relatively smooth margins.[3] Neither isotretinoin nor cryotherapy would be effective in treating patients with acne scars.

128. E. There is no evidence from clinical studies that the restriction of foods such as chocolate, nuts, shellfish, iodized salt, cheese, fatty foods, colas, or any other foods adversely affect acne.[4]

129. C. A good skin care program is essential in the management of acne. Vigorous washing and scrubbing may actually worsen the condition. If the patient's skin is particularly oily, washing up to three times per day with a mild soap and water is optimal.[1]

Patients should learn to leave acne lesions alone. Picking or other manipulations will only increase the probability of rupture of the acne lesion into the dermis. This, subsequently, will result in more inflammation, and possibly more scarring.[1]

As acne patients usually have oily skin, moisturizers are usually not indicated. If, however, an agent that produces significant drying of the skin is used, a moisturizer may be required. If a moisturizer is to be used, it should be oil-free. Examples of oil-free moisturizers include Neutrogena Hand Cream, Norwegian Formula, Johnson and Johnson All Purpose Dry Skin Cream, and Complex 15.

130. C. The most frequently used topical agent for the treatment of acne vulgaris is benzoyl peroxide. As well as acting as an antibiotic agent against Propionbacterium acnes, it also acts as a drying and desquamating agent, and as an agent that promotes superficial peeling and loosens comedones.[1] Because of its drying and desquamating properties, benzoyl peroxide is often irritating to sensitive or relatively dry skin.

Benzoyl peroxide products are available in acetone or water-based lotions, creams, gels, and washes in 2.5%, 5%, and 10% concentrations. Gels tend to be more effective than lotions or creams.[1] Acetone bases should be used only on excessively oily skin. Water-based products are ideal for delicate or even dry skin. Benzoyl peroxide is usually applied in the morning after washing.

Tretinoin (Vitamin A acid) is another good first-line agent in the treatment of acne.[1] Tretinoin, which is available in a gel or a cream, normalizes follicular keratinization and loosens horn cells. Although the gel is more effective, it can cause excessive peeling or drying. Tretinoin is usually applied at night and is begun at a concentration of 0.01%.

An excellent combination is the use of benzoyl peroxide gel in the morning and tretinoin gel at night.

131. A. Antibiotics are often as effective when applied topically as when given in low-dose oral form. Erythromycin, tetracycline, and clindamycin are all available in topical lotion form. These products, when applied to a clean skin surface with a sponge applicator twice daily are effective in decreasing the level of P. acnes.[1] The destructive hydrolytic enzymes and chemotactic factors that are present in P. acnes are thus decreased and inflammation is reduced. Gentamicin is not available in a topical lotion and is not effective in treating acne vulgaris.

132. C. The oral antibiotics of choice in the treatment of acne are erythromycin and tetracycline.[1] Clindamycin is a major cause of pseudomembranous colitis and is not used systemically for acne treatment. Chloramphenicol is associated with aplastic anemia and is not appropriate for acne treatment.

133. E. Oral isotretinoin (Accutane) is now the treatment of choice for severe, recalcitrant nodulocystic acne.[1] It is the only drug that works against all components of acne genesis. It is not only active against P. acnes, but it impedes comedogenesis and significantly inhibits sebum production.[1] This drug is able to prevent scarring and also improve existing scars.

Isotretinoin is a well-established teratogen.[1] Pregnancy must be excluded before initiation of treatment. All women of childbearing potential who use the drug must use an adequate birth control method (preferably the oral contraceptive pill). Because of the severe CNS defects seen in offspring of women who have taken the drug during pregnancy, abortion should be strongly considered should pregnancy occur during treatment.

Elevated serum triglycerides and liver enzymes are often seen in patients taking isotretinoin.[1]

Therefore, baseline levels should be drawn before therapy is commenced. Although serum cholesterol may be minimally elevated, the major change in cholesterol metabolism on isotretinoin is a decrease in the level of high density lipoprotein cholesterol.

Intralesional corticosteroid injections are also effective for severe nodulocystic acne.[1]

SUMMARY OF THE CLASSIFICATION AND MANAGEMENT OF ACNE VULGARIS

Classification:

I. Obstructive:
    closed comedones (whiteheads)
    open comedones (blackheads)

II. Inflammatory:
    papules, pustules, nodules, cysts, scars

Treatment:

I. General measures:
    1. gentle face washing
    2. avoidance of manipulation of acne lesions
    3. use water-based cosmetics only
    4. use oil-free moisturizers only
    5. eat well balanced diet

II. Specific management:
    A. Obstructive acne
       1. benzoyl peroxide
       2. tretinoin (Retin-A)
       3. comedo extraction
    B. Inflammatory acne
       1. antibiotics—topical, systemic
       2. benzoyl peroxide
       3. tretinoin
       4. intralesional corticosteroid injection
    C. Resistant cases and severe nodulocystic acne
       1. isotretinoin (Accutane)
       2. topical antibiotics
       3. systemic antibiotics
       4. intralesional corticosteroid injections

References

1. Quan M. Management of acne vulgaris. Am Fam Physician 1988; 38(2): 207–217.

2. Olsen TG. Therapy of acne. Med Clin North Am 1982; 66:851–871.

3. Watson W, Kaye RL, Klein A, Stegman S. Injectable collagen: a clinical overview. Cutis 1983; 31: 543–546.

4. Rosenberg EW, Kirk BS. Acne diet reconsidered. Arch Dermatol 1981; 117: 193–195.

PROBLEM 16: A 35-YEAR-OLD FEMALE WITH DIFFUSE MUSCULOSKELETAL PAIN

A 35-year-old female patient presents with a chronic aching pain in her cervical, shoulder, pectoral, and proximal lumbosacral areas. As well, she complains of a chronic headache, disturbed sleep, and generalized fatigue. When questioned, she describes swelling, numbness, and morning stiffness. On examining her musculoskeletal system you find no evidence of joint swelling, warmth, or deformity. However, you find multiple tender areas over her back and upper extremities.

SELECT THE ONE BEST ANSWER TO THE FOLLOWING QUESTIONS:

134. The most likely diagnosis in this patient is:
     a) polymyalgia rheumatica
     b) masked depression
     c) fibromyalgia
     d) diffuse musculoskeletal pain NYD
     e) early rheumatoid arthritis

135. Which one of the following is NOT usually a site of tenderness in the disorder described above?
     a) rectus abdominis muscle
     b) supraspinatus tendon
     c) lateral epicondyle of the humerus
     d) trapezius muscle
     e) middle gluteus muscle

136. Which of the following conditions should be considered in the differential diagnosis of the condition described above?
    a) psychogenic rheumatism
    b) malingering
    c) masked depression
    d) a and b
    e) all of the above

ANSWER THE FOLLOWING QUESTIONS ACCORDING TO THE CODE:

A: 1, 2, and 3 are correct
B: 1 and 3 are correct
C: 2 and 4 are correct
D: Only 4 is correct
E: All of the above are correct

137. Which of the following laboratory investigations should be performed in the patient described in question 134?
    1) ESR
    2) rheumatoid factor with titer
    3) ANA
    4) CBC

138. Which of the following treatment modalities is(are) indicated in the treatment of the disorder discussed above?
    1) nonsteroidal anti-inflammatory drugs
    2) muscle relaxants
    3) tricyclic antidepressants
    4) corticosteroids

ANSWERS

134. C. This patient has fibromyalgia. Fibromyalgia is characterized by chronic, diffuse achiness or stiffness affecting three or more areas for more than 3 months; tender points at multiple locations; the absence of other conditions to explain musculoskeletal symptoms; and other symptoms including chronic headache, disturbed sleep, generalized fatigue, and a subjective sensation of swelling, numbness, or morning stiffness.[1]

Fibromyalgia, which is 10 times more common in women than in men, is usually diagnosed between the ages of 35 and 65 years.[2]

Rheumatoid arthritis is unlikely because of the lack of objective evidence of joint warmth, swelling or deformity, and the multiple tender soft-tissue areas. Laboratory evaluation, however, is necessary to exclude an inflammatory condition.

Polymyalgia rheumatica occurs in an older age group and will be discussed in another section of this book.

Diffuse musculoskeletal pain NYD is not a diagnosis.

A primary diagnosis of masked depression should always be considered when vague, somatic complaints are accompanied by sleep disturbance and fatigue. The multiple tender areas, however, are not usually seen in masked depression.

135. A. Fibromyalgia is associated with tender points at multiple characteristic locations.[1] These locations include the supraspinatus tendon, costochondral junction, lateral epicondyle of the humerus, the iliac chest, the greater trochanteric bursa of the femus, the medial fat pad of the knee, the splenius muscle of the head, the nuchal ligament, the trapezius muscle, the infraspinatus tendon, the rhomboid muscle, the erector spinae of the lumbar spine, the middle gluteus muscle, and the piriform muscle.[2] The rectus abdominus is not included.

The sensitivity of tender points can be assessed by measuring the exact amount of pressure applied over a certain anatomic site. This is measured by a dolorimeter.[2]

136. E. Fibromyalgia must be distinguished from psychogenic rheumatism, malingering, and masked depression.

Masked depression, as discussed earlier, does not usually present with the distinct multiple tender areas seen in fibromyalgia.

Fibromyalgia must be differentiated from psychogenic rheumatism and malingering. In the latter two conditions, patients may report tenderness over almost every area palpated or pressed on by the examiner, or may exhibit different patterns of tenderness on serial examinations.[2]

137. E. Generalized aches and pains are characteristic of many conditions. The differential diagnosis may include certain metabolic disorders, inflammatory conditions, infections, anatomic problems, and neurologic conditions.

Certain investigations including ESR, rheumatoid factors with titer, ANA, and CBC should probably be performed in all patients suspected of having fibromyalgia.[2] Additional laboratory tests including urinalysis, serum liver and muscle enzyme determinations, thyroid function studies, radiographic procedures, and nuclear medicine scanning may be necessary if the symptoms appear to target a particular anatomic area or organic system.[2] Electromyography and nerve conduction studies may be indicated when numbness, tingling, or burning sensations are present.[2]

138. A. Treatment of fibromyalgia begins with education and reassurance. Patients should be encouraged to participate in their own care. Support from family members is essential. Stress reduction by means of relaxation techniques, biofeedback, and hypnotherapy may be helpful.[2] Pharmacologic treatment includes the nonsteroidal antiinflammatory drugs, tricyclic antidepressants, and muscle relaxants such as cyclobenzaprine.[2]

Physical therapy modalities such as massage, acupressure, ultrasound, hot packs, and "spray-and-stretch" treatments may be helpful.

If the treatment modalities discussed above are not effective, the injection of a local anesthetic, with or without a corticosteroid, may help break the pain-spasm-pain cycle.[2]

Systemic corticosteroids and narcotic analgesics are not appropriate for the treatment of fibromyalagia.

SUMMARY OF THE DIAGNOSIS AND TREATMENT OF FIBROMYALGIA

1. **Diagnosis:** chronic diffuse achiness or stiffness, multiple tender points, headache, chronic fatigue, sleep disturbance, numbness or swelling

2. **Differential diagnosis:** psychogenic rheumatism, malingering, masked depression and other major inflammatory conditions. Absence of other conditions to explain musculoskeletal symptoms must be established.

3. **Treatment:** reassurance about benign nature of condition, relaxation therapy, biofeedback, NSAIDs, tricyclic antidepressants, muscle relaxants, physical therapy, injection of local anesthetic/corticosteroid

References

1. Goldenberg DL. Fibromyalgia syndrome: an emerging but controversial condition. JAMA 1987; 257(20):2782–2787.

2. Romano T. The fibromyalgia syndrome: it's the real thing. Postgrad Med 1988; 83(5): 231–243.

PROBLEM 17: A 40-YEAR-OLD OBESE MALE WITH AN ACUTELY INFLAMED LEFT GREAT TOE

A 40-year-old obese male presents to the office after waking up with an acutely swollen left great toe. This is his first episode of such an attack.

On examination, the patient's temperature is 38.5° C. His blood pressure is 170/110 mm Hg. He has an erythematous, tender, swollen left great toe. There is extensive swelling and erythema of the left foot, and the whole foot is tender. No other abnormalities are found on physical examination.

SELECT THE ONE BEST ANSWER TO THE FOLLOWING QUESTIONS:

139. The most likely diagnosis in this patient is:
    a) acute cellulitis
    b) acute gouty arthritis
    c) acute rheumatoid arthritis
    d) acute septic arthritis
    e) acute osteomyelitis

140. Which of the following statements regarding the condition described in question 139 is false?

a) the condition is more common in males than in females
b) fever is unusual
c) greater than 50% of the initial attacks of this condition are confined to the first metatarsophalangeal joint
d) peripheral leukocytosis may be found
e) involvement is usually asymmetric

141. For the condition described in the patient in question 139, the diagnostic test of choice is:
    a) a plasma level
    b) a random urine determination

c) a 24-hour urine determination
d) a synovial fluid analysis
e) a Gram stain plus culture and sensitivity

142. The most common metabolic abnormality associated with the condition described above is:
a) increased production of uric acid
b) decreased renal excretion of uric acid
c) increased production of metabolites of uric acid
d) decreased renal excretion of metabolites of uric acid
e) none of the above

143. The drug of choice for the initial management of the patient described in question 139 is:
a) indomethacin
b) colchicine
c) acetaminophen
d) aspirin
e) phenylbutazone

144. The drug of choice for the prevention of future attacks of the condition described in question 139 is:
a) allopurinol
b) probenecid
c) sulfinpyrazone
d) indomethacin
e) none of the above

145. The treatment of choice for asymptomatic hyperuricemia is:
a) probenecid
b) sulfinpyrazone
c) allopurinol
d) a or b
e) none of the above

ANSWER THE FOLLOWING QUESTION ACCORDING TO THE CODE:

A: 1, 2, and 3 are correct
B: 1 and 3 are correct
C: 2 and 4 are correct
D: Only 4 is correct
E: All of the above are correct

146. Which of the following conditions is associated with the condition described in this patient?
1) obesity
2) alcoholism
3) hypertension
4) diabetes mellitus

147. Which of the following statements regarding pseudogout is(are) true?
1) pseudogout is characterized by the deposition of calcium pyrophosphate crystals in articular cartilage
2) the most commonly affected joint is the knee
3) diagnosis is made by aspiration of joint fluid, which contains rhomboidal crystals that are positively birefringent
4) hypothyroidism may predispose to pseudogout

ANSWERS

139. B. The most likely diagnosis in this patient is acute gouty arthritis. The patient usually develops an acute pain in a joint of the lower extremity, most commonly the first metatarsophalangeal joint. The pain often wakes the patient from sleep. The pain is usually described as crushing or excruciating.[1]

The joint rapidly becomes erythematous, swollen, warm, and extremely tender. The skin surrounding the joint is usually tense and shiny. The swelling in acute gout often extends well beyond the joint itself and may involve the entire foot (or other part of the extremity). This swelling, due to periarticular edema, makes the differentiation from septic arthritis or cellulitis difficult. The patient often presents with a limp and is unable to bear weight on the affected extremity.

140. B. Fever may occur in patients with gout, especially in patients with polyarticular disease.[2] The temperature may reach 39.5° C.

The metatarsophalangeal joint is the location of the acute attack in over 50% of patients experiencing their first attack.[2] Therefore, most first attacks are asymmetric. If untreated, involvement of other joints of the foot may occur simultaneously or follow rapidly. Acute gout may also involve bursae, or tendon sheaths.

Leukocytosis may be seen. Tophi are occasionally seen with the first attack. Usually, however, there is a time interval (often 10 years or more) between the initial attack and the appearance of a gouty tophus.[2]

Gout is more common in males than in females. In females, it most often occurs following the menopause.

141. D. Gout is definitely diagnosed by the demonstration of negatively birefringent, needle-shaped crystals under a polarizing microscope. This should be attempted in all patients suspected of having gout.[2] Although an elevated serum uric acid concentration is usually seen with acute gout, it is not as sensitive or specific a test for gout as the demonstration of crystals. The diagnosis of septic arthritis can be ruled out by appropriate stains and cultures of the same specimen of synovial fluid.

142. B. The most common metabolic abnormality associated with gout is decreased renal excretion of uric acid.[1] This may be either primary or secondary to a number of causes such as chronic renal disease, acute ethanol ingestion, or diuretic therapy. The most common cause of overproduction of uric acid is a myeloproliferative or lymphoproliferative disorder.

143. A. Colchicine was, until recently, the drug of choice in the treatment of acute gout. This agent, however, has many gastrointestinal side effects that limit its usefulness. NSAIDs such as indomethacin 50 mg t.i.d. are the drugs of choice in most settings at this time.[3] The NSAIDs should ideally be given for 1–2 weeks until treatment aimed at decreasing the uric acid pool is begun.

Aspirin, taken in small doses, can actually aggravate the problem. Acetaminophen has no anti-inflammatory activity and is not indicated in the acute treatment of gout. Phenylbutazone is an excellent anti-inflammatory agent but has now been associated with bone marrow suppression and aplastic anemia.

Prednisone or other corticosteroids can be used to treat patients with acute gout who have not responded to other therapies and patients in whom the other agents are contraindicated.[3]

144. A. The drug of choice for preventing future attacks of gout is allopurinol.[3] Allopurinol's method of action is both as a xanthine oxidase inhibitor, and as an inhibitor of denovo purine production. Allopurinol may be given in a single daily dose of 300 mg/day, although some patients still require 300–600 mg/day in divided doses.

Probenecid and sulfinpyrazone are uricosuric agents.[3] Probenecid is the drug of second choice. These drugs block the renal tubular reabsorption of both filtered urate and secreted urate. Sulfinpyrazone, a drug related to phenylbutazone, is rarely indicated in the treatment of hyperuri-

cemia.[3] In patients in whom acute gouty arthritis is secondary to another factor such as a thiazide diuretic or ethanol, the offending agent should be discontinued before long-term drug therapy is considered. It is reasonable to consider long-term treatment after 2 or 3 attacks of gout; one attack is probably insufficient to warrant long term therapy.

145. E. Asymptomatic hyperuricemia does not warrant treatment, as only 10% of asymptomatic patients eventually develop gout.[4] The risk/benefit ratio is against treatment unless the patient has a history of uric acid stones, hyperuric calcium stones, or gouty attacks.

Patients with hyperuricemia should be advised to decrease meat (purine) intake, decrease alcohol intake, and decrease or discontinue medications such as diuretics or ASA.

146. E. The incidence of acute and chronic gout is increased in patients with hypertension, diabetes mellitus, alcoholism, obesity, and hypertriglyceridemia.[2]

147. E. Chondrocalcinosis is defined as the presence of calcium-containing salts in articular cartilage. It is usually diagnosed radiologically. Chondrocalcinosis may be familial and is more common in patients with hyperparathyroidism, hypothyroidism, diabetes mellitus, and true gout. Pseudogout refers to acute, recurrent, and sometimes chronic arthritis that occurs in patients (usually over the age of 60 years) as a result of chondrocalcinosis of the affected joint.

Pseudogout is diagnosed by the presence of positively birefringent calcium pyrophosphate crystals in joint aspirates.

Treatment of pseudogout is directed at treatment of the primary condition. NSAIDs, however, are helpful in the treatment of acute attacks.

SUMMARY OF THE DIAGNOSIS AND TREATMENT OF GOUT

1. **Symptoms:** acute onset of pain in joint of lower extremity, most commonly metatarsophalangeal joint.

   Associated tenderness, erythema, and swelling of the surrounding tissues is common

2. **Pathophysiology:** most often associated with decreased renal excretion of uric acid

3. **Diagnosis:** although clinical history and elevated uric acid support the diagnosis, the diagnosis is definitively established by aspiration of joint fluid and demonstration of uric acid crystals using a polarizing microscope.

4. **Treatment:**
    acute attack: indomethacin is the drug of choice
        prophylaxis against recurrent attacks: allopurinol is drug of choice
        asymptomatic hyperuricemia: no treatment is usually indicated

References

1. Kelley W, Palella T. Gout and other disorders of purine metabolism. In: Braunwald W, Isselbacher K, Petersdorf R, Wilson J, Martin J, Fauci A, eds. Harrison's principles of internal medicine. 11th Ed. New York: McGraw-Hill, 1987: 1623–1632.

2. Krane S. Crystal-induced joint disease. In: Rubenstein E, Federman D, eds. Scientific American medicine. New York: Scientific American Medicine Inc, 1986: 15(IX); 1–15.

3. Klearman M, Pereira M. Arthritis and rheumatologic diseases. In: Dunagan W, Ridner M, eds. Manual of medical therapeutics. 26th Ed. Boston: Little, Brown, 1989: 453–456.

4. Dallman J. The joints and connective tissue. In: Taylor R, ed. Family medicine: principles and practice. 3rd Ed. New York: Springer-Verlag, 1988: 356.

PROBLEM 18: A 51-YEAR-OLD FEMALE ENTERING THE MENOPAUSE

A 51-year-old female presents to your office for a routine health assessment. On functional inquiry you discover that her menstrual periods ceased 3 months ago. You ask her whether or not she has heard of osteoporosis. She states that she has, but states that she doesn't wish preventive treatment as she has heard that it causes cancer. You are now about to enter into a discussion with her regarding the prevention and treatment of osteoporosis.

SELECT THE ONE BEST ANSWER TO THE FOLLOWING QUESTIONS:

148. Osteoporosis is defined as:
    a) an increased turnover of calcium in newly formed bone
    b) a failure to deposit inorganic mineral in newly formed organic bone matrix
    c) a lack of calcium in newly formed bone
    d) a decrease in bone mass in the absence of a mineralization defect
    e) a decrease in both bone mass and matrix in both trabecular and cortical bone

149. Osteoporosis is divided into two subtypes, Type I and Type II. Which of the following bone sites is not associated with Type II osteoporosis?
    a) vertebra
    b) femoral neck
    c) proximal humerus
    d) proximal tibia
    e) pelvis

150. Which of the following is not an established risk factor for osteoporosis?
    a) postmenopausal status
    b) sedentary lifestyle
    c) cigarette smoking
    d) obesity
    e) excessive alcohol intake

ANSWER THE FOLLOWING QUESTIONS ACCORDING TO THE CODE

A: 1, 2, and 3 are correct
B: 1 and 3 are correct
C: 2 and 4 are correct
D: Only 4 is correct
E: All of the above are correct

151. Which of the following are established therapies for the prevention of osteoporosis?
    1) Vitamin D supplementation
    2) calcium supplementation
    3) sodium fluoride
    4) estrogen

152. Your 51-year-old patient has presented her fears that the prevention of osteoporosis may be associated with the development of cancer. Which of

the following statements regarding estrogen replacement therapy are true?

1) if used unopposed, estrogen replacement therapy may be associated with an increased risk of endometrial cancer
2) if used in conjugation with progesterone there appears to be no increased risk of developing endometrial cancer
3) estrogen replacement therapy must be initiated with the equivalent of at least 0.625 mg of conjugated estrogen
4) estrogen users have been found to have a lower all-cause mortality than non-users.

ANSWERS

148. D. Osteoporosis and osteomalacia are often confused. Osteoporosis is defined as a decrease in bone mass in the absence of a mineralization defect. Osteomalacia defines a group of diseases characterized by a failure to deposit the inorganic mineral phase in the newly formed organic bone matrix.[1] None of the other definitions apply.

149. A. Type I osteoporosis, which occurs primarly in postmenopausal women, is characterized by a decrease in trabecular bone mass. Trabecular bone is most common in the vertebral bodies and in the distal forearm, and is associated with fractures in these areas.[1] Type II osteoporosis, which is characterized by a decrease in both cortical and trabecular bone, occurs in both sexes in the seventh decade of life or later. It is most commonly associated with fractures in the femoral neck, proximal humerus, proximal tibia, and pelvis.[1]

150. D. The established risk factors for osteoporosis include postmenopausal status, low skeletal mass, poor musculature, sedentary lifestyle, cigarette smoking, the Caucasian race, and excessive alcohol intake.[1,2] Obesity appears to be somewhat protective.[1]

151. D. Only estrogen has been shown in double-blind, placebo-controlled trials to prevent postmenopausal osteoporosis and subsequent fractures.[3] Estrogen should be given in the oral form (equivalent to 0.625 mg of conjugated estrogen per day).[3] Although it is reasonable to suggest that transdermal estrogen should prevent osteoporosis, there is no convincing data to confirm this.[3] It seems premature to advise estrogen replacement

therapy for all postmenopausal women.[4] A rational approach would be to consider estrogen replacement therapy for those women at risk for osteoporosis who have recently entered the menopause. The optimal length of time of treatment is unknown.

The role of calcium in the prevention of osteoporosis is unclear.[3] A high calcium intake may reduce the rate of cortical bone loss, but not trabecular bone loss. In addition, the benefit of calcium in preventing osteoporotic fractures is not known.[3]

In spite of contradictory and inconclusive evidence it seems reasonable to recommend a calcium intake of approximately 1500 mg/day in postmenopausal women.[3] Every effort should be made to increase dietary calcium, thus lessening the need for supplements.

As sodium fluoride has many side effects, it is currently recommended that it be reserved for experimental use.[4] Vitamin D alone has not been shown to improve calcium balance.[4]

Regular exercise, discontinuing cigarette smoking, and avoiding excessive alcohol intake are all reasonable preventive measures.

152. E. Estrogen replacement therapy may be associated with an increased risk of endometrial cancer.[3] A progesterone added to the estrogen regimen is protective.[3] A minimum dose of 0.625 mg conjugated estrogen should be given.[3] One study suggested a relative risk in all-cause mortality of 0.37 for estrogen users, regardless of their gynecologic status.[5]

A reasonable preventive regimen would be 0.625 mg of conjugated estrogen on days 1–25 of each calendar month with progesterone 10 mg added from days 16–25. The rest of the month should be hormone free.

SUMMARY OF OSTEOPOROSIS

1. **Definition:** A decrease in bone mass in the absence of a mineralization defect

2. **Classification:**
    Type I: Location—vertebra and distal forearm. Type of bone—trabecular.
    Type II: Location—femoral neck, proximal humerus, proximal tibia, pelvis. Type of bone: trabecular and cortical

3. **Prevention:**

    estrogen: proven—0.625 mg days 1–25 with progesterone 10 mg days 16–25

    calcium: unproven but may be reasonable (1500 mg/day total intake)

    sodium fluoride and Vitamin D: Use not established at the present time

    regular exercise, discontinuing smoking, and avoiding excessive alcohol may be beneficial and should be recommended

References

1. Krane S, Holick M. Metabolic bone disease. In: Braunwald E, Isselbacher K, Petersdorf R, Wilson J, Martin J, Fauci A, eds. Harrison's principles of internal medicine. 11th Ed. New York: McGraw-Hill, 1987: 1889–1900.

2. Garcia J. Mineral, parathyroid, and metabolic bone diseases. In: Dunagan W, Ridner M, eds. Manual of medical therapeutics. 26th Ed. Boston: Little, Brown, 1988: 431–435.

3. Consensus development conference: prophylaxis and treatment of osteoporosis. Br Med J 1987; 295: 914–915.

4. Goldbloom R, Battista R. The periodic health examination: 1. Introduction. Can Med Assoc J 1988; 138: 617–625.

5. Bush TL, Cowan LD, Barrett-Conner E, et al. Estrogen and all-cause mortality. Preliminary results from the lipid research clinics program follow-up study. JAMA 1983; 249: 903–906.

PROBLEM 19: A 25-YEAR-OLD COLLEGE STUDENT WITH A FEVER AND A SORE THROAT

A 25-year-old college student presents with a 3-week history of fatigue, malaise, fever, chills, and sore throat.

On physical examination, the patient has a temperature of 39° C. There is pharyngeal hyperemia and edema and marked exudates are seen in both tonsillar areas. There is significant cervical lymphadenopathy present.

You suspect infectious mononucleosis.

SELECT THE ONE BEST ANSWER TO THE FOLLOWING QUESTIONS:

153. Of the following clinical features of acute infectious mononucleosis, the least common is:
   a) splenomegaly
   b) hepatomegaly
   c) fever
   d) exudative tonsillitis
   e) generalized lymphadenopathy

154. Which one of the following findings is so specific for infectious mononucleosis that serologic testing becomes unnecessary?
   a) combination of fever, tonsillitis, and generalized lymphadenopathy
   b) splenomegaly
   c) lymphocytosis
   d) lymphocyte atypia of more than 40%
   e) none of the above

155. Which one of the following statements regarding infectious mononucleosis is false?
   a) infectious mononucleosis is caused by the Epstein-Barr virus
   b) kissing is the most common mode of transmission of infectious mononucleosis
   c) greater than 90% of all adults are carriers of the virus that causes infectious mononucleosis
   d) in young children, fever and pharyngitis from primary infectious mononucleosis may be clinically indistinguishable from upper respiratory tract infections caused by other viruses, mycoplasma, or streptococci
   e) bacterial throat culture is not necessary in patients suspected of having infectious mononucleosis

156. Which one of the following statements regarding serologic testing for infectious mononucleosis is false?
   a) the rapid heterophile antibody test is 95% sensitive
   b) the rapid heterophile antibody test is 95% specific
   c) in acute primary infection, anti-EA (early antigen) titers are usually low
   d) in acute primary infection, IgM VCA (IgM viral capsid antigen) titers are high
   e) after several months, the anti-EBNA (Epstein-Barr nuclear antigen) titers become high

157. The treatment of choice for uncomplicated acute infectious mononucleosis is:
    a) penicillin
    b) prednisone
    c) penicillin plus prednisone
    d) penicillin plus high dose ASA
    e) none of the above

ANSWER THE FOLLOWING QUESTIONS ACCORDING TO THE CODE:

A: 1, 2, and 3 are correct
B: 1 and 3 are correct
C: 2 and 4 are correct
D: Only 4 is correct
E: All of the above are correct

158. Which of the following signs commonly occur in acute infectious mononucleosis ?
    1) palatine petechiae
    2) splenomegaly
    3) periorbital edema
    4) generalized lymphadenopathy

159. Which of the following are complications of acute infectious mononucleosis?
    1) pneumonitis
    2) pericarditis
    3) meningoencephalitis
    4) Bell's palsy

160. Which of the following statements is (are) true regarding chronic mononucleosis?
    1) chronic mononucleosis does not exist
    2) most patients with chronic mononucleosis eventually recover
    3) patients with true chronic mononucleosis usually do not demonstrate significant elevations of antibody titers to EB virus
    4) chronic mononucleosis is characterized by recurrent episodes of weakness, fatigue, myalgia, arthralgia, pharyngitis, or fever

ANSWERS

153. B. The least common clinical feature is hepatomegaly. The major clinical features of acute symptomatic infectious mononucleosis include fever, exudative tonsillitis, generalized lymphadenopathy, splenomegaly, and palatine petechiae.

154. D. A lymphocyte count in which more than 40% of lymphocytes are atypical is so specific for infectious mononucleosis that further serologic testing, including either a heterophil antibody titer or a "spot test" for heterophil antibodies is unnecessary.[2]

155. E. Infectious mononucleosis is caused by the Epstein-Barr virus.

    The usual mode of transmission of the virus is through infected saliva (kissing). Most adults (>90%) have been infected with Epstein-Barr virus and are carriers.

    Infectious mononucleosis is usually distinguishable from other viral infections in older children and adults. In younger children, however, it may be difficult to distinguish from other respiratory tract infections including those caused by other viruses, mycoplasma, or streptococci.[3]

    Bacterial throat culture should be done in patients with significant pharyngitis to exclude concomitant beta-hemolytic streptococcal infection.

156. C. With lymphocyte atypia >40%, no further testing is required.

    The heterophil antibody test is 95% sensitive and 95% specific for infectious mononucleosis. If this test does not support your clinical impression, further testing may be necessary.

    Serologic testing for EBV infection includes determining antibody titers to latently infected (anti-EBNA), early replication cycle (anti-EA), or later replication cycle (anti-VCA) viral proteins. Acute infectious mononucleosis produces high EA and IgM VCA titers, and low IgG VCA and EBNA titers. In recovering patients, the IgG VCA titer is high; and the EA, IgM, and EBNA titers are low. With time, the EBNA titer also becomes high.[3]

157. E. Symptomatic treatment including bed rest, the avoidance of strenuous exercise (because of the danger of splenic rupture), and analgesics are the only treatments necessary in acute uncomplicated mononucleosis.[3] Antibiotics are unnecessary unless a streptococcal pharyngitis coexists. Antibiotics (especially ampicillin) will produce a skin rash in most patients with infectious mononucleosis. Corticosteroids may occasionally be useful in the treatment of pharyngeal swelling and severe odonyphagia.

158. E. All of the symptoms listed in this question occur in acute infectious mononucleosis. See the critique of question 153.

159. E. The complications of acute infectious mononucleosis include meningoencephalitis, Guillain-Barré syndrome, Bell's palsy, pneumonitis, pericarditis, myocarditis, and the syndrome of inappropriate secretion of antidiuretic hormone.[3]

160. C. There are rare cases of chronic progressive primary EBV infection in young adults.[3] These patients have severe acute mononucleosis and persistent clinical manifestations including lymphadenopathy, and visceral organ involvement.

Most patients with chronic progressive EBV infection eventually recover without specific treatment. Persistent active EBV infection has been proposed as the cause of a syndrome that has become known as "adult neurasthenia."[3] This illness is characterized by weakness, fatigue, myalgia, arthralgia, pharyngitis, and fever. The role of EBV in this syndrome can only be substantiated when the antibody titers to EBV-specific antigens differ significantly from those of normal infected adults.[3]

SUMMARY OF THE DIAGNOSIS AND TREATMENT OF INFECTIOUS MONONUCLEOSIS

1. **Causative agent**: Epstein-Barr virus

2. **Incubation period**: 2–5 weeks

3. **Symptoms and signs**: a syndrome consisting of malaise, fever, exudative tonsillitis, lymphadenopathy, pharyngitis, enlarged tonsillar or cervical lymph nodes, splenomegaly, and palatine petechiae

4. **Diagnosis:**
   i) lymphocyte atypia
   ii) positive heterophil antibody titer
   iii) antibodies to EBV antigens:
   acute: anti-EA, anti-IgM VCA titers high
   convalescent: anti-IgG VCA titer high
   recovered: anti-IgG VCA and anti-EBNA high

5. **Treatment:**
   Symptomatic treatment is sufficient in most cases; corticosteroids with severe pharyngeal swelling and odynophagia

6. Chronic mononucleosis is rare. Diagnosis must be substantiated by antibody evidence of chronic infection.

References

1. McSherry J. Diagnosing infectious mononucleosis. Am Fam Physician 1985; 32(4): 129–132.

2. Ho-Yen D. Is the serological diagnosis of infectious mononucleosis always necessary? Br Med J (Clin Res) 1983; 287: 1187–1188.

3. Kieff E. Infectious mononucleosis. In: Wyngaarden J, Smith L, eds. Cecil textbook of medicine. 18th Ed. Philadelphia: WB Saunders, 1988: 1786–1788.

PROBLEM 20: A 32-YEAR-OLD FEMALE WITH FEVER, WEIGHT LOSS AND CHRONIC DIARRHEA

A 32-year-old female presents to the office with a 6-month history of loose bowel movements. These loose bowel movements have been associated with bloody diarrhea. She has lost 30 pounds in that period of time. For the last 3 weeks she has had an intermittent fever.

On examination, the patient looks ill. Her blood pressure is 100/70 mm Hg. Her pulse is 96 and regular. She has generalized abdominal tenderness.

Sigmoidoscopy examination reveals a friable mucosa, with multiple bleeding points.

SELECT THE ONE BEST ANSWER TO THE FOLLOWING QUESTIONS:

161. The most likely diagnosis in this patient is:
    a) irritable bowel syndrome
    b) Crohn's disease
    c) ulcerative colitis
    d) bacterial dysentery
    e) amebiasis

162. Investigations for the patient described in question 161 should include:
    a) a barium enema
    b) a colonoscopy
    c) a GI series and follow-through
    d) a and b
    e) all of the above

163. Which of the following may be useful in the management of the acute condition described in question 161?
    a) hydrocortisone enemas
    b) systemic corticosteroids
    c) adrenocorticotropic hormone (ACTH)
    d) a and b
    e) a, b, and c

164. Which of the following statements regarding the use of sulfasalazine in the condition described above is FALSE?
    a) sulfasalazine is structurally related to both aspirin and sulfa drugs
    b) sulfasalazine has been shown to be effective in maintaining a remission in the condition described above
    c) sulfasalazine is effective in treating the acute condition described above
    d) sulfasalazine may impair folic acid absorption

165. Which of the following statements regarding the long-term prognosis of the patient described in question 161 is FALSE?
    a) following an initial attack, 10% of patients go into remission lasting up to 15 years
    b) following an initial attack, 75% of patients experience intermittent exacerbations for many years
    c) following an initial attack, 10% of patients continue to have active disease until surgical intervention is undertaken
    d) following an initial attack, 5% of patients die within 1 year
    e) none of the above statements are false

ANSWER THE FOLLOWING QUESTION ACCORDING TO THE CODE:

A: 1, 2, and 3 are correct
B: 1 and 3 are correct
C: 2 and 4 are correct
D: Only 4 is correct
E: All of the above are correct

166. Which of the following are(is) complications of the condition described above?
    1) toxic megacolon
    2) colonic cancer
    3) stricture
    4) iritis

SELECT THE ONE BEST ANSWER TO THE FOLLOWING QUESTIONS:

167. A 25-year-old male presents with an 18-month history of chronic abdominal pain. The patient has seen several physicians, and he has been diagnosed as having "nervous stomach," "irritable bowel syndrome," and "depression." Associated with this abdominal pain for the last 3 months has been nonbloody diarrhea, anorexia, and a weight loss of 20 pounds. He has just developed a painful area near the anus.

On examination, the patient has diffuse abdominal tenderness. He looks thin and unwell. He has a tender, erythematous area in the right perirectal region.

The most likely diagnosis in this patient is:
    a) irritable bowel syndrome
    b) Crohn's disease
    c) ulcerative colitis
    d) bacterial dysentery
    e) amebiasis

168. Which one of the following investigations is the most sensitive test for confirming the diagnosis in this patient?
    a) sigmoidoscopy
    b) colonoscopy
    c) barium enema
    d) CT scan of the abdomen
    e) MRI scan of the abdomen

169. Which of the following drugs is the most appropriate initial therapy for the patient discussed in question 167?
    a) prednisone
    b) sulfasalazine

c) metronidazole
d) 6-mercaptopurine
e) none of the above

ANSWER THE FOLLOWING QUESTION ACCORDING TO THE CODE:

A: 1, 2, and 3 are correct
B: 1 and 3 are correct
C: 2 and 4 are correct
D: Only 4 is correct
E: All of the above are correct

170. Which of the following statements regarding complications of the condition discussed in the patient described in question 167 is(are) true?
1) rectal fissures, rectocutaneous fistulas, or perirectal abscesses are common complications
2) arthritis is sometimes seen as a complication and may even precede the gastrointestinal symptoms
3) erythema nodosum and pyoderma gangrenosum are sometimes seen in patients with this condition
4) patients with this condition are not at increased risk of developing colorectal cancer

ANSWERS

161. C. The most likely diagnosis in this patient is ulcerative colitis.

Ulcerative colitis usually presents with abdominal pain and the passage of bright red blood per rectum. The symptoms in mild disease may be nonspecific.[1] Tenesmus is often present.

Systemic symptoms such as fatigue, weight loss, fever, and chills suggest severe disease.

Sigmoidoscopy usually reveals friability (with easy bleeding) and granularity.

Crohn's disease is usually not associated with rectal bleeding. Crohn's disease will be discussed in a subsequent question.

Bacterial dysentery may produce similar symptoms, but the symptoms do not last for 6 months.

Amebiasis is often indistinguishable from ulcerative colitis,[1] but would not last for 6 months.

Watery diarrhea is often a component of the irritable bowel syndrome. Bloody diarrhea, however, does not occur.

162. D. Barium enema and colonoscopy should be performed in this patient. Sigmoidoscopy should precede both of these procedures.[1]

Barium enema findings include the loss of haustra foreshortening and gross ulcers at the mucosal margin. Although the rectal and the distal colon are the most common sites of involvement, patients with more severe disease may have involvement of the entire colon.[1]

Colonoscopy identifies the extent of disease, and also allows biopsies to be taken.

A GI series and follow-through would not add any useful information to the investigation of a patient strongly suspected of having ulcerative colitis.

163. E. Patients with acute ulcerative colitis are usually treated with either topical corticosteroids (corticosteroid enemas) or systemic corticosteroids if significant systemic symptoms are present.[1,2] Patients with severe disease may also be given ACTH.

If topical corticosteroids are used, an enema containing 100 mg of hydrocortisone is usually given daily for 2 to 3 weeks.

If systemic corticosteroids are used, the usual initial dosage for severe disease is 20–40 mg/day.[2] This dosage can then be gradually tapered.

If corticosteroid therapy does not ameliorate symptoms, a trial of ACTH should be considered.[3]

Patients with severe disease require hospitalization, nasogastric tube insertion, and intravenous fluids and electrolytes. A nasogastric tube should be inserted and fluids and electrolytes given intravenously in order to restore extracellular volume and maintain electrolyte balance.[1] A systemic corticosteroid, such as prednisolone or ACTH should be administered.

164. C. Sulfasalazine is structurally related to both aspirin and the sulfa drugs.

Sulfasalazine is effective in maintaining a remission after an acute episode of ulcerative colitis has been controlled.

Sulfasalazine may increase gastrointestinal distress in patients with acute colitis, and thus, it should not be prescribed.

Sulfasalazine may impair folic acid metabolism, and a folic acid supplement is indicated in patients taking the drug.

165. E. None of the above statements are false. Following an initial attack of ulcerative colitis, 10% of

patients go into remission lasting up to 15 years, 75% of patients have intermittent exacerbations for many years, 10% of patients have continually active disease, and 5% of patients die within 1 year of the initial attack.[3]

Of all patients with ulcerative colitis of any severity, 25% of patients will undergo total proctocolectomy within 5 years of the first attack.[3]

166. E. Colonic complications of ulcerative colitis include toxic megacolon, perforation, colorectal cancer, stricture, and hemorrhage. Extracolonic complications include skin disease (erythema nodosum and pyoderma gangrenosum), aphthous ulcers, iritis, arthritis, and liver disease.[3]

167. B. This patient has Crohn's disease. Pathologically, Crohn's disease involves an inflammation of all layers of the bowel. Associated anorectal complications including fistulas, fissures, and perirectal abscesses may occur.[1] The peak incidence of Crohn's disease is about 30 years of age; most cases occur between the ages of 20 and 40.

Crohn's disease often follows an indolent course; the diagnosis, therefore, is often delayed.

Crohn's disease often presents as mild chronic abdominal pain, mild nonbloody diarrhea, anorexia, weight loss, and fatigue.[1] Pain is often confined to the lower abdomen and is of an aching or cramping quality. This can lead to a misdiagnosis of irritable bowel syndrome.

None of the other choices listed in this question would produce such long-standing symptomatology.

168. C. A barium enema examination is the most important single diagnostic procedure in the confirmation of the diagnosis in a patient with Crohn's disease.[1] Crohn's disease often presents as segmental involvement of two or more colonic areas; between these areas is normal colon, most commonly in the ascending colon. Because of the transmural involvement, certain characteristic radiologic features including a defect protruding into the lumen ("thumbprinting") is often seen.[3]

Sigmoidoscopy will miss Crohn's disease in 30–50% of patients. Colonoscopy is more sensitive than sigmoidoscopy but will again not show the transmural involvement.

CT scan and MRI scanning are not investigations that are commonly employed in the diagnosis of Crohn's disease.

169. A. The drug of choice for the induction of remission in patients with Crohn's disease is prednisone.[2] As in ulcerative colitis, this dosage can often be tapered after a few weeks. Sulfasalazine (4–6 g/day in four divided doses) is effective in producing a remission in 40% of patients.[3] In contrast to ulcerative colitis, sulfasalazine is not effective in maintaining a remission in Crohn's disease.

Metronidazole and 6-mercaptopurine are also sometimes used in some patients with active Crohn's disease, but they are not first-line agents.

170. A. Rectal fissures, rectocutaneous fistulas, or perirectal abscesses occur in up to 50% of patients with Crohn's disease at some time during their illness.

Extracolonic complications of Crohn's disease occur in 10% of patients with the disease. These include arthritis (which in fact may precede the gastrointestinal symptoms), iritis, erythema nodosum, pyoderma gangrenosum, and aphthous ulcers.[3]

The risk of colorectal cancer is much less frequent in patients with Crohn's disease than in patients with ulcerative colitis; however, patients who have had the disease for more than 15 years are at increased risk of malignancy.

SUMMARY OF THE DIAGNOSIS AND TREATMENT OF INFLAMMATORY BOWEL DISEASE

1. **Ulcerative colitis:**
   Symptoms: passage of mucus or blood per stools associated with constipation, tenesmus, weight loss and abdominal pain
   Investigations: sigmoidoscopy, biopsy, barium enema and colonscopy
   Treatment:
   Acute: hydrocortisone enemas, oral prednisone, or ACTH.
   Prophylactic agent for maintenance of remission: sulfasalazine.
   Surgery (hemicolectomy) should be considered for prevention of colorectal cancer in patients with long-standing disease

2. **Crohn's disease:**
   Symptoms: abdominal pain with nonbloody diarrhea, anorexia, weight loss, and fatigue
   Investigations: barium enema is most sensitive investigation

Treatment: prednisone 20–40 mg/day for acute condition

Sulfasalazine is not indicated as long-term prophylaxis for prevention of recurrences.

Results of surgery are generally disappointing.

References

1. Glickman R. Inflammatory bowel disease. In: Braunwald E, Isselbacher K, Petersdorf R, Wilson J, Martin J, Fauci A, eds. Harrison's principles of internal medicine. New York, McGraw-Hill, 1987: 1277–1290.

2. Cort D, Shuman R. Gastroenterologic diseases. In: Dunagan W, Ridner M, eds. Manual of medical therapeutics. 26th Ed. Boston: Little, Brown, 1989: 299–302.

3. Gray G. Inflammatory bowel disease. In: Rubenstein E, Federman D, eds. Scientific American medicine. New York: Scientific American Medicine Incorporated, 1988: 4(IV): 1–16.

PROBLEM 21: A 30-YEAR-OLD FEMALE WITH LOWER ABDOMINAL PAIN

A 30-year-old female presents to the office with a 6-month history of lower abdominal pain associated with bloating, increased flatulence, and alternating diarrhea and constipation. She states that she can sometimes pass up to three loose bowel movements per day, and then will go for two or three days without a bowel movement. Occasionally, there is mucus associated with the bowel movements. The patient has never noticed any blood. The symptoms are at times of stress.

On physical examination, the abdomen is soft. There appears to be very mild generalized tenderness. The patient looks well.

Laboratory investigations reveal a normal CBC, normal urinalysis, and a normal sigmoidoscopy.

SELECT THE ONE BEST ANSWER TO THE FOLLOWING QUESTIONS:

171. The most likely diagnosis for this patient is:
   a) nervous stomach
   b) ulcerative colitis
   c) Crohn's disease
   d) irritable bowel syndrome
   e) none of the above

172. Which of the following statements regarding the condition described above is FALSE?
   a) the typical location is in the lower abdomen
   b) defecation frequently relieves the pain
   c) there is often a feeling of incomplete emptying of the rectum
   d) the abdomen is usually not tender
   e) bowel action is often irregular

173. Which of the following investigations is (are) indicated in the patient described above?
   a) complete blood count and erythrocyte sedimentation rate
   b) sigmoidoscopy
   c) barium enema
   d) a and b
   e) all of the above

174. The condition described above is often associated with:
   a) diverticulosis
   b) chronic appendicitis
   c) chronic cholecystitis
   d) chronic pancreatitis
   e) none of the above

175. Which of the following treatments have been found to be beneficial in the treatment of irritable bowel syndrome?
   a) phenobarbitol
   b) antispasmodics
   c) high fiber diet
   d) antihistamines
   e) none of the above

ANSWERS

171. D. This patient has irritable bowel syndrome (IBS). Irritable bowel syndrome can be defined as a syndrome consisting of: (1) abdominal pain and/or altered bowel habit (diarrhea or constipation) for over 3 months and (2) no evidence of gastrointestinal pathology or other organic disease to explain the symptoms.[1-3] Irritable bowel syndrome may be confused with depression,

anxiety disorder, somatization disorder, or adjustment disorder.[3]

Ulcerative colitis and Crohn's disease are considered in another chapter in this book.

Nervous stomach is not a diagnosis.

172. D. Irritable bowel syndrome usually presents with abdominal pain, which may be alleviated by a bowel movement or by the passing of gas. Bowel movements are often irregular, and there is often a feeling of incomplete emptying following a bowel movement. Pain is more common in the lower abdomen than the upper abdomen. Tenderness, especially in the area of the sigmoid colon, is common.[3]

173. D. In a patient with typical irritable bowel symptoms, lack of physical findings, a normal hemoglobin, and a normal ESR, the sensitivity and specificity for the diagnosis may be as high as 83% and 97% respectively.[3] A sigmoidoscopy is also recommended in all patients.[3] Patients over the age of 50 should probably have a barium enema examination as well.[3] In a patient with diarrhea, stools for culture and sensitivity, and ova and parasites are also recommended.[3]

174. A. Diverticulosis is often associated with IBS. This may be due to muscle hypertrophy on the left side of the colon. It is often difficult to distinguish diverticular disease from irritable bowel syndrome.[3]

Appendicitis, cholecystitis, pancreatitis, and other abdominal conditions have no known association with IBS.

175. C. Explanation of the origin and benign nature of the symptoms is the most important aspect of treatment.[4] A good doctor-patient relationship is essential to successful treatment.[4]

High fiber diet has been shown, in many studies, to be of benefit to patients with IBS.[4] This is, however, still controversial.

Medications including phenobarbitol, antispasmodics, antihistamines, and others have not been demonstrated to be effective in the treatment of this syndrome.[4]

SUMMARY OF THE DIAGNOSIS AND MANAGEMENT OF IRRITABLE BOWEL SYNDROME

1. **Definition:** A syndrome consisting of abdominal pain and/or altered bowel habits (diarrhea or constipation) persisting for over 3 months and not associated with any evidence of gastrointestinal pathology or other organic disease to explain the symptoms.

2. **Etiology:** Unknown. Probably has both behavioral or psychologic components, as well as gastrointestinal motility component.[3]

Irritable bowel syndrome is a common diagnosis. It may be responsible for 10% of visits to family physicians, 50% of visits to gastroenterologists,[5] and many unnecessary operations. It is easily confused with depression, anxiety, somatization disorder, and adjustment disorder.

3. **Diagnostic workup:** history, physical examination, CBC, ESR, and sigmoidoscopy on all patients. Barium enema in those patients over 50; and stool for culture, ova, and parasites in those patients with diarrhea.

4. **Treatment:** Explanation about the benign nature of the condition, with a good doctor-patient relationship is the most important aspect of treatment. High fiber diet may be beneficial. Other drugs have not been shown to be helpful.

References

1. Alpers DH. Irritable bowel; still more questions than answers. Gastroenterology 1981; 80: 1068–1069.

2. Ford MJ. Invited review. The irritable bowel syndrome. J Psychosom Res 1986; 30: 399–410.

3. Crouch M. Irritable bowel syndrome. Prim Care 1988; 15(1): 99–110.

4. Collins S. The irritable bowel syndrome. Can Med Assoc J 1988;138(15): 309–315.

5. Switz DM. What the gastroenterologist does all day. Gastroenterology 1976; 70: 1048–1050.

PROBLEM 22: A 40-YEAR-OLD EXECUTIVE WHO SMOKES 3 PACKS OF CIGARETTES A DAY

A 40-year-old executive who smokes three packs of cigarettes per day presents for his routine health assessment. He states that he would like to quit smoking, but is having some difficulty. He has tried three times previously. He has a family history of premature cardiovascular disease.

SELECT THE ONE BEST ANSWER TO THE FOLLOWING QUESTIONS:

176. Current evidence suggests that coronary artery disease is strongly related to cigarette smoking. What percentage of deaths from coronary artery disease is thought to be due directly to cigarette smoking?
    a) less than 5%
    b) 10%
    c) 20%
    d) 25%
    e) 30–40%

177. Which of the following malignancies IS NOT associated with cigarette smoking?
    a) carcinoma of larynx
    b) carcinoma of esophagus
    c) carcinoma of bladder
    d) carcinoma of the colon
    e) carcinoma of the pancreas

178. With regard to "passive smoking," which of the following statements is FALSE?
    a) spouses of patients who smoke are not at an increased risk of carcinoma of the lung
    b) "sidestream smoke" contains more carbon monoxide than "mainstream smoke"
    c) infants of mothers who smoke absorb measurable amounts of their mothers' cigarette smoke
    d) children of parents who smoke have an increased prevalence of bronchitis and pneumonia
    e) the most common symptom arising from exposure to passive smoking is eye irritation

179. Which of the following factors is the MOST IMPORTANT factor in determining the success of a quit-smoking program?
    a) the wish of the patient to quit smoking
    b) nicotine containing chewing gum
    c) the inclusion of a behavior modification program in the program
    d) physician advice to quit smoking
    e) repeated office visits

ANSWER THE FOLLOWING QUESTIONS ACCORDING TO THE CODE:

A: 1, 2, and 3 are correct
B: 1 and 3 are correct
C: 2 and 4 are correct
D: Only 4 is correct
E: All of the above are correct

180. Which of the following diseases is(are) directly associated with cigarette smoking?
    1) peripheral arterial occlusive disease
    2) peptic ulcer
    3) oral cancer
    4) periodontal disease

181. You attempt to educate the patient described in this problem about the immediate consequences of smoking cessation. Which of the following are immediate consequences of smoking cessation?
    1) improved ability to breathe
    2) increased sense of smell
    3) increased sense of taste
    4) decreased heart rate

182. Which of the following interventions have been shown to be successful in helping patients quit smoking?
    1) physician advice
    2) behavior modification aids
    3) nicotine containing chewing gum
    4) a switch to very low nicotine cigarettes

183. Which of the following statements regarding nicotine containing chewing gum is(are) CORRECT?
    1) smokers should stop smoking completely before they start using the gum
    2) nicotine containing chewing gum should not be used for longer than 2 months
    3) nicotine containing chewing gum should be chewed slowly and intermittently
    4) nicotine containing chewing gum is contraindicated in patients with peptic ulcer disease

ANSWERS

176. D. Twenty-five percent of deaths from coronary artery disease are directly attributable to smoking.[1] The incidence of myocardial infarction and death from coronary heart disease is 70% higher in cigarette smokers than in nonsmokers. In the United States, 18% of all deaths are due to cigarette smoking.[2]

177. D. The only cancer listed which is not associated with cigarette smoking is cancer of the colon.

In addition to cancer of the lung (25% of all cancer deaths), smoking is associated with cancer of the larnyx, cancer of the esophagus, cancer of the bladder, cancer of the kidney, cancer of the pancreas, and oral cancer.[1]

Other diseases and conditions associated with smoking include the atherosclerotic diseases (angina, myocardial infarction, abdominal aneurysm, peripheral vascular disease); chronic obstructive pulmonary disease; peptic ulcer disease; periodontal disease; and perinatal conditions (increased perinatal mortality, reduced birth weight, and SIDS).[1]

178. A. Tobacco smoke in the environment is derived from either mainstream smoke (exhaled smoke), or sidestream smoke (smoke arising from the burning end of a cigarette). Sidestream smoke contains a higher concentration of potentially dangerous gas-phase constituents including carbon monoxide.[1]

Infants of mothers who smoke absorb measurable amounts of cigarette smoke. As well, there is an increased prevalence of bronchitis and pneumonia in infants and children whose parents smoke.[2]

The most common symptom arising from exposure to passive smoking is eye irritation. Other significant symptoms are headaches, nasal symptoms, and cough. Exposure to tobacco smoke also precipitates or aggravates allergic attacks in persons with respiratory allergies.

Spouses of patients who smoke are at increased risk of developing lung cancer and coronary artery disease.[2]

179. A. The most important factor in determining the success of a quit-smoking program is the desire of the patient to quit.[2] If the patient is not interested in quitting, the probability of success is very low. Physician advice to quit, behavior modification aids, nicotine containing chewing gum, and repeated office visits are all important. They are, however, unlikely to have any impact unless the patient wants to quit.

180. E. See critique of question 177.

181. E. There are many immediate consequences of smoking cessation. These include an improved ability to breathe, an improved sense of smell, an improved sense of taste, a considerable saving of money, increased energy, fresh breath, an odor-free environment, decreased risk of passive smoking on family and co-workers, better insurance rates, improved lung cleansing through ability to cough and improved ciliary activity, improved coronary and peripheral circulation, decreased heart rate, reduced blood carbon monoxide levels, reduced perspiration, improved exercise tolerance, improved ability to perform physical work, and lower grocery bills.[2]

182. A. A smoking cessation program has the greatest chance of success when it contains multiple components. Physician advice, behavior modification aids[2,3] nicotine chewing gum, setting a quit date, and frequent follow-up visits are all important components of the program.[2] A switch to low nicotine cigarettes, however, has not been shown to be effective.[2] Smokers will simply inhale more of the cigarette to try and achieve the same effect.

183. B. Guidelines for the use of nicotine containing chewing include: (1) smokers should stop smoking completely before they start using the gum; (2) nicotine gum is more effective if combined with a behavior modification program; (3) the gum should be chewed slowly and intermittently to allow the nicotine to be absorbed; and (4) the gum should be used for at least 3 months (to decrease the probability of relapse).[2]

Contraindications to nicotine containing chewing gum include pregnancy, nursing, and recent myocardial infarction.[2] Peptic ulcer disease is not a recognized contraindication to nicotine gum.

SUMMARY OF PHYSICIAN INTERVENTION IN SMOKING CESSATION

1. Identify all patients who smoke in your practice
2. Present the health consequences of smoking
3. Present the health benefits of cessation
4. Assess and develop the desire to modify smoking behavior
5. Develop and formalize a patient-centered plan for change
6. Establish a quit date and have the patient sign a contract
7. Utilize nicotine containing chewing gum as an adjunct
8. Utilize behavior-modification techniques as outlined by the American Lung Association
9. Implement maintenance strategies as outlined by the American Lung Association
10. Continue surveillance for relapse prevention and plan modifications as needed

From Green H. et al: Cigarette smoking: the physician's role in cessation and maintenance. J Gen Intern Med 1988; 3:75-

References

1. Holbrook J. Tobacco. In: Braunwald E, Isselbacher K, Petersdorf R, Wilson J, Martin J, Fauci A, eds. Harrison's principles of internal medicine. 11th Ed. New York: McGraw-Hill, 1987: 855–859.

2. Greene H, Goldberg R, Ockene J. Cigarette smoking: the physician's role in cessation and maintenance. J Gen Intern Med 1988;3:75–87.

3. Bass F. Helping patients to quit smoking. Can Fam Physician 1989; 35: 1497–1502.

PROBLEM 23: A 24-YEAR-OLD MALE WITH A "SKIN RASH" AFTER EXPOSURE TO COLD

A 24-year-old male presents to your office with a 3-month history of a "skin rash" after exposure to cold water or cold air. The patient describes the onset of a pruritic, raised skin rash after walking 2 or 3 blocks in cold weather, or after exposure to cold water. The rash begins 10 minutes after exposure to cold, and persists for 2 or 3 hours.

SELECT THE ONE BEST ANSWER TO THE FOLLOWING QUESTIONS:

184. The most likely diagnosis in this patient is:
    a) cholinergic urticaria
    b) cold-induced urticaria
    c) chronic urticaria NYD
    d) cold-induced eczematoid dermatitis
    e) cold-induced cryoglobulinemia

185. To confirm the diagnosis in the patient described in question 184 you should:
    a) order a complete immunologic work-up
    b) give the patient a trial of an antihistamine
    c) ask the patient to come into the office immediately after the next attack occurs
    d) apply an ice cube to the skin for 3 to 5 minutes
    e) perform a skin biopsy

186. Which of the following medications is most commonly associated with a skin reaction similar to the reaction experienced by the patient in question 184?
    a) penicillin
    b) codeine
    c) tetracycline
    d) erythromycin
    e) aspirin

187. A patient is being desensitized for house dust, house dust mite, cat fur, and dog dander. He has been receiving allergy shots for the past 6 months. After being given his last allergy shot he collapses while leaving the office. You notice a large wheal at the site of injection, numerous smaller wheals forming all over his body, and swelling of his lips. At this time, you should:
    a) call for the paramedics
    b) administer epinephrine
    c) administer dopamine
    d) administer diphenylhydramine
    e) b and d

188. A 6-year-old boy presents to your office with his mother. He has just developed multiple wheals and lip swelling. With appropriate treatment, the reaction begins to subside. On questioning the mother you discover that the child has just eaten a peanut-containing chocolate bar. The mother states that the child has had previous reactions to peanuts, but they have been milder (a few hives at the most). At this time you would advise the mother to:
    a) relax, a reaction of this severity is unlikely to happen again
    b) limit the intake of peanuts to one or two at a time
    c) avoid any further eating of peanuts or contact with peanuts
    d) avoid any further eating of peanuts or contact with peanuts; obtain a preloaded syringe containing adrenaline to carry with the child at all times
    e) relax, the relationship with the peanuts is purely coincidental

189. A 28-year-old nurse presents to your office with a swollen left eyelid. She has been working on the chemotherapy service and recalls rubbing her eye after administering a chemotherapeutic agent to a patient. She states that she washed her hands well before rubbing her eye. Which of the following statements about this patient is true?
    a) it is unlikely that there is a relationship between the chemotherapeutic agent and her swollen left eyelid
    b) the chemotherapeutic agent is probably a contact allergen in this nurse
    c) drugs are uncommon causes of contact sensitivity
    d) this is probably an idiosyncractic reaction
    e) an immediate job transfer to another service not using chemotherapy is indicated

ANSWER THE FOLLOWING QUESTION ACCORDING TO THE CODE:

A: 1, 2, and 3 are correct
B: 1 and 3 are correct
C: 2 and 4 are correct
D: Only 4 is correct
E: All of the above are correct

190. Which of the following may be indicated in a patient with chronic urticaria?
    1) hydroxyzine
    2) cyproheptadine
    3) cimetidine
    4) doxepin

ANSWERS

184. B. This patient has cold-induced urticaria.

Cold, heat (sunlight), and pressure are the main physical factors that can trigger urticaria.[1]

The etiology of cold urticaria is unknown. The lesions, which must often appear after the rewarming phase of cold exposure, usually remain for 1–2 hours.[1] Anaphylactic shock may occur.

Secondary cold urticaria, which is associated with circulating cryoglobulins, is rare compared to the idiopathic form.

Cholinergic urticaria is another common type of physical urticaria. The lesions of cholinergic urticaria, which are induced by sweating (heat, exercise, and anxiety), are small (2 to 3 mm). Cooling the skin helps diminish the reaction.[1]

Solar urticaria occurs after exposure to ultraviolet light of specific wavelengths.

Although cold, dry weather can produce an eczematoid dermatitis, the acute history is not compatible with this diagnosis.

185. D. The diagnosis can be confirmed by applying an ice cube to the skin for 3 to 5 minutes. This should produce a wheal and flare response in a patient with cold urticaria.[1] If the "ice cube" test is positive, further diagnostic tests are unnecessary.

Although an antihistamine will treat the reaction, it will not establish a diagnosis.

A skin biopsy is not indicated in this type of skin lesion.

186. A. Penicillin is the most common drug causing allergic (urticarial) drug reactions. Urticarial reactions to drugs are often cross-reactive; this property depends on the molecular structure of the drug. Because the beta-lactam ring is shared by ampicillin, cloxacillin, and the cephalosporins, the potential for an allergic reaction following exposure to any antibiotic with a beta-lactam ring is present.[1,2]

Because it may take several weeks for antibodies to form, an allergic reaction may not occur for several weeks following initiation of therapy.

Sulfonamides and aspirin are also common causes of urticarial reactions.[2]

Codeine and other narcotic drugs may cause urticaria by nonimmunologically stimulating the release of histamine.

Although tetracycline and erythromycin may trigger urticarial reactions, allergic reactions are less frequent with these drugs than with penicillin.

Often, many drugs are taken concurrently. This makes the identification of the offending drug difficult. As well, especially in children, the infection itself may precipitate an urticarial response, further complicating the diagnosis.

187. E. Allergy shots may cause anaphylaxis.[3] When a patient is receiving immunotherapy, he is already hypersensitive to the injected allergen. Allergic reactions following allergy shots include urticaria, asthma, rhinitis, and anaphylaxis.[1] The initial manifestation is usually a large wheal at the injection site itself.

Immediate treatment with subcutaneous epinephrine and intramusclar diphenylhydramine is indicated. In this case, an intravenous tube should also be established. Angioedema (as manifested by lip swelling) involves edema of the deeper dermis and subcutaneous tissues.

A mistake in the dosage of desensitizing allergen is often the cause of the allergic reaction. In this patient, a tourniquet should be temporarily applied about the site of injection to limit absorption of the allergen.

Physicians who administer allergy shots must be prepared and have the necessary equipment to treat anaphylactic reactions.[3]

Family physicians should not consider desensitizing a patient for allergies until all other measures have failed. Getting rid of the cat or dog, or installing an electronic air filter should certainly be considered first. Also, patients should wait at least 20 minutes after an allegy shot and have the area of injection inspected by the physician before they leave the office.

188. D. Foods can cause severe, and even fatal, allergic reactions. The most common food allergens are peanuts, true nuts, fish, shellfish, milk, and eggs.[1] Because of multiple ingredients, it is often difficult to determine the exact food triggering the reaction.

Once the association is made, all contact with the food (not just eating) must be avoided. Even a food odor can trigger a severe allergic reaction.

In this case, the mother should be advised to obtain a preloaded syringe containing adrenalin. This should be carried with the child at all times. In cases of severe food allergy, this can be life-saving.

189. B. This is an example of contact sensitivity. Contact sensitivity to medications, chemicals, and foods is common.[1] Physicians, nurses, and pharmacists are at risk for contact sensitivity to medications. As well, latex rubber is a known cause of urticaria; this can be a problem for either the patient or the surgeon.

In this patient, after appropriate treatment, special care should be taken when handling chemotherapeutic agents. If a further reaction occurs, it would then be appropriate to consider transfer to another service.

190. E. Urticaria can be classified as either acute or chronic. The treatment of acute urticaria has already been discussed.

Chronic urticaria, by definition, is urticaria occurring at least once per week for at least six weeks. The cause of chronic urticaria can frequently not be found.[1]

Chronic urticaria may best be controlled by taking an antihistamine daily. Hydroxyzine, cyproheptadine, diphenylhydramine, or chlorotripolon are commonly used. Doxepine is effective in cold urticaria induced by ice-water challenge and in chronic idiopathic urticaria.[1]

The combination of a histamine$_1$ receptor antagonist, hydroxyzine, and a histamine$_2$ receptor antagonist, cimetidine has been found to be more effective than the H_1 antagonist alone in chronic idiopathic urticaria.[1] Sedation is often a limiting side effect with most of the currently available H_1 antihistamines. Terfenadine and astemizole which are nonsedating, have demonstrated efficacy in chronic urticaria.[1]

Severe cases of chronic idiopathic urticaria may require prednisone for control of symptoms.[1]

SUMMARY OF DIAGNOSIS AND TREATMENT OF URTICARIA

1. **Acute:** less than 6 weeks
   Chronic: greater than 6 weeks

2. **Main categories of urticaria:**
   a) drug allergy
   b) contact sensitivity
   c) food allergy
   d) external physical factors
      i) cold-induced urticaria
      ii) cholinergic urticaria
      iii) solar urticaria

3. **Treatment:**
    a) elicit cause if possible
    b) acute treatment: epinephrine subcutaneous, diphenylhydramine intramuscular
    c) Chronic urticaria: combination of H_1 and H_2 receptor blockers, doxepin, corticosteroids in severe cases
    d) prevention of life-threatening reaction: carry injectable epinephrine if significant food allergy

References

1. Wagner W. Urticaria—a challenge in diagnosis and treatment. Postgrad Med 1988; 83(5): 321–329.

2. Wood A, Oates J. Adverse reactions to drugs. In: Braunwald E, Isselbacher K, Petersdorf R, Wilson J, Martin J, Fauci A, eds. Harrison's principles of internal medicine. 11th Ed. New York: McGraw-Hill, 1987: 352–358.

3. Gillette R, Lustig J. The immunologic system. In: Taylor R, ed. Family medicine: principles and practice. 3rd Ed. New York: Springer-Verlag, 1988: 397–398.

PROBLEM 24: A 45-YEAR-OLD MALE WITH A HEADACHE

A 45-year-old male presents with a 4-week history of recurrent headaches that wake him up in the middle of the night. The headaches have been occurring every night, and lasting approximately 1 hour. The headaches are described as a deep burning sensation centered behind the left orbit. It is excruciating and is associated with lacrimation, facial flushing, nasal discharge, and conjunctivitis.

On examination, his blood pressure is 120/70 mm Hg. His pulse is 96 and regular. There is a left ptosis and left pupillary constriction.

SELECT THE ONE BEST ANSWER TO THE FOLLOWING QUESTIONS:

191. The most likely cause of this patient's headache is:
    a) subarachnoid hemorrhage
    b) tension-migraine syndrome
    c) atypical migraine
    d) cluster headache
    e) left-sided cerebrovascular accident

192. Which of the following statements regarding the headache of the patient described in question 191 is FALSE?
    a) oxygen may be useful in the treatment of the acute attack
    b) ergotamine may be used as a prophylactic drug in the condition described above
    c) methylsergide may be used as a prophylactic drug in the condition described above
    d) lithium carbonate may be used as a prophylactic drug in the condition described above
    e) none of the above statements are false

193. A 32-year-old female presents with a 2-year history of recurrent headaches. These headaches occur once a week and often last 8–12 hours. The headaches are almost always confined to the left side of the head and are associated with malaise, nausea and vomiting, and photophobia. She has

been using acetaminophen without significant relief.

On examination, her blood pressure is 100/70 mm Hg. Her neurological examination is within normal limits. The optic fundi are normal.

The most likely diagnosis in this patient is:
a) classic migraine
b) common migraine
c) tension headache
d) cluster headache
e) nervous headache

194. With respect to migraine headache, which of the following statements is INCORRECT?
    a) during a migraine attack extracranial vasodilation is followed by intracranial vasoconstriction
    b) the neurologic symptoms preceding the headache are caused by intracranial arterial constriction and cerebral ischemia
    c) alteration of arterial tone is associated with liberation of vasoactive substances including catecholamines, histamines, serotonin, kinins, neuropeptides, and prostaglandins
    d) the pounding headache is presumed to be related to neurogenic vasodilatation and a sterile inflammatory response generated by the interaction of these substances with blood vessels and nerves

195. The treatment of choice for acute migraine headache is:
   a) meperidine
   b) acetylsalicylic acid
   c) an ergot alkaloid
   d) haloperidol
   e) morphine sulfate

ANSWER THE FOLLOWING QUESTION
ACCORDING TO THE CODE:

A: 1, 2, and 3 are correct
B: 1 and 3 are correct
C: 2 and 4 are correct
D: Only 4 is correct
E: All of the above are correct

196. Which of the following medications is(are) useful
for the prophylaxis of migraine headache?
   1) amitriptyline
   2) cyproheptadine
   3) propranolol
   4) nifedipine

SELECT THE ONE BEST ANSWER TO THE
FOLLOWING QUESTION:

197. A 35-year-old male presents with a 6-month history of recurrent headaches. These headaches
occur almost daily, and usually begin in the late
afternoon. The headaches are described by the
patient as "a vice around my head."

   The headaches are not associated with nausea,
vomiting, or malaise. The patient does, however,
describe some "dizziness" and "light-headedness"
with these headaches.

   On examination, the patient's blood pressure is
100/70 mm Hg. His optic fundi are normal. There
are no neurological abnormalities.

   The most likely diagnosis in this patient is:
   a) classic migraine
   b) common migraine
   c) tension headache
   d) cluster headache
   e) nervous headache

ANSWER THE FOLLOWING QUESTIONS
ACCORDING TO THE CODE:

A: 1, 2, and 3 are correct
B: 1 and 3 are correct
C: 2 and 4 are correct

D: Only 4 is correct
E: All of the above are correct

198. The treatment(s) of choice for the patient described
in question 197 is(are):
   1) a prostaglandin synthetase inhibitor
   2) relaxation techniques
   3) a tricyclic antidepressant
   4) an aspirin-codeine combination

199. A 75-year-old female presents to your office with
a severe left-sided temporal headache. She
describes a tender area in the left temple. She also
describes pain in the jaw while chewing. This
headache has been present for the past 3 days.

   On physical examination, her blood pressure is
170/100 mm Hg. Her neurologic examination is
normal. There is moderate tenderness in the area
of the left temple.

   Which of the following statements regarding
this patient is(are) true?
   1) this probably represents a late-onset migraine
   2) simple analgesics should be prescribed before
      embarking on any extensive investigation
   3) this headache is unlikely to be associated with
      significant complications
   4) an erythrocyte sedimentation rate should be
      ordered immediately

200. Which of the following statements regarding the
investigation of headaches is(are) true?
   1) patients with a chronic classic or common
      migraine rarely require more than a careful
      history and physical examination
   2) patients with chronic tension headache rarely
      require more than a careful history and physi-
      cal examination
   3) the EEG is almost never useful in the diagnosis
      of headache
   4) radioisotope brain scanning is no longer indi-
      cated in investigation of a patient with head-
      ache

ANSWERS

191. D. This patient has a cluster headache. Cluster
headaches often awaken a patient from sleep and
may recur at the same time each day or night for
weeks at a time.

   Cluster headache, which usually occurs in
males, is described as a deep, burning, or stabbing
pain. It is often excruciating; the patient may even
be suicidal. The associated symptoms of cluster

headaches, usually ipsilateral to the pain include lacrimation, facial flushing, and nasal discharge. The eye is often red; conjunctival vessels are dilated, and ptosis and pupillary constriction often occur.

Cluster headache is thought to be a migraine variant. Oxygen therapy may be beneficial in an acute attack. Cluster headache may be prevented by ergotamine, methysergide, prednisone, or lithium.

The other common causes of headache will be discussed in subsequent questions.

192. E. See critique of question 191.

193. B. This patient has a common migraine headache. Migraine headaches are unilateral, throbbing, recurrent headaches that are often associated with nausea and/or vomiting, and photophobia.

Migraine headaches tend to be familial and are more common in women. Migraine headaches may be precipitated by stress, excessive sleeping, menstruation, pregnancy, oral contraceptives, certain medications (especially vasodilators), and certain foods (especially red wine, chocolate, nuts, and aged cheese).[1,2]

Classic migraine is a migraine headache that is preceded by definite symptoms of neurologic dysfunction. These neurologic symptoms include visual scotomata, unilateral paresthesias, aphasia, hemiparesis, and hemisensory deficits.

Tension headache will be discussed in a subsequent question.

Nervous headache is not a diagnosis.

194. A. During a migraine attack, intracranial vasoconstriction is followed by extracranial vasodilation. The neurologic symptoms preceding the painful phase are caused by intracranial arterial constriction and cerebral ischemia, and pain is related to dilatation of the extracranial and some intracranial arteries. Alteration of arteriolar tone is associated with liberation of vasoactive substances including catecholamines, histamines, serotonin, kinins, neuropeptides, and prostaglandins. The pounding headache is presumed to be related to neurogenic vasodilatation and a sterile inflammatory response generated by the interaction of these substances with blood vessels and nerves.[1]

195. C. The treatment of choice in acute migraine headache is an ergot alkaloid (ergotamine). Ergotamine can be given orally (1 mg to be repeated up to 4 mg), sublingually (2 mg to be repeated up to 6 mg), by oral inhalation, parenterally, or by rectal suppository. Ergotamine abolishes the headache by causing extracranial vasoconstriction. Nausea, vomiting, and epigastric discomfort are signs of toxicity.[1,3]

The combination of ergotamine with an antiemetic such as metoclopramide will often increase the efficacy of the treatment of the acute attack.

196. E. The drugs useful in the prophylactic treatment of migraine headaches include: (1) propranolol or other beta blockers, (2) amitriptyline or other tricyclic antidepressant, (3) cyproheptadine, (4) a calcium-channel blocker such as nifedipine or verapamil, (5) an ergot preparation with or without belladona, and (6) methysergide.[1,3]

197. C. This patient has a "tension" or muscle contraction headache. Tension headaches are often described as a steady, aching, "vice-like" sensation that encircles the entire head. Tension headaches are often accompanied by tight and tender muscles at the site of maximal pain, often in the posterior cervical, frontal, or temporal muscles. Tension headaches are recurrent and often brought on by stress.[1,2]

In many patients, it is difficult to distinguish a tension headache from a common migraine headache. Patients often present with headaches that have features of both tension and migraine headaches.

The pathogenesis of tension headache is unclear. It may be related to the release of vasoactive substances that also occur in migraine headaches. This may explain why it is often difficult to separate the two syndromes.[1]

198. A. Causal factors for tension headache must be identified first. Incorrect posture, significant stress, or other factors must be corrected.

Relaxation techniques, tricyclic antidepressants, and nonsteroidal anti-inflammatory drugs are all useful treatments. Narcotic analgesics should be avoided. Therefore, the prescription of an aspirin-codeine combination or any other more potent narcotic analgesic is inappropriate.[1]

199. D. This patient has temporal arteritis (giant cell arteritis) until proven otherwise. When an elderly patient presents with a new-onset headache, temporal arteritis must be excluded. This patient presents with a unilateral headache with a tender

temporal area. This probably represents the inflamed temporal artery.

The most significant complication is sudden unilateral blindness due to occlusion of the terminal branches of the ophthalmic artery. This is a completely preventable complication.[4]

Temporal arteritis is often associated with polymyalgia rheumatica. Hypothyroidism may also be associated with temporal arteritis.[5]

The erythrocyte sedimentation rate is a highly sensitive test in a patient you suspect of having temporal arteritis. The ESR is usually elevated above 50 mm/hr, and may exceed 100 mm/hr.

The treatment of choice for a patient with temporal arteritis is high-dose prednisone. When cranial arteritis is diagnosed or even suspected, treatment should be started immediately with at least 50 mg of prednisone. If the diagnosis is confirmed, treatment should be continued for at least 4 weeks before gradual reduction is instituted. If ocular complications have occurred, treatment should continue for 1–2 years.[4]

200. E. As headache is such a common disorder, and the excessive application of expensive and highly technical laboratory procedures to the diagnosis and management of benign headache is not only expensive, but also epidemiologically unsound, the following principles should apply to the investigation of headache.[1]

1. Patients with migraine headache or tension headache rarely require more than a careful history and physical examination.

2. Headaches of recent origin or progression deserve investigation. This is especially true of headaches that have a consistently focal distribution, headaches that follow trauma, or headaches that begin after the age of 30 years. CT or MRI scanning is recommended.

3. The electroencephalogram (EEG) is almost never helpful in the diagnosis of headache.

4. Skull x-rays are useful only when abnormalities involving the base of the brain are suspected, or immediately following head trauma.

5. Diagnostic lumbar puncture should be performed in any patient with a headache that is (a) accompanied by fever or (b) is explosive or the most severe headache ever suffered. Lumbar puncture should, if possible, be deferred until after CT scanning in other forms of acute headache, especially if the patient has a stiff neck.

6. CT scanning and MRI scanning are the diagnostic modalities of choice in the evaluation of acute headache in which serious pathology is suspected.

SUMMARY OF THE DIAGNOSIS AND TREATMENT OF HEADACHE

1. **Symptomatology:**
Common migraine: recurrent headaches, usually unilateral, pulsating in character, associated with nausea, vomiting, and photophobia.

Classic migraine: neurologic symptoms precede or accompany the migraine headache

Cluster headache: Short-lived attacks of severe, acute, and intense unilateral head pain; often associated with rhinorrhea, lacrimation, ptosis, and Horner's syndrome

Tension headache: recurrent headache, due to muscle contraction that is often described as a "vice around my head."

Tension-migraine syndrome: a headache that has characteristics of both tension headache and migraine headache.

2. **Investigations:** Usually a good history and physical examination will suffice. More extensive testing is not epidemiologically sound in most cases.

3. **Treatment:**
Migraine headache: ergot preparation is treatment of choice. Prophylactic agents include amitriptyline (or other tricyclic antidepressant), propranolol (or other beta blocker), cyproheptadine, low-dose ergot, methysergide, and calcium-channel blockers.

Cluster headache: Oxygen therapy may be used for the acute attack. Prophylactic medications during the cluster period include ergotamine, methylsergide, prednisone, and lithium.

Tension headache: relaxation techniques, nonsteroidal anti-inflammatory agents, tricyclic antidepressants

References

1. Posner J. Headache and other head pain. In: Wyngaarden J, Smith L, eds. Cecil textbook of medicine. Philadelphia: WB Saunders, 1988: 2128–2136.

2. Ferrante J, Middleton D. Headache. In: Taylor R, ed. Family medicine: principles and practice. 3rd Ed. New York: Springer-Verlag, 1988: 108–110.

3. Applegate C, Fox P. Neurologic emergencies in internal medicine. In: Dunagan W, Ridner M, eds. Manual of medical therapeutics. 26th Ed. Boston: Little, Brown, 1989: 476–478.

4. Fauci A. The vasculitis syndromes. In: Braunwald E, Issel-bacher K, Petersdorf R, Wilson J, Martin J, Fauci A, eds.

Harrison's principles of internal medicine. 11th Ed. New York: McGraw-Hill, 1987: 1443.

5. Wiseman P, Stewart K, Rai G. Hypothyroidism in poly-myalgia rheumatica and giant cell arteritis. Br Med J 1989; 298: 647–648.

PROBLEM 25: A 50-YEAR-OLD MALE WITH ASCITES

A 50-year-old male is brought into your office by his wife. His wife states that for the past several months he has experienced extreme weakness and fatigue. In addition, he has lost 35 pounds during the last 4 months. During the last few weeks the patient has eaten hardly anything. When you question the patient he states that his wife is "overreacting."

On physical examination, the patient has a significantly enlarged abdominal girth. There is a level of shifting dullness present. The patient's liver edge is felt 6 cm below the right costal margin. It has a nodular edge. In addition, spider nevi are present on the upper part of the body. There is palmar erythema noted, and a flapping tremor is elicited.

SELECT THE ONE BEST ANSWER TO THE FOLLOWING QUESTIONS:

201. Which of the following statements regarding this patient's condition is false?
    a) the most likely diagnosis is cirrhosis of the liver
    b) this condition is probably associated with alcohol abuse
    c) jaundice is an uncommon sign in the disorder described above
    d) approximately 33% of patients with a history of alcohol abuse will go on to develop alcoholic hepatitis
    e) approximately 50% of patients with this condition (in an advanced stage) will die within 2 years

202. A 25-year-old male with a history of heavy alcohol intake presents to your office for a periodic health assessment. He states that "his appetite has been off," and he has had generalized abdominal pain for the last 3 weeks.

    On examination, there is no clinical jaundice. There is tenderness present in the right upper quadrant of the abdomen. The liver edge is palpable 5 cm below the right costal margin. You suspect alcoholic hepatitis.

    Which of the following statements about alcoholic hepatitis is FALSE?
    a) Laënnec's cirrhosis develops in approximately 10% of patients with alcoholic hepatitis
    b) serum bilirubin may often be 10–20 times the normal level

    c) serum ALT is almost always lower than serum AST
    d) hepatomegaly is seen in 80–90% of patients with alcoholic hepatitis
    e) a mortality rate of 10–15% is seen in acute alcoholic hepatitis

203. The most common cause of cirrhosis is:
    a) hepatitis A
    b) hepatitis B
    c) non-A, non-B hepatitis
    d) alcoholic hepatitis
    e) cytomegalovirus

204. The ascites that accompanies cirrhosis should be treated by:
    a) sodium restriction
    b) water restriction
    c) spironolactone
    d) a and c
    e) a, b, and c

205. A 25-year-old school teacher presents with nausea, vomiting, anorexia, aversion to her usual two pack a day smoking habit, and right upper quadrant pain. She has been sick for the past 3 days. Two of the students in her class have come down with similar symptoms. She has had no exposure to blood products and has no other significant risk factors for sexually transmitted disease.

    On examination her sclera are icteric and her liver edge is tender. She looks acutely ill.

    The most likely diagnosis in this patient is:
    a) hepatitis A
    b) hepatitis B

c) non-A, non-B hepatitis
d) atypical infectious mononucleosis
e) none of the above

206. Which of the following tests is the most sensitive in confirming the diagnosis suspected in question 205?
    a) anti-HAV-IgG
    b) anti-HAV-IgM
    c) hepatitis A core antigen
    d) anti- HB core antigen
    e) anti- non-A, non-B hepatitis antigen

207. An infant is born to a mother who is HBsAg (hepatitis B surface antigen) positive. Which of the following statements regarding this infant is true?
    a) no prophylaxis against hepatitis B needs to be undertaken in this infant
    b) this infant should have one dose of hepatitis B immunoglobulin administered
    c) this infant should have one dose of hepatitis B vaccine administered
    d) this infant should have one dose of hepatitis B immunoglobulin and a complete 3-dose immunization of hepatitis B vaccine administered

ANSWER THE FOLLOWING QUESTIONS ACCORDING TO THE CODE:

A: 1, 2, and 3 are correct
B: 1 and 3 are correct
C: 2 and 4 are correct
D: Only 4 is correct
D: All of the above are correct

208. Initial screening for hepatitis B should include which of the following antigen/antibody tests?
    1) anti-HBs
    2) anti-HBc
    3) HBeAg
    4) HBsAg

209. Which of the following laboratory tests is (are) usually abnormal in a patient with acute viral hepatitis?
    1) serum AST
    2) serum bilirubin
    3) serum ALT
    4) serum alkaline phosphatase

210. Clinical manifestations of cirrhosis include:
    1) fatigue
    2) jaundice
    3) splenomegaly
    4) hypoalbuminemia

211. Indications for the use of hepatitis B vaccine include:
    1) health care personnel
    2) hemodialysis patients
    3) patients requiring frequent blood transfusions
    4) male homosexuals

212. Which of the following types of viral hepatitis is(are) associated with the development of chronic active hepatitis?
    1) hepatitis B
    2) non-A, non-B hepatitis
    3) delta hepatitis
    4) hepatitis A

ANSWERS

201. C. This patient has cirrhosis of the liver.

Most cases of cirrhosis of the liver are directly attributable to alcohol abuse.

Symptoms of early cirrhotic liver disease include weakness, fatigue, and weight loss. In advanced disease, anorexia, nausea, and vomiting may occur. Abdominal pain is also often present.[1] Other symptoms include loss of libido, gynecomastia, and in women, menstrual irregularities.[1]

The liver is usually enlarged, palpable, and firm. In advanced cirrhosis it may actually shrink.[1] Dermatologic manifestations include spider nevi, palmer erythema, telangiectases of exposed area, and sometimes evidence of vitamin deficiencies (glossitis and cheilosis).[1] Although jaundice is rarely an initial sign, it usually develops later. Other later developing signs include ascites, pleural effusion, peripheral edema, purpuric lesions, asterixis, tremor, delirium, and coma.[1] Fever, splenomegaly, and superficial venous dilatation on the abdomen and thorax may also occur.[1]

Approximately 33% of chronic alcoholics will go on to develop alcoholic hepatitis. Many of these develop subsequent cirrhosis. There appears to be a genetic predisposition to the development of these complications.

Fifty percent of patients with advanced cirrhosis will be dead in 2 years; 65% will be dead in 5 years. Hematemesis, jaundice, and ascites are unfavourable signs.[1]

202. A. Only about 33% of chronic alcoholics develop significant alcoholic liver disease. Alcoholic hepatitis is the first clinical manifestation of this change.[1]

The symptoms of alcoholic hepatitis include anorexia, nausea, weight loss, emesis, fever, and abdominal pain.[1]

Hepatomegaly is seen in 80–90% of patients. Other signs include jaundice, ascites, splenomegaly and spider angiomas.[1]

Laboratory abnormalities in alcoholic hepatitis include hyperbilirubinemia and elevated serum transaminases. The ratio of AST to ALT is often 2/1 or greater. This can differentiate alcoholic hepatitis from viral hepatitis. Other laboratory abnormalities include elevated alkaline phosphatase, low serum albumin, and a prolonged prothrombin time.[1]

The prognosis of alcoholic hepatitis is variable; many patients only develop a mild illness. There is, however, a 10–15% mortality for the acute event.

Treatment of alcoholic hepatitis involves cessation of alcohol consumption, increased calorie and protein intake, and vitamin supplementation.[2]

Laënnec's cirrhosis develops in approximately 50% of patients surviving alcoholic hepatitis, and in the other half varying degrees of hepatic fibrosis develop.

203. D. The most common cause of cirrhosis is alcoholic hepatitis.[1]

Hepatitis A does not progress to chronic active hepatitis and subsequent cirrhosis. Ten percent of patients with hepatitis B infection and 40% of patients with non-A, non-B hepatitis infection go on to chronic persistent and chronic active hepatitis and possible subsequent cirrhosis.

Cytomegalovirus infection does not go on to produce cirrhosis.

204. D. The ascites that accompanies cirrhosis should be treated by salt restriction (<500 mg Na/day), bed rest, and diuretic therapy.[2] Water restriction is usually not necessary.

Ascites is maintained by increased levels of aldosterone, which causes intense sodium and water retention. Spironolactone is a drug that decreases aldosterone production, and it is the agent of choice in treating ascites. Amiloride or triamterene can be used in patients who do not tolerate aldosterone.

Peritoneovenous shunting (Laveen shunt, Denver shunt) is used for intractable ascites.

Paracentesis is not recommended as a form of treatment because the fluid that is removed rapidly reaccumulates.

205. A. This patient most likely has hepatitis A. This infection may occur sporadically or in epidemics;[1] transmission is usually via the oral-fecal route.

Hepatitis A usually presents with general malaise, myalgia, arthralgia, abdominal pain, nausea, vomiting, and severe anorexia out of proportion to the degree of illness.[1] Aversion to smoking is common.[1]

Hepatitis B and non-A, non-B hepatitis are unlikely due to the absence of risk factors. Although infectious mononucleosis may involve the liver, the diagnosis of hepatitis A is much more likely.

206. B. Acute infection with hepatitis A is confirmed by the demonstration of IgM antibodies to hepatitis A virus (IgM-anti HAV).[1] These antibodies persist for approximately 12 weeks. IgG antibodies to hepatitis A virus are only diagnostic of previous exposure.

Hepatitis A does not possess a recognizable core or surface antigen; these tests apply to hepatitis B. Antibodies to HB core antigen have nothing to do with hepatitis A. Anti-non-A, non-B hepatitis antigen does not exist.

207. D. Infants of mothers who are HBsAg positive should have one dose of hepatitis B immune globulin (HBIG) and a complete three-dose series of Hepatitis B vaccine administered. This regimen is 85–90% effective in preventing chronic antigenemia in the infant.[3]

208. C. Hepatitis B antigen and antibody tests are a continuing source of confusion because of the number of tests available. Initial screening for hepatitis B should include HBsAg and anti-HBc. These two tests will identify most cases of acute hepatitis B. There is a "window" period between the clearance of HBsAg and the appearance of anti-HBs. This period can last for 4–6 weeks, and during this time the only marker for hepatitis B is anti-HBc. If acute hepatitis B is suggested from the initial screening, then further tests including the following should be done:
1) HBeAg: The presence of this antigen indicates a highly contagious state or a chronic infection.

2) anti-HBe: The presence of this antibody indicates low infectivity and predicts later seroconversion or resolution of hepatitis B.

3) anti-HBs: The presence of this antibody indicates past hepatitis B infection and current immunity.[1,4]

209. E. In acute viral hepatitis, the serum transaminases (AST and ALT), serum bilirubin, and alkaline phosphatase are elevated.[1,3,4]

210. E. The clinical manifestations of cirrhosis have been discussed in the critique of question 201. Hypoalbuminemia is also common due to the accumulation of ascitic fluid.[1]

211. E. Hepatitis B vaccine should be offered to persons at high risk and continued exposure to hepatitis B infection. The previous hepatitis B vaccine was a noninfectious, formalin-inactivated fragment of the hepatitis B surface antigen that induced formation of anti-HBs. Hepatitis B vaccines that are manufactured using DNA-recombinant technology are now available. Persons at high risk for acquiring hepatitis B include all health care personnel, hemodialysis patients, patients requiring frequent blood transfusions, employees and residents of institutions for the mentally handicapped, male homosexuals, intravenous drugs users, and sexual contacts of chronic HBs Ag carriers.[4] All of these individuals should be immunized with hepatitis B vaccine.

212. A. Chronic active hepatitis, which may lead to cirrhosis of the liver, liver cell failure, and hepatocellular carcinoma is associated with hepatitis B, delta hepatitis, and non-A, non-B hepatitis. Hepatitis A does not lead to chronic active hepatitis. Chronic active hepatitis appears to be a particularly high risk in patients who have the delta agent associated with hepatitis B.[3,4]

SUMMARY OF THE DIAGNOSIS AND TREATMENT OF HEPATITIS AND CIRRHOSIS

1. **Essentials of diagnosis of viral hepatitis:**
   a) anorexia, nausea, vomiting, malaise, symptoms of upper respiratory tract infection, aversion to smoking
   b) fever, enlarged, tender liver; jaundice
   c) normal to low white blood cell count; abnormal liver functions tests, especially AST and ALT

2. **Types of viral hepatitis:**
   Hepatitis A: sporadic infection or epidemic.
   treatment: symptomatic
   diagnosis: transaminase elevation, IgM-anti HAV
   prevention: gamma globulin
   Hepatitis B: usually transmitted by blood or blood products. Particularly common in intravenous drug users.
   treatment: symptomatic
   diagnosis: transaminase elevation, HBsAg, anti-HBc
   prevention: hepatitis B hyperimmunoglobulin after exposure, hepatitis B vaccine
   Non-A, non-B hepatitis: usually transmitted by blood or blood products. Most common type of post-transfusion hepatitis.
   treatment: symptomatic
   Delta hepatitis: the delta agent is only found in association with hepatitis B. It is particularly likely to lead to chronic active hepatitis, and its complications including cirrhosis, liver cell failure, and hepatocellular carcinoma.

3. **Alcoholic hepatitis and cirrhosis:**
   Alcoholic hepatitis: the symptoms of alcoholic hepatitis closely resemble the symptoms of viral hepatitis. The serum ALT is almost always less than the serum AST. Patients who develop alcoholic hepatitis are at high risk of developing cirrhosis of the liver.
   Cirrhosis of the liver: weakness, fatigue, weight loss, anorexia, hepatomegaly, spider nevi, palmar erythema, asterixis, tremor, and ascites are common symptoms. Patients may develop hepatic encephalopathy.
   treatment: lactulose for hepatic encephalopathy, Na restriction, diuretics (spironolactone) for ascites, Laveen shunt
   Common complications: upper gastrointestinal bleeding from varices, hemorrhagic gastritis, or gastroduodenal ulcers. Liver failure, hepatic encephalopathy, hepatorenal syndrome.

References

1. Knauer C, Silverman S. Alimentary tract and liver. In: Schroeder S, Krupp M, Tierney L, McPhee S, eds.

Current medical diagnosis and treatment. Norwalk: Appleton and Lange, 1989: 398–411.

2. Regenstein F. Hepatic diseases. In: Dunagan W, Ridner M, eds. Manual of medical therapeutics. 26th Ed. Boston: Little, Brown, 1989: 310–323.

3. Dienstag J, Wands J, Koff R. Acute hepatitis. In: Braunwald E, Isselbacher K, Petersdorf R, Wilson J, Martin J, Fauci A, eds. Harrison's principles of internal medicine. 11th Ed. New York: McGraw-Hill, 1987: 1325–1335.

4. Schreeder M. Viral hepatitis. Prim Care 1988; 15(1): pp 157–173.

PROBLEM 26:   A 38-YEAR-OLD FEMALE WITH SWEATING, PALPITATIONS, NERVOUSNESS, IRRITABILITY, AND TREMOR

A 38-year-old female presents with a 3-month history of sweating, palpitations, nervousness, irritability, insomnia, tremor, frequent stools, and a 10-pound weight loss. She denies anorexia.

On examination, her blood pressure is 160/70 mm Hg. Her pulse is 120 and regular. She demonstrates mild proptosis; a smooth, diffusely enlarged, nontender, thyroid gland; and a loud S1 and S2 with an ejection systolic murmur heard along the left sternal edge.

SELECT THE ONE BEST ANSWER TO THE FOLLOWING QUESTIONS:

213. The most likely diagnosis in this patient is:
    a) Graves' disease
    b) Hashimoto's thyroiditis
    c) atypical pheochromocytoma
    d) toxic nodular goiter
    e) toxic adenoma

214. The single most useful test to be performed in this patient at this time would be:
    a) serum T4
    b) free T4
    c) 24-hour urine for free catecholamines, VMA, and metanephrines
    d) serum TSH
    e) functional thyroxine index

215. The treatment of choice for the patient described in question 213 is:
    a) propylthiouracil
    b) methimazole
    c) subtotal thyroidectomy
    d) radioactive iodine
    e) none of the above

216. A 25-year-old female is seen for a complete physical assessment. Her past history is unremarkable; she is feeling well at present and is currently taking the oral contraceptive pill.

    No abnormalites are found on physical examination. A routine T-4 level done is elevated at 13 μg/dl (169 nmol/L). The most likely explanation for the elevated T-4 level is:

    a) thyrotoxicosis
    b) toxic nodular goiter
    c) an elevated thyroid binding globulin (TBG) level
    d) laboratory error
    e) none of the above

217. The differentiation of hyperthyroidism due to thyrotoxicosis from hyperthyroidism due to thyroiditis is best made by:
    a) thyroid antibody level
    b) radioactive iodine uptake (I-131 uptake)
    c) thyroid scan
    d) level of elevation of serum T4
    e) level of thyroglobulin level

218. A 28-year-old female is seen in your office for a complete physical assessment. She is asymptomatic. On physical examination, she is found to have a 3 cm nodule in the left lobe of the thyroid gland.

    The first investigation that should be performed in this patient is:
    a) serum T4
    b) serum TSH
    c) radioactive iodine scan
    d) thyroid ultrasound
    e) no investigation

219. The most common cause of hypothyroidism is:
    a) autoimmune thyroiditis
    b) post I-131 hypothyroidism
    c) iodine deficiency
    d) idiopathic hypothyroidism
    e) post-thyroidectomy hypothyroidism

220. A 65-year-old male presents with a 6-month history of lethargy, weakness, psychomotor retardation, cold intolerance, constipation, hair loss, and weight gain. You suspect hypothyroidism. Which of the following tests will provide the most useful information for diagnosing hypothyroidism?
    a) serum T3
    b) serum T4
    c) free thyroxine index
    d) thyroid binding globulin
    e) serum TSH

ANSWER THE FOLLOWING QUESTION ACCORDING TO THE CODE:

A: 1, 2, and 3 are correct
B: 1 and 3 are correct
C: 2 and 4 are correct
D: Only 4 is correct
E: All of the above are correct

221. Which of the following statements regarding the treatment of the patient described in question 221 is(are) true?
    1) optimal therapy can be determined by measurement of the serum TSH level
    2) until the TSH is normal, full replacement has not been established
    3) patients with significant cardiac disease and elderly patients should be treated cautiously
    4) dessicated thyroid is the treatment of choice

ANSWERS

213. A. This patient has Graves' disease, the most common cause of hyperthyroidism.

Graves' disease usually presents with symptoms of sweating, palpitations, nervousness, irritability, insomnia, tremor, diarrhea, and weight loss.

Physical signs include a diffuse nontender goiter, tachycardia, systolic hypertension, loud heart sounds, and a cardiac murmur. A bruit is sometimes heard over the thyroid gland. Proptosis, with a straight ahead stare and lid lag are frequently seen. Occasionally, patients present with severe exophthalmos accompanied by ophthalmoplegia, follicular conjunctivitis, chemosis, and even loss of vision. Additional features may include dermopathy, pretibial myxedema, clubbing, and acropachy.[1]

Graves' disease is thought to be an autoimmune disease, and antibodies are present in serum. Toxic nodular goiter and toxic adenoma are other causes of hyperthyroidism. Their presentation, however, is much more subtle than Grave's disease and is generally not confused with this condition.

Hashimoto's thyroiditis is a cause of hypothyroidism rather than hyperthyroidism. Its presentation will be discussed in a subsequent question.

Atypical pheochromocytoma is not a serious diagnostic consideration.

214. A. The single most useful test to be performed in this patient at this time would be a serum T4. To confirm clinically obvious hyperthyroidism, measurement of the serum T4 level is the simplest test.

Patients who are taking drugs would alter thyroxine-binding proteins. A simultaneous resin T3 uptake is needed to calculate the free T4 level. This is sometimes called the functional thyroxine index. Free T4 can also be measured directly. This, however, is significantly more expensive.[2]

Serum TSH is most useful in the detection of hypothyroidism. However, a very sensitive radioimmunoassay that has recently been developed for TSH will provide significant information in many thyroid disorders.

215. D. The treatment of choice for this patient at this time is probably radioiodine. The antithyroid drugs propylthiouracil and methimazole, are probably the initially preferred treatment for young women (<30 years) with mild disease and a small goiter. If there is a recurrence, radioiodine should be administered. For any men older than 21 years, and for women older than 30 years, radioactive iodine is probably the treatment of choice.[2]

Subtotal thyroidectomy is effective for patients who are apprehensive about radioiodine treatment, and who are not suitable candidates for drug therapy.[2]

The acute symptoms that this patient presented with are probably best managed by administration of a beta blocker until radioactive iodine treatment is complete.

Subsequent hypothyroidism following radioiodine therapy is not uncommon; frequent thyroid function testing should follow.[2]

216. C. The most likely explanation for the elevated T4 level in this patient is an elevated TBG level secon-

dary to the estrogen component of the oral contraceptive pill.[2] TBG is increased in patients on the oral contraceptive pill, patients taking estrogen supplementation, and patients with infectious hepatitis. TBG is decreased in patients with chronic liver disease, nephrotic syndrome, hypoproteinemia from other causes, and those on androgen therapy.

217. B. The differentiation of hyperthyroidism due to thyrotoxicosis (Graves' disease) from hyperthyroidism due to thyroiditis is best made by radioactive iodine uptake (I-131 uptake).[3] Normal radioiodine uptake is below 25%. The I-131 uptake is significantly elevated in Graves' disease and moderately elevated in toxic nodular goiter. In subacute thyroiditis, autoimmune thyroiditis, or factitious hyperthyroidism it is low.[3]

218. C. The first investigation that should be performed in this patient is a radioactive thyroid scan to determine whether this is a "hot nodule" or a "cold nodule."[1] With "hot nodules," no other testing is necessary unless the patient is hyperthyroid. If the nodule is cold, ultrasound should differentiate a cystic lesion from a mixed or solid lesion. Cystic lesions may be treated by simple drainage; mixed lesions or solid lesions should be further investigated by aspiration cytology and fine-needle biopsy. Aspiration cytology and fine-needle biopsy will decrease surgical intervention rates.[2] Aspiration cytology and fine needle biopsy may even eliminate the need for thyroid scanning.

219. A. The most common cause of hypothyroidism is autoimmune thyroiditis or Hashimoto's thyroiditis. The patient with Hashimoto's thyroiditis may be initially hyperthyroid, but usually progresses to a hypothyroid state. Symptoms of hypothyroidism include fatigue, lethargy, constipation, cold intolerance, dry skin, hair loss, weight gain, edema, headache, arthralgias, hoarseness, amenorrhea, bradycardia, and hypotension. A painless goiter is frequently found on physical examination.[1-3]

220. E. The most useful test for diagnosing hypothyroidism is the serum TSH level. TSH is elevated in almost all cases of primary hypothyroidism. If hypothyroidism is suspected, both TSH and T4 determinations should be performed.[2]

221. A. Serum TSH level will determine optimal thyroid replacement therapy. With adequate replacement, the serum TSH should be normal.

Thyroxine is the preferred therapeutic agent,[4] though dessicated thyroid and triodothyroxine can return TSH to normal.

SUMMARY OF THE DIAGNOSIS AND TREATMENT OF THYROID DYSFUNCTION

1. **Hyperthyroidism:**
Causes:
a) Graves' disease
b) toxic nodular goiter
c) toxic adenoma
Investigations:
a) serum T4 to confirm clinically obvious hyperthyroidism
b) if patient is taking drugs or has a disease state that alters thyroid binding globulin (TBG) a T3-resin uptake should be included
c) when the goal is to exclude hyperthyroidism the most sensitive test is T3 by RIA[2]
d) radioiodine scan is still the investigation of choice in a patient with a thyroid nodule.
Fine needle aspiration and ultrasound are useful in investigation of the "cold nodule"
Treatment:
Graves' disease: female under 30—antithyroid drugs (propylthiouracil, methimazole). Males and females over 30: radioiodine
Toxic goiter: subtotal thyroidectomy or radioiodine

2. **Hypothyroidism:**
Cause: Almost exclusively caused by Hashimoto's thyroiditis.
Investigations: serum TSH is most sensitive test in diagnosing primary hypothyroidism. Serum T4 and antithyroid antibodies should be included.
Treatment: Levothyroxine

References

1. Ingbar S. Diseases of the thyroid. In: Braunwald E, Isselbacher K, Petersdorf R, Wilson J, Martin J, Fauci A, eds. Harrison's principles of internal medicine. 11th Ed. New York: McGraw-Hill, 1987: 1732–1741.

2. Federman D. Thyroid. In: Federman D, Rubenstein E, eds. Scientific American medicine. New York: Scientific American Medicine Incorporated, 1987; 3 (I): 1–23.

3. Baker C, McFarland K. Endocrinology. In: Rakel R, ed. Textbook of family practice. 3rd Ed. Philadelphia: WB Saunders, 1984: 963–974.

4. Saltman R, Goldberg A. Endocrine and lipid disorders. In: Dunagan W, Ridner M, eds. Manual of medical therapeutics. 26th Ed. Boston: Little, Brown, 1989 :398–401.

PROBLEM 27: A 24-YEAR-OLD COLLEGE STUDENT WITH PNEUMONIA

A 24-year-old college student presents with a 3-day history of dry, hacking cough that initially was nonproductive but which has become productive of scant, white sputum. The patient also complains of malaise, headache, fever and arthralgias.

Physical examination reveals a temperature of 39 °C and a few scattered rales in both lung bases. Chest x-ray reveals patchy perihilar and bilateral lower lobe infiltrates.

222. The most likely organism responsible for this patient's illness is:
   a) *Streptococcus pneumoniae*
   b) *Klebsiella pneumoniae*
   c) *Mycoplasma pneumoniae*
   d) influenza A
   e) *Haemophilus influenzae*

223. The treatment of choice for the patient discussed in question 221 is:
   a) penicillin
   b) amoxicillin
   c) erythromycin
   d) gentamicin
   e) carbenicillin

224. A 55-year-old female, previously healthy, and recovering from an episode of bronchitis suddenly develops a shaking chill followed by a high fever, pleuritic chest pain, and cough productive of purulent rusty sputum. On examination, the patient appears acutely ill, with a respiratory rate of 30/minute and chest splinting is present. Bronchial breath sounds are heard in the left lower lobe. Chest x-ray reveals a consolidation present in the left lower lobe. The most likely organism responsible for this patient's illness is:
   a) *Streptococcus pneumoniae*
   b) *Klebsiella pneumoniae*
   c) *Mycoplasma pneumoniae*
   d) influenza A
   e) *Haemophilus influenzae*

225. The treatment of choice for the patient described in question 224 is:

   a) penicillin
   b) erythromycin
   c) tetracycline
   d) gentamicin
   e) chloramphenicol

226. A 75-year-old alcoholic with a history of chronic obstructive lung disease is admitted to hospital suffering from fever, shortness of breath, chest pain, and cough productive of purulent sputum and blood. Physical examination reveals a temperature of 39° C, a respiratory rate of 28/minute, and bronchial breath sounds heard in the right upper lobe. Chest x-ray confirms a right upper lobe pneumonia. The most likely organism responsible for this patient's illness is:
   a) *Streptococcus pneumoniae*
   b) *Klebsiella pneumoniae*
   c) *Mycoplasma pneumoniae*
   d) influenza A
   e) *Haemophilus influenzae*

227. The drug(s) of choice for the patient described in question 226 is(are):
   a) erythromycin
   b) cephalothin
   c) penicillin
   d) gentamicin
   e) b and d

228. A 23-year-old male presents to your office for assessment of "a severe cold." He has had nasal congestion, coryza, and a productive cough for the last 6 days. The sputum was initially clear but has

become purulent in the last 24 hours. He has no fever.

On examination, the patient's temperature is 37.5° C. There are a few rhonci heard in both lung fields. His ears are clear. His throat appears slightly hyperemic. There are no cervical lymphadeno-pathy.

The chest x-ray shows accentuation of bronchial wall markings, but no infiltrate.

The most likely diagnosis in this patient is:
a) chronic bronchitis
b) acute bronchitis
c) early viral pneumonia
d) the common cold
e) atypical pneumonia

ANSWER THE FOLLOWING QUESTIONS ACCORDING TO THE CODE:

A: 1, 2, and 3 are correct
B: 1 and 3 are correct
C: 2 and 4 are correct
D: Only 4 is correct
E: All of the above are correct

229. The most appropriate treatment(s) for the patient discussed in question 228 include:
1) a cough suppressant
2) a broad-spectrum antibiotic
3) an expectorant
4) hydration and steam or mist inhalation

230. Which of the following statements regarding sputum cytology in the diagnosis of pneumonia is(are) true?
1) sputum cytology is essential to the accurate diagnosis of pneumonia
2) a good sputum specimen should contain more than 25 squamous cells/LPF
3) a good sputum specimen should contain many polymorphonuclear leukocytes
4) a Gram stain of a sputum specimen is a waste of time

231. Which of the following is(are) common symptoms or signs of viral pneumonia?
1) sudden onset of shaking chill
2) tachycardia
3) tachypnea
4) interstitial infiltrate on the chest x-ray

ANSWERS

222. C. This patient has Mycoplasma pneumonia. Mycoplasma pneumonia is a common respiratory tract illness in young adults. The most common respiratory symptom is a dry, hacking, usually nonproductive cough. Systemic symptoms include malaise, headache, and fever. Rash, serous otitis media, and joint symptoms occasionally accompany the respiratory symptoms.

Physical findings are usually unremarkable. Auscultation of the chest usually reveals only scattered rhonchi or fine localized rales. The chest x-ray, on the other hand, often reveals fine or patchy lower lobe or perihilar infiltrates. The WBC is often elevated (10,000 to 15,000/mm^3). Cold agglutinins are nonspecific, and negative in one-third of cases. The diagnosis is confirmed by acute and convalescent mycoplasma complement fixation titers.[1]

Clinically and radiologically, pneumonia caused by adenovirus is often difficult to differentiate from mycoplasma. *H. influenzae* is a common cause of pneumonia in children and sometimes occurs in debilitated patients. It is uncommon in young, healthy adults.

The other options listed in the question are discussed in subsequent sections of this problem.

223. C. The treatment of choice for Mycoplasma pneumonia is erythromycin or tetracycline for 10 days.[1]

224. A. This patient presents with a classical history of pneumococcal pneumonia. *Streptococcus pneumoniae* (pneumococcus) is the most common cause of pneumonia in the adult population.

Pneumococcal pneumonia usually presents with a shaking rigor, followed by fever, pleuritic chest pain, and cough with purulent or rusty sputum. Viral upper or lower respiratory tract infections may precede pneumococcal pneumonia.

In elderly or debilitated patients, the presentation may be atypical. Fever may be low grade, behavior disturbances may seem more significant than respiratory symptoms, and cough may not be prominent. Patients appear acutely ill, frequently with dyspnea and chest splinting. Signs of consolidation are frequently present.[2]

An elevated WBC with a left shift is common. Chest x-ray usually shows disease confined to one lobe (frequently a lower lobe), but several lobes may be involved with either consolidation or bronchopneumonia. Gram stain of the sputum should show polymorphonuclear leukocytes and "lancet shaped" gram-positive diplococci. Sputum cultures should be obtained, but up to 40% of patients with bacteremic pneumococcal pneumonia will have negative sputum cultures. Therefore, blood cultures should be obtained in all patients.

225. A. The treatment of choice for this patient is penicillin G. With this patient's clinical picture including a respiratory rate of 30/minute and chest splinting, IV penicillin is indicated. Humidified oxygen is also indicated. Amoxicillin and erythromycin could be used in place of penicillin G but would not be first-line drugs. Gentamicin and carbenicillin are not indicated for the treatment of pneumococcal pneumonia.[2]

226. B. The most likely cause of pneumonia in an elderly, debilitated alcoholic is a gram-negative organism; most commonly *Klebsiella pneumoniae*. It is frequently nosocomial. Although the presentation may be similar to pneumococcal pneumonia, the upper lobes are more frequently involved. Sudden onset is common. Pleuritic chest pain and hemoptysis are common features. Sputum is thick, and often bloody. Other important causes of pneumonia in elderly patients include other gram-negative organisms such as *E.coli*, *H.influenzae* as well as gram-positive organisms such as *Streptococcus pneumoniae* and *Staphylococcus*.[3]

227. E. The treatment of choice until culture results are available is a combination of antibiotics that covers *Klebsiella, E.coli, H.influenzae, Streptococcus pneumoniae*, and *Staphylococcus*. A good combination is a beta-lactam antibiotic like cephalothin and an aminoglycoside like gentamicin in divided doses.[3] In a debilitated or immunocompromised patient, an aminoglycoside combined with an extended spectrum penicillin like piperacillin would be optimal.

228. B. This patient has acute bronchitis. Acute bronchitis is an inflammation of the bronchi that is usually secondary to a viral upper respiratory tract infection. Infection of the bronchi causes inflammation with increased respiratory secretions. Symptoms of the common cold may precede acute bronchitis by several days. Cough may become productive of mucupurulent or purulent sputum.

The most common physical finding is diffuse rhonci. The respiratory rate is usually normal.

Although accentuation of bronchial wall markings may be seen on chest x-ray, no infiltrate is seen.

Chronic bronchitis is discussed in another section of this book. The absence of an infiltrate on the chest x-ray excludes the diagnosis of pneumonia.

The patient started out with "the common cold," but this has progressed to the complication of acute bronchitis.[4]

229. D. Treatment of acute bronchitis in the otherwise healthy patient is supportive. The primary treatment should include hydration and steam or mist inhalation, rest, cessation of cigarette smoking, and an antipyretic.

Cough suppressants and expectorants are overutilized, and in many cases, useless medications. In the uncompromised patient they have little, if any, role.

Broad-spectrum antibiotics should not be prescribed routinely; rather, a risk/benefit ratio should be determined for each patient. If the patient has chronic bronchitis, or is in another way debilitated, they may be appropriate.

Oral bronchodilators may be helpful if bronchospasm is present.[4]

230. B. Sputum cytology is essential to an accurate diagnosis of pneumonia. Saliva or nasopharyngeal secretions are of little value in determing the etiology of pneumonia, since colonization with gram-negative bacilli and other organisms is frequent.

If greater than 25 squamous epithelial cells are seen/LPH, the specimen is considered inadequate for culture because it represents normal flora. The ideal sputum specimen contains fewer than 10 squamous epithelial cells/LPF and many polymorphonuclear leukocytes.[5]

A Gram stain of a sputum specimen is a useful adjunct in the diagnosis of pneumonia.

231. D. Viral and bacterial pneumonias have different presenting signs and symptoms. Viral pneumonias often present with a gradual onset, absence of a shaking chill, absence of tachycardia and tachypnea, and absence of chest pain. The cough associated with viral pneumonia is prominent, and the fever is typically low-grade. The sputum is scant and mucoid, and consolidation on the chest x-ray is unusual. Generally, the chest x-ray shows

a diffuse, bilateral, infiltrate. Leukocytosis may occur, especially in the early period, but is generally not present. The most common viral agent responsible for pneumonia in the adult population is adenovirus.

SUMMARY OF THE DIAGNOSIS AND TREATMENT OF PNEUMONIA IN THE ADULT

1. **Symptoms and signs:**
    Bacterial: fever, chills (sudden onset of shaking chill in pneumococcal pneumonia), pleuritic chest pain, purulent sputum, tachycardia, tachypnea, bronchial breath sounds
    Viral/atypical: gradual onset, general malaise, headache, prominent cough, few if any abnormalities on examination of the lungs

2. **Laboratory diagnosis:**
    a) sputum specimen: <25 epithelial cells/LPF, many polymorphonuclear leukocytes
    b) Gram stain is essential.
    c) blood cultures should be done.
    d) chest x-ray: lobar consolidation is typical in bacterial pneumonia, although diffuse infiltrates do occur. Bilateral interstitial infiltrate is commonly seen with atypical (usually Mycoplasma) or viral pneumonia.
    e) WBC count: frequently elevated in bacterial pneumonia, seldom elevated in atypical or viral pneumonia

3. **Treatment:**
    Viral pneumonia: symptomatic
    Mycoplasma pneumoniae: erythromycin or tetracycline

Pneumococcal pneumonia: penicillin
Gram-negative pneumonia: third generation, cephalosporin/aminoglycoside
Legionella: erythromycin
Immunocompromised patient: aminoglycoside plus extended-spectrum penicillin

4. **Prevention:**
    Consider influenza vaccine and pneumococcal vaccine in high risk groups

References

1. Clyde W. Mycoplasma infections. In: Braunwald E, Isselbacher K, Petersdorf R, Wilson J, Martin J, Fauci A, eds. Harrison's principles of internal medicine. 11th Ed. New York: McGraw-Hill, 1987: 757–759.

2. Austrian R. Pneumococcal infections. In: Braunwald E, Isselbacher K, Petersdorf R, Wilson J, Martin J, Fauci A, eds. Harrison's principles of internal medicine. 11th Ed. New York: McGraw-Hill, 1987: 533–537.

3. Schaberg D, Turck M. Diseases caused by gram-negative enteric bacilli. In: Braunwald E, Isselbacher K, Petersdorf R, Wilson J, Martin J, Fauci A, eds. Harrison's principles of internal medicine. 11th Ed. New York: McGraw-Hill, 1987: 583–585.

4. Rodnick J, Gude J. The respiratory system. In: Taylor R, ed. Family medicine: principles and practice. 3rd Ed. New York: Springer-Verlag, 1988: 214–215.

5. Plorde J. The diagnosis of infectious diseases. In: Braunwald E, Isselbacher K, Petersdorf R, Wilson J, Martin J, Fauci A, eds. Harrison's principles of internal medicine. 11th Ed. New York: McGraw-Hill, 1987: 460.

PROBLEM 28:   A 65-YEAR-OLD MALE WITH A NEW ONSET SEIZURE

A 65-year-old male is brought to the emergency department after suffering a "seizure" while eating a meal in a restaurant. His wife states that this is his first seizure. Apparently, the patient developed convulsive jerking in his right arm and leg that lasted approximately 5 minutes. There was no loss of consciousness.

The only other significant medical problem that the patient has had is chronic bronchitis. He has smoked 2 packs of cigarettes a day for the past 40 years.

On examination, the neurologic examination is completely normal. The patient appears drowsy. His blood pressure is 150/100 mm Hg, and his pulse is 96 and regular.

SELECT THE ONE BEST ANSWER TO THE FOLLOWING QUESTIONS:

232. The seizure described in this patient is:

a) a simple partial seizure
b) a complex partial seizure
c) an absence seizure
d) a tonic-clonic (grand mal) seizure

e) a myoclonic seizure

233. The most common cause of a new onset seizure in a patient of this age is:
a) idiopathic
b) a metabolic problem
c) head trauma
d) an old stroke
e) a brain tumor

234. Which of the following medications would not be a drug of first choice for the prevention of further seizures in the patient described above?
a) phenytoin
b) carbamazepine
c) phenobarbital
d) valproic acid
e) ethosuximide

235. A 22-year-old male is brought into the emergency room by his wife. While he was raking leaves in the back yard, he suddenly lost consciousness, became rigid, and fell to the ground. His respiration temporarily ceased. This lasted for approximately 45 seconds. This was followed by a period of jerking of all four limbs of the body that lasted for 2–3 minutes. The patient then became unconsious for 3–4 minutes according to his wife.

On examination, the patient is drowsy. There is a large laceration present on his tongue, and a small laceration present on his lip. The neurological examination is otherwise normal. The vital signs are normal.

The seizure described in this case is:
a) a simple partial seizure
b) a complex partial seizure
c) an absence seizure
d) a grand mal (tonic-clonic) seizure
e) a myoclonic seizure

236. Which of the following medications would not be a drug of first choice for the prevention of further seizures in the patient described in question 235?
a) phenytoin
b) carbamazepine
c) phenobarbital
d) primidone
e) ethosuximide

237. A mother presents to your office with her 12-year-old daughter. The mother states that for the past 6 months she (and the girl's teacher) have frequently noted the child staring into space. This lack of concentration usually only lasts 30–45 seconds. Sometimes, there appears to be brief twitching of all limbs during this brief period of time.

The child's neurologic examination is normal.

The most likely cause of this patient's symptoms are:
a) simple partial seizures
b) complex partial seizures
c) absence seizures
d) myoclonic seizures
e) none of the above

238. All of the following medications may be useful in the treatment of the patient's condition described in question 237 except:
a) valproic acid
b) clonazepam
c) ethosuximide
d) phenytoin

ANSWER THE FOLLOWING QUESTIONS ACCORDING TO THE CODE:

A: 1, 2, and 3 are correct
B: 1 and 3 are correct
C: 2 and 4 are correct
D: Only 4 is correct
E: All of the above are correct

239. Which of the following statements regarding beginning and stopping antiepileptic therapy is(are) true?
1) antiepileptic therapy can safely be discontinued after a seizure-free interval of 1 year
2) antiepileptic medication should be started on every patient who has a seizure
3) antiepileptic medication should be begun with a combination of two or more antiepileptic agents
4) the decision to stop antiepileptic medication should be guided by the results of the electroencephalogram

240. Which of the following investigations is(are) useful in the evaluation of a patient with seizures?
1) EEG
2) MRI scan
3) CT scan
4) skull x-ray

241. Which of the following statements regarding the diagnosis and treatment of status epilepticus is(are) true?

1) poor compliance with the anticonvulsant drug regimen is the most common cause of tonic-clonic status epilepticus
2) the mortality rate of status epilepticus may be as high as 20%
3) the establishment of an airway is a first priority in the management of status epilepticus
4) intravenous diazepam is the drug of first choice in the immediate management of status epilepticus

ANSWERS

232. A. The seizure described in this patient is a simple partial seizure.

The symptoms of simple seizures include focal motor symptoms, or somotasensory symptoms that spread or "march" to other parts of the body. Other symptoms include special sensory symptoms that involve visual, auditory, olfactory, or gustatory regions of the brain; and autonomic symptoms or signs. Psychologic symptoms, often accompanied by impaired level of consciousness, can occur.[1]

Complex partial seizures are partial seizures in which consciousness is impaired.

The other types of seizures will be considered in other questions in this chapter.

The origin of this seizure should be confirmed by EEG. If a focal disturbance is substantiated by EEG, a CT or MRI scan should be ordered.

233. E. The most common cause of a new onset seizure in this patient is a brain tumor. A primary bronchogenic carcinoma with a secondary brain metastasis would be the most likely cause of a new onset seizure in a 65-year-old heavy cigarette smoker with COPD. The common causes of new onset seizures by age are:[2]
a) less than 10 years:
   i) idiopathic
   ii) congenital
   iii) birth injury
   iv) metabolic
b) 10–40 years of age:
   i) idiopathic
   ii) head trauma
   iii) preexisting focal brain disease
   iv) drug withdrawal
c) greater than 40 years:
   i) brain tumor
   ii) old stroke
   iii) trauma

234. E. Partial seizures can be treated effectively with phenytoin, carbamazepine, phenobarbital, primidone, and valproic acid. Treatment with one drug is preferable to combination therapy.[1]

Ethosuximide is not a good choice for the treatment of partial seizures. It is primarly indicated in the petit mal (absence seizures).

235. D. This patient has had a grand mal (tonic-clonic) seizure. Tonic-clonic seizures are often associated with a sudden loss of consciousness. The tonic phase is followed by a clonic phase characterized by generalized body musculature jerking. Following this is a stage of flaccid coma.[1]

Associated manifestations include tongue or lip biting, urinary or fecal incontinence, and other injuries.

An aura may precede a generalized seizure.

236. E. As in partial (focal) seizures, the drugs of choice are phenytoin, carbamazepine, phenobarbital, primidone, and valproic acid. Ethosuximide is not an effective drug in the treatment of grandmal seizures.[1]

237. C. This patient presents with typical absence (petit mal) seizures. Petit mal seizures may present with impairment of consciousness, sometimes accompanied by mild clonic, tonic, or atonic or autonomic symptoms.[1] These seizures, often very brief in duration, interrupt the current activity and are characterized by a description of the patient "staring into space."

Petit mal seizures that begin in childhood are terminated by the beginning of the third decade of life.

A bilaterally synchronous and symmetric 3-Hz spike-and-wave pattern is seen.[1]

238. D. Petit mal seizures can be effectively treated with ethosuximide, valproic acid, or clonazepam. Phenytoin is not an effective treatment for petil mal seizures.[1]

239. D. The decision to treat or not treat an initial seizure should include (1) details of the seizure, (2) adequate laboratory data including measurement of glucose, electrolytes, alcohol, and other toxins, and (3) the presence of EEG evidence of epileptic activity at least 2 weeks after the seizure. Careful reevaluation and monitoring is essential.

A consideration of discontinuation of medication can be made after a seizure-free period of 4 years. This decision should be confirmed by a lack of seizure activity on EEG.[1]

240. A. Laboratory investigations for a patient with an initial seizure should include a complete blood count, blood glucose determination, liver and renal function tests, and a serologic test for syphilis.[1]

Initial and periodic electroencephalography is mandatory. CT or MRI scanning should be performed in patients with focal neurologic symptoms or signs, focal seizures, or electroencephalographic findings indicating a focal disturbance.[1]

A chest x-ray should be performed in all patients who are cigarette smokers, as a primary lung neoplasm with secondary brain metastases producing cerebral edema and seizures is not uncommon.

A plain x-ray of the skull or skull series is unlikely to produce any useful diagnostic information.

241. E. Status epilepticus is a medical emergency, with a mortality rate of up to 20% and a high incidence of neurologic and mental sequelae in survivors.

Status epilepticus may be caused by poor compliance with medication, alcohol withdrawal, intracranial infection, neoplasm, a metabolic disorder, or a drug overdose. Prognosis depends on length of time from onset of seizure activity to effective treatment.

The management of status epilepticus includes establishing an airway, giving 50% dextrose in case of hypoglycemia, giving IV diazepam and IV phenytoin, and treating resistant cases with IV phenobarbitol.[3,4]

SUMMARY OF THE DIAGNOSIS, INVESTIGATION, AND MANAGEMENT OF EPILEPSY

1. **Classification:**
Partial seizures:
a) simple partial seizures
b) complex partial seizures
Generalized seizures:
a) petit mal (absence) seizures
b) tonic-clonic (grand mal) seizures
c) myoclonic seizures
d) tonic, clonic, or atonic seizures

2. **Diagnosis and investigation:**
a) characteristic pattern of seizure
b) EEG
c) CT or MRI
d) blood profile including CBC, blood glucose, liver function, renal function, and a serologic test for syphilis

3. **Treatment:**
a) carefully evaluate whether or not the patient needs antiepileptic treatment after the first seizure
b) drugs for generalized tonic-clonic (grand mal) or partial (focal) seizures include phenytoin, carbamazepine, phenobarbitol, primidone, and valproic acid
c) drugs for absence (petit mal) seizures include ethosuximide, valproic acid, and clonazepam

d) once antiepileptic drug therapy is initiated, it should be continued for at least 4 years. Patients should be carefully selected for discontinuation of therapy.

4. **Status epilepticus:**
Treatment: 50% dextrose, IV diazepam, IV phenytoin, and sometimes IV phenobarbital.

References

1. Aminoff M. Epilepsy. In: Schroeder S, Krupp M, Tierney L, and McPhee, S, eds. Current medical diagnosis and treatment. Norwalk: Appleton and Lange, 1989: 611–615.

2. Pohowalla P, Hogen V, McIntyre H. Evaluation of the patient with new onset seizures. Prim Care 1984; 11(4): 625–642.

3. Dichter M. The epilepsies and convulsive disorders. In: Braunwald E, Isselbacher K, Petersdorf R, Wilson J, Martin J, Fauci A, eds. Harrison's principles of internal medicine. 11th Ed. New York: McGraw-Hill, 1987: 1921–1930.

4. Delgado-Escueta AV, Wasterlain C, Treiman DM, et al. Current concepts in neurology: management of status epilepticus. N Engl J Med 1982; 306: 1337.

PROBLEM 29: A 51-YEAR-OLD MALE WITH EPIGASTRIC PAIN

A 51-year-old male presents with a 6-month history of epigastric pain that begins several hours after meals and is relieved by foods or antacids. The pain often wakes him up in the middle of the night. The pain is intermittent and is described as a dull ache. There is no radiation of the pain.

On examination, the patient has a slightly tender epigastrium. The examination is otherwise normal.

SELECT THE ONE BEST ANSWER TO THE FOLLOWING QUESTIONS:

242. The most likely diagnosis in this patient is:
    a) gastric carcinoma
    b) duodenal ulcer
    c) irritable bowel syndrome
    d) acute cholecystitis
    e) nervous stomach

243. Which of the following statements regarding the patient described in question 242 is FALSE?
    a) an upper gastrointestinal series is the diagnostic procedure of choice
    b) cigarette smoking may aggravate the condition
    c) alcohol does not aggravate the condition
    d) the patient should be placed on a bland diet
    e) this condition may be aggravated by the ingestion of certain medications

244. The patient discussed is prescribed antacid therapy for his condition. Which of the following statements regarding antacid therapy in the treatment of the condition described above is FALSE?
    a) antacids should be given 1 hour and 3 hours after meals and before bedtime
    b) antacids in tablet form are just as effective as antacids in liquid form
    c) magnesium hydroxide may produce diarrhea and hypokalemia
    d) aluminum hydroxide may produce constipation
    e) antacid treatment should continue for 4–6 weeks

245. The patient described in question 242 is placed on antacid therapy for the appropriate time interval. His symptoms recur 2 months after stopping therapy. Which of the following is the most appropriate course of action at this time?
    a) repeat the upper gastrointestinal series
    b) perform fiberoptic gastroscopy
    c) begin antacid therapy again
    d) select another anti-ulcer agent for therapy
    e) c or d

ANSWER THE FOLLOWING QUESTIONS ACCORDING TO THE CODE:

A: 1, 2, and 3 are correct
B: 1 and 3 are correct
C: 2 and 4 are correct
D: Only 4 is correct
E: All of the above are correct

246. Which of the following statements regarding the role of drugs and alcohol in peptic ulcer disease is(are) true?
    1) the incidence of peptic ulcer is increased in patients who take indomethacin or other NSAIDs
    2) alcohol has been established to be an ulcerogenic agent
    3) corticosteroids are ulcerogenic when taken in moderate doses
    4) aspirin is a gastric irritant that produces erosions and probably predisposes individuals to ulcer development when taken in doses of 1.2 to 2.4 g/day

247. Which of the following statements regarding cimetidine is(are) TRUE?
    1) cimetidine is an H1 histamine receptor antagonist
    2) cimetidine may be combined with antacids to increase the efficacy of treatment
    3) recurrence of peptic ulcer after 6 weeks of cimetidine therapy is unusual
    4) cimetidine is usually given in a dose of 800–1200 mg/day for active peptic ulcer disease

248. With which of the following drugs does cimetidine interact?
    1) warfarin
    2) doxepin
    3) diazepam
    4) theophyllines

249. Which of the following statements regarding the therapy for peptic ulcer disease is(are) true?

1) the H2 receptor antagonists have been shown to be superior to antacids for the treatment of peptic ulcer
2) ranitidine and famotidine have been shown to be superior to cimetidine for the treatment of peptic ulcer
3) pirenzepine has been shown to be superior to the H2 receptor antagonists for the treatment of peptic ulcer
4) all current available modalities for the treatment of peptic ulcer appear to be equally efficacious

250. Which of the following statements regarding the diagnosis and treatment of gastric ulcer is(are) correct?
1) the pain of gastric ulcer, like duodenal ulcer, is typically relieved by food
2) anorexia, nausea, and vomiting are much more common in patients with gastric ulcer than in patients with duodenal ulcer
3) gastric ulcers generally heal at the same rate as duodenal ulcers
4) fiberoptic gastroscopy should follow the identification of a gastric ulcer on an upper GI series

ANSWERS

242. B. This patient has the typical symptoms of a duodenal ulcer.

Duodenal ulcer is characterized by a deep, aching recurrent pain that is usually located in the midepigastrium. It is often relieved by food or antacids and aggravated by aspirin, coffee, or other irritants. Nocturnal pain is common.[1]

Anorexia, weight loss, and vomiting are infrequent associated symptoms of duodenal ulcer. The occurrence of these symptoms should lead one to suspect a gastric ulcer, or a more sinister cause, such as gastric carcinoma.

Irritable bowel syndrome and acute cholecystitis are described elsewhere in this book. Nervous stomach is not a diagnosis.

243. D. An upper gastrointestinal series is the diagnostic procedure of choice in this patient.[1] It will identify a duodenal ulcer in 80–90% of cases. If a gastric ulcer is seen endoscopy should be carried out to rule out a malignant ulcer.

Cigarette smoking has been shown to aggravate peptic ulcer disease and delay healing. Patients who smoke also have an increaed probability of recurrence.[1]

Aspirin and other nonsteroidal anti-inflammatory drugs can aggravate or produce a peptic ulcer.[1] Alcohol does not predispose to peptic ulceration.[1]

Bland diets or other special diets should not be prescribed; they may actually increase acid production.[1]

244. B. Antacid therapy is still a good first treatment for peptic ulcer disease, although the H2 receptor antagonists are replacing them as drugs of first choice.[2] Antacids should generally be given 1 hour and 3 hours after meals and at bedtime.

Most antacids are combinations of aluminum hydroxide and magnesium hydroxide. Magnesium hydroxide tends to produce diarrhea with possible subsequent hypokalemia. Aluminum hydroxide tends to be constipating. When these two compounds are combined the side effects often cancel each other.[2] Calcium carbonate, which is the active component in a number of antacids, may lead to hypercalcemia and the milk-alkali syndrome.[2]

Antacid therapy given in the liquid form has a much greater acid binding capacity than when given in the tablet form. The liquid form is therefore the preferred formulation.[2] Antacid therapy should be continued for 4–6 weeks to allow adequate healing time for the ulcer.

245. E. Peptic ulcer disease is a recurrent disease, with 60–90% of patients relapsing within 12 months, regardless of the type of therapy initially prescribed.[1] If recurrent symptoms are identical to previous episodes, no diagnostic tests need to be run and treatment can be restarted immediately. You have the option of restarting the same treatment regimen used previously or using another agent. In the case of the patient discussed in this case either restarting antacids or beginning therapy with an H2 receptor antagonist or cytoprotective agent would be appropriate.

246. D. Nonsteroidal anti-inflammatory drugs, including indomethacin and phenylbutazone, are commonly believed to predispose to or cause duodenal ulcer disease.[1] These drugs are gastric irritants, but the incidence of peptic ulcer disease among patients who have taken them for long periods of time is not significantly increased.[1]

Corticosteroids do not appear to be ulcerogenic in moderate dosage, even though they increase gastric acid secretion.[1] When potent cortico-steroids like dexamethasone are taken, an H2 receptor antagonist is recommended as prophylactic therapy against peptic ulcer disease.

Aspirin predisposes to gastric erosions and ulcer development, even when in doses as low as 1.2–2.4 g/day.[1] The healing rate of ulcers in smokers is significantly lengthened, especially when the patient is already taking aspirin.[1]

247. C. Cimetidine is an H2 histamine receptor antagonist that is now the most commonly prescribed treatment for peptic ulcer disease. The total daily dose of cimetidine for peptic ulcer disease is 800–1200 mg/day, divided into 2–4 doses, and given for 4–6 weeks.[1,2] This will produce healing in 90% of patients.

In resistant peptic ulcer disease, combination therapy with an H1 blocker may increase efficacy of treatment.

Peptic ulcer disease is a recurrent disease. Relapse rates may be as high as 80–90% during a period of 5–10 years, but the disease frequently becomes quiescent after 10–15 years.

248. E. Cimetidine delays hepatic microsomal metabolism of any drug that is primarly excreted by the liver. Examples of these drugs include the anticoagulant warfarin, all drugs in the tricyclic antidepressant group (including doxepin), diazepam and all of its derivatives, and all drugs in the theophylline class. Because of the delay of excretion induced by cimetidine, the dose of the other agents has to be adjusted accordingly.[1]

249. D. All currently available modalities for the treatment of peptic ulcer appear to be equally effective.[3] Antacids such as Maalox and Mylanta; the H2 receptor antagonists cimetidine, ranitidine, and famotidine; the cytoprotective agents sucralfate and misoprostol, and the anticholinergic agent pirenzepine appear to produce similar healing rates in peptic ulcer.

A new class of agents, the proton pump inhibitors, may be useful in resistant cases of peptic ulcer disease. The prototype, omeprazole,[4] is, however, at this time only indicated for the treatment of severe reflux esophagitis.

250. C. Gastic ulcers are less common than duodenal ulcers. Recurrence rates are less (50%), and the recurrence usually develops at the same site as the original ulcer.[1]

Patients with gastric ulcers usually experience abdominal pain that is typically relieved by antacids. The ingestion of food, however, aggravates rather than alleviates symptoms in approximately 50% of gastric ulcer patients. Anorexia, weight loss, nausea, and vomiting are also more common in patients with gastric ulcer.

Diagnosis of gastric ulcer by GI series should be followed by fiberoptic bronchoscopy, as 5% of gastric ulcers are malignant.[1]

Gastric ulcers heal more slowly than duodenal ulcers.[1] As with duodenal ulcers, all the modes of therapy discussed previously appear to be equally effective. Gastroscopy should be repeated after 8 weeks of therapy to confirm healing.[1]

SUMMARY OF THE DIAGNOSIS AND MANAGEMENT OF PEPTIC ULCER DISEASE

1. **Symptoms:**
   Duodenal ulcer: midepigastric pain, relieved by the ingestion of food or antacids. Nocturnal pain.

   Peptic ulcer: midepigastric pain, relieved by antacids but often aggravated by food. Anorexia, weight loss, nausea, and vomiting are frequently associated

2. **Differential diagnosis:** cholecystitis, pancreatitis, appendicitis, carcinoma of the stomach (gastric ulcer), ischemic bowel disease in the elderly

3. **Investigations:**
   a) no investigation may be appropriate if the symptoms suggest duodenal ulcer and resolution of symptoms takes place within 4 to 6 weeks on medical therapy.
   b) upper GI series
   c) gastroscopy (if gastric ulcer shown on GI series)

4. **Treatment:**
   H2 receptor antagonists:
      cimetidine
      ranitidine
      famotidine
      antacids (1 and 3 hours after meals and upon retiring)
   Cytoprotective agents:
      sucralfate
      misoprostol
   Anticholinergics:
      pirenzepine

Proton pump inhibitors:

Omeprazole may be an important treatment in the future

References

1. Gray G. Peptic ulcer disease. In: Federman D, Rubenstein E, eds. Scientific American medicine. New York: Scientific American Medicine Incorporated, 1988: 4(II): 1–15.

2. Cort D, Shuman R. Gastroenterologic diseases. In: Dunagan W, Ridner M, eds. Manual of medical therapeutics. 26th Ed. Boston: Little, Brown, 1989: 290–295.

3. Knauer C, Silverman S. Peptic ulcer. In: Schroeder S, Krupp M, Tierney L, McPhee S, eds. Current medical diagnosis and treatment. Norwalk: Appleton and Lange, 1989: 365–370.

4. Omeprazole. Med Lett 1990; 32(813): 19–20.

PROBLEM 30: A 35-YEAR-OLD FEMALE WITH FATIGUE

A 35-year-old female presents with a 4-month history of fatigue. Her past history is unremarkable apart from heavy menstrual periods during the last year. She is not taking any medications.

On physical examination, the patient looks pale. Her blood pressure is 90/70 mm Hg.

Her hemoglobin is measured at 9.5 g/dl.

SELECT THE ONE BEST ANSWER TO THE FOLLOWING QUESTIONS:

251. The most likely diagnosis in this patient is:
    a) iron-deficiency anemia
    b) pernicious anemia
    c) hemolytic anemia
    d) folate deficiency
    e) hypothyroidism

252. The treatment of choice for the patient described in question 251 is:
    a) naproxen 375 mg b.i.d. during the last 2 weeks of the menstrual cycle
    b) ferrous sulfate 300 mg o.d. to t.i.d.
    c) vitamin B$_{12}$ 100 μg every 2 days decreasing to 100 μg monthly
    d) levothyroxine 100 μg o.d.
    e) a and b

253. The most sensitive test for the detection of iron deficiency anemia is:
    a) serum iron
    b) serum iron binding capacity
    c) serum ferritin
    d) serum transferrin
    e) reticulocyte count

254. A 55-year-old male presents for a periodic health assessment. His only complaint is that he has been feeling quite fatigued for the past 3 months.

On physical examination, the patient looks pale. His blood pressure is 100/80 mm Hg. His pulse is 96 and regular. The rest of the physical examination is normal.

A complete blood count reveals a hemoglobin of 100 g/L. His blood picture reveals a decreased mean corpuscular hemoglobin concentration (MCHC) and a mean corpuscular volume (MCV).

Until proven otherwise, the most likely cause of this blood picture is:
    a) a lymphoma
    b) a gastrointestinal malignancy
    c) lack of intrinsic factor
    d) dietary deficiency of folic acid
    e) dietary lack of iron

255. A 78-year-old female presents to your office complaining of a "lack of energy" that began 8 months ago.

On examination, she has marked pallor. Her hemoglobin level is 75 g/L. A peripheral blood smear shows hypochromasia and microcytosis. Her previous hemoglobin level 1 year ago was 13.0 g/dl.

The most likely cause of this patient's anemia is:
    a) malnutrition
    b) pernicious anemia
    c) folic acid deficiency
    d) gastrointestinal bleeding
    e) hypothyroidism

256. The anemia of chronic disease is most often:
    a) hypochromic and normocytic
    b) hypochromic and microcytic
    c) normochromic and macrocytic
    d) normochromic and normocytic
    e) hyperchromic and macrocytic

ANSWER THE FOLLOWING QUESTIONS ACCORDING TO THE CODE:

A: 1, 2, and 3 are correct
B: 1 and 3 are correct
C: 2 and 4 are correct
D: Only 4 is correct
E: All of the above are correct

257. Which of the following disorders is(are) often associated with anemia?
    1) rheumatoid arthritis
    2) non-Hodgkin's lymphoma
    3) renal failure
    4) liver failure

258. A 75-year-old female presents to your office with a 4-month history of fatigue, paresthesias, weakness, and unsteady gait.

    On examination, her skin is pale with a hint of jaundice. She has a number of neurologic findings including patchy impairment of touch and temperature sensation, loss of vibration and position sense, a positive Romberg sign, hyperreflexia and a bilaterally positive Babinski sign. Her hemoglobin is 6.8 g/dl. Which of the following statements is(are) TRUE about this patient's condition?
    1) this patient has a hemolytic anemia
    2) oval macrocytes will be seen on the peripheral smear
    3) a CT scan of the brain should be performed
    4) a Schilling test should be performed to confirm the diagnosis

SELECT THE ONE BEST ANSWER TO THE FOLLOWING QUESTIONS:

259. The treatment of choice for the patient described in question 258 is:
    a) folic acid 5 mg/day
    b) ferrous sulfate 300 mg t.i.d.
    c) vitamin B_{12} 200 μg/day intramuscularly indefinitely
    d) vitamin B_{12} 500 μg/day intramuscularly indefinitely

    e) none of the above

260. Which of the following statements regarding folic acid deficiency anemia is false?
    a) folic acid deficiency anemia is a macrocytic anemia
    b) hypersegmented neutrophils are often seen on the peripheral blood smear
    c) the most common cause of folic acid deficiency anemia is an inadequate dietary intake
    d) folic acid deficiency is uncommon in alcoholics
    e) reduced folate levels are usually seen in red blood cells and in serum

ANSWERS

251. A. This patient has iron deficiency anemia. This is the most common cause of anemia. In this patient, the most likely cause of her anemia is excessive blood loss during her menstrual periods.[1]

    Pernicious anemia, folate deficiency, hemolysis, and hypothyroidism are all forms of or conditions associated with anemia; however, they are not nearly as common as iron deficiency.

252. E. The treatment of choice in this patient is ferrous sulfate 300 mg o.d. to t.i.d. to replace the iron loss during menstruation[1] and an antiprostaglandin agent such as naproxen 375 mg b.i.d. to decrease prostaglandin production and subsequent menstrual blood loss.[2] It may only be necessary to use the ferrous sulfate for 1–2 months; at that time the patient can be taken off iron and remain on the prostaglandin synthetase inhibitor.

253. C. The most sensitive test for the diagnosis of iron deficiency anemia is the serum ferritin level.[1] In iron deficiency anemia, the serum ferritin level usually falls first. Thereafter, total iron binding capacity (TIBC) increases, and serum iron levels gradually decrease. The transferrin saturation will also decrease at this time. The reticulocyte count is not useful in assessing the degree of iron deficiency.

254. B. Until proven otherwise, iron deficiency anemia in a middle-aged or elderly male is due to gastrointestinal blood loss;[1] the most sinister cause of this is a gastrointestinal maligancy. This patient should have fecal occult blood determinations, followed by an air-contrast barium enema and a colonoscopy. If all of these investigations are nor-

mal, the upper GI tract should be investigated by gastroscopy.

Dietary iron deficiency or dietary folic acid deficiency is extremely unusual in a male.

A lymphoma is more likely to produce a normochromic, normocytic picture than a hypochromic, microcytic picture.

Bleeding hemorrhoids may also produce iron-deficiency anemia in middle-aged males.

Vitamin B_{12} deficiency due to lack of intrinsic factor would present as a macrocytic rather than a microcytic anemia.

255. D. This patient's hypochromic-microcytic blood picture, coupled with a drop in hemoglobin from 13.0–7.5 g/dl in 1 year is almost certainly due to blood loss from a gastrointestinal malignancy or other bleeding source. The discussion in question 254 regarding iron deficiency anemia in males also applies to females past the menopause. The other common cause of iron deficiency anemia in elderly patients is malnutrition.[1]

Pernicious anemia would be the most common megaloblastic anemia in elderly individuals. Folic acid deficiency and anemia due to hypothyroidism are also seen in the elderly.

256. D. The anemias associated with chronic disease are most often normochromic and normocytic.[3]

257. E. Anemia may be associated with many chronic diseases including infectious, inflammatory, neoplastic, cardiovascular, endocrinologic, hepatic, and renal disorders.[1] These disorders include non-Hodgkin's lymphoma, rheumatoid arthritis, chronic renal failure, chronic liver disease. The anemia of chronic disease is the second most common anemia (second only to iron deficiency anemia).

258 . C. This patient has pernicious anemia. Pernicious anemia results from a deficiency of vitamin B_{12}. Vitamin B_{12} deficiency results from a lack of intrinsic factor, a protein secreted by gastric parietal cells.[1]

Patients with pernicious anemia often have neurologic symptoms. These symptoms result from involvement of the dorsal and lateral columns of the spinal cord.

The blood picture of pernicious anemia is a megaloblastic anemia characterized by an increase in the MCV, an oval shape to the macrocytes, and hypersegmented neutrophils.

Pernicious anemia can be confirmed by the Schilling test.[1]

The treatment of Vitamin B_{12} deficiency is intramuscular B_{12}, beginning at 200 µg/day for the first week, 200 µg weekly for the first month, and 200 µg/month thereafter.[1]

This form of anemia does not have a hemolytic component and the neurologic symptoms will resolve without further investigation (such as CT scan) or treatment.

259. E. None of the above. See critique of question 258.

260. D. Folic acid deficiency is most commonly seen in alcoholics, cancer patients, and elderly patients.[1] The most common cause of folate deficiency is inadequate dietary intake.

Folic acid deficiency anemia is also a macrocytic anemia. Patients with folic acid deficiency anemia have normal Vitamin B_{12} levels.

Patients with folic acid deficiency should be treated with 1 mg/day of folic acid.

SUMMARY OF THE DIAGNOSIS AND TREATMENT OF COMMON ANEMIAS

1. **Iron deficiency anemia:**
   a) most common form of anemia
   b) most common cause in premenopausal women is excessive menstrual flow. Iron deficiency anemia in males or in postmenopausal females should be considered to be from GI blood loss until proven otherwise.
   c) iron deficiency anemia is usually microcytic. Hypochromia is seen in most advanced cases
   d) serum ferritin level less than 12 µg/L is most sensitive test for iron deficiency
   Treatment: ferrous sulfate

2. **Anemia of chronic disease:**
   a) seen in many diseases including chronic renal, hepatic, endocrinologic, and cardiovascular diseases.
   b) most often is normochromic-normocytic
   Treatment: effective treatment of the disease itself

3. **Vitamin B_{12} deficiency anemia:**
   a) macrocytic anemia with macro-ovalocytes and hypersegmented neutrophils on the peripheral blood smear.
   b) due to lack of instrinic factor to promote absorption of Vitamin B_{12} in the GI tract

c) diagnosed by Vitamin B_{12} level less than 74 pmol/L (100 pg/ml) and confirmed by Schilling test

Treatment: Vitamin B_{12}

4. **Folic acid deficiency anemia:**
   a) macrocytic anemia with macro-ovalocytes and hypersegmented neutrophils on peripheral blood smear
   b) normal serum Vitamin B_{12} level
   c) reduced folate level in red blood cells or serum
   d) most common cause is inadequate dietary intake

Treatment: folic acid 1 mg/day

References

1. Linker C. Anemias. In: Schroeder S, Krupp M, Tierney L, McPhee S, eds. Current medicial diagnosis and treatment. Norwalk: Appleton and Lange, 1989: 295–303.

2. Phillips D, Gearhart J. The female reproductive system. In: Taylor R, ed. Family medicine: principles and practice. 3rd Ed. New York: Springer-Verlag, 1988: 308.

3. Kusher J. Hypochromic anemias. In: Wyngaarden J, Smith L, eds. Cecil textbook of medicine. 18th Ed. Philadelphia: WB Saunders, 1988: 892–900.

PROBLEM 31: A 35-YEAR-OLD FEMALE WITH A RASH ON HER LEFT WRIST

A 35-year-old female presents to your office for assessment of a skin rash that has been present on her left wrist for 2 months. The rash is constant.

The patient has had no previous dermatologic problems. Her health has been otherwise well.

On examination, the patient has a dry, excoriated rash around the left wrist. This appears to coincide with the metal band of a new wristwatch, which she purchased 2 months ago.

SELECT THE ONE BEST ANSWER TO THE FOLLOWING QUESTIONS:

261. The most likely cause of this patient's skin rash is:
    a) nummular eczema
    b) lichen simplex chronicus
    c) allergic contact dermatitis
    d) irritant contact dermatitis
    e) idiopathic eczema

262. The most definitive therapy for the patient's skin rash described in question 261 is:
    a) low-potency topical corticosteroid
    b) medium-potency topical corticosteroid
    c) high-potency topical corticosteroid
    d) alternate day prednisone
    e) none of the above

263. A 58-year-old female presents to the office with a "skin rash" that has been present on both legs for the past 3 months. She has a history of bilateral varicose veins that have been stripped and injected bilaterally.

    On examination there are significant superficial varicose veins bilaterally. There is a brawny, edematous, red, hyperpigmented, petechial, scar-ring and weeping eruption present maximally around the medial malleoli bilaterally and distal one-third of the lower leg. The rest of the physical examination is normal.

    The most likely diagnosis in this patient is:
    a) stasis dermatitis
    b) lichen simplex chronicus
    c) nummular eczema of both lower legs
    d) idiopathic eczema
    e) none of the above

264. The treatment regimen for the patient described in question 263 may include all of the following except:
    a) systemic corticosteroids
    b) topical corticosteroids
    c) support hose
    d) wet compresses
    e) weight loss

265. A 25-year-old female presents with a 6-month history of a "skin rash" on her arms and legs. She states that the rash is "slightly itchy."

    On examination, the patient has a number of coin-shaped patches that are comprised of an erythematous, macular, papular rash that have thickened in some areas. The rest of the dermatologic examination is normal.

The most likely diagnosis in this patient is:
a) idiopathic eczema
b) lichen simplex chronicus
c) nummular eczema
d) allergic contact dermatitis
e) irritant contact dermatitis

266. A 31-year-old male with schizophrenia is brought into your office by his mental health worker. Apparently, small pink creatures from outer space began to land on his skin 6 months ago. He found that the only way to dislodge them was to vigorously scratch his skin. Antipsychotic medication has been unable to control his hallucinations.

On examination, the patient has an erythematous, macular, papular, lichenified eruption on the nape of his neck, his lower legs, his groin, and his arms. The rest of the dermatologic examination is normal.

The most likely diagnosis in this patient is:
a) nummular eczema
b) lichen simplex chronicus
c) idiopathic eczema
d) atopic dermatitis
e) fixed drug eruption secondary to antipsychotic medication

267. A 42-year-old professor presents to your office for assessment of a facial skin rash that he has had for several months. He has seen six other physicians who have prescribed various forms of topical corticosteroid therapy. None of the treatments have worked. The patient states that the rash if often made worse by drinking alcohol, drinking coffee, and eating hot, spicy foods. At these times, the patient will often become flushed.

On examination, the patient has a diffuse erythematous, macular, papular, eruption over the central portion of the face. The rest of the examination is within normal limits except for a blood pressure reading of 150/100 mm Hg.

The most likely diagnosis in this patient is:
a) pheochromocytoma
b) carcinoid syndrome
c) rosacea
d) systemic lupus erythematosus
e) seborrheic dermatitis

268. A 51-year-old female presents to your office for assessment of a skin lesion on her nose. The lesion has been present for the past 4 months. Apparently,

it has not changed in appearance since she first noticed it. She is, however, quite concerned about the lesion.

On examination, the patient has a 4 mm, circular, slightly raised lesion present in the center of her nose.

At this time, you should :
a) tell the patient to quit worrying about it and return to your office in 6 months if it is still present
b) administer a trial of topical antibiotic therapy
c) administer a trial of topical corticosteroid therapy
d) biopsy the skin lesion
e) cauterize the lesion just to be on the safe side

ANSWER THE FOLLOWING QUESTIONS ACCORDING TO THE CODE:

A: 1, 2, and 3 are correct
B: 1 and 3 are correct
C: 2 and 4 are correct
D: Only 4 is correct
E: All of the above are correct

269. Which of the following is(are) drugs that have been implicated in the development of drug eruptions?
1) penicillin
2) ampicillin
3) trimethoprim-sulfamethoxazole
4) furosemide

270. Which of the following is(are) recognized complications of topical corticosteroid therapy?
1) peptic ulceration
2) cushinoid appearance
3) osteoporosis
4) skin atrophy

ANSWERS

261. C. This patient has an allergic contact dermatitis due to the nickel component of her new wristwatch.

Contact dermatitis may be allergic or irritant. Irritant dermatitis occurs when a substance produces a direct toxic effect on the skin.[1] Many substances, including acids, solvents, alkalis, and detergents may produce an irritant dermatitis.

Allergic contact dermatitis occurs as a delayed hypersensitivity reaction to any one of a number of substances.[1] Common examples of allergic contact dermatitis include nickel and poison ivy. Lichen simplex chronicus and nummular eczema will be discussed in subsequent questions.

262. E. The most definitive therapy for the skin rash described in the patient in question 261 is to remove the source of the irritation (the nickel watchband). Topical corticosteroid therapy[2] will suppress the inflammation, but will not irradicate the condition. Oral corticosteroids are not indicated in the treatment of allergic contact dermatitis unless the inflammation is severe and extensive.

263. A. This patient has stasis dermatitis. Stasis dermatitis is an eczematous eruption of the lower legs secondary to venous imcompetence in the lower extremities.[1] Stasis dermatitis presents as a brawny, erythematous, hyperpigmented, and sometimes weepy reaction. The most common location is the medial malleolus or distal one-third of the lower leg.[1]

264. A. Stasis dermatitis can be effectively treated by the use of supportive hose while the patient is ambulatory, weight reduction, and by the use of topical corticosteroids[2] and wet compresses such as aluminum acetate. Infected stasis ulcers should be treated with topical agents such as fucidic acid. Neomycin should not be used, as it may cause a secondary allergic dermatitis. Systemic corticosteroids are rarely, if ever, indicated in the treatment of stasis dermatitis.

265. C. This patient has nummular eczematous dermatitis. Nummular eczematous dermatitis presents as coin-shaped patches on the extensor surfaces of the arms and legs.[1] The lesions usually begin as vesicles and papules that eventually thicken. They are erythematous and may resemble a fungal infection. Pruritis is common. Many factors including dry skin, frequent bathing, and certain irritating substances may contribute to nummular eczema.

Topical corticosteroids and moisturizing lotions are very effective in treating the condition. A bath emollient may also be extremely effective.

266. B. This patient has lichen simplex chronicus or "neurodermatitis." Neurodermatitis presents as a lichenified, eczematous eruption that results from constant scratching. Pruritis often precedes the scratching, and an "itch-scratch" cycle is established. Neurodermatitis is most frequently found on the neck, the lower legs, and the groin. Scaling and excoriation may occur.[1]

Treatment consists of explaining to the patient the cause and the need to stop rubbing (which in this case is unlikely to be successful), and the use of topical corticosteroids and systemic antihistamines.[1] On occasion, direct intralesional steroid injection will be necessary to break the itch-scratch cycle. For this patient, the most important aspect of treatment is probably to try to get rid of the visual hallucinations with more appropriate antipsychotic therapy.

267. C. This patient has rosacea. Rosacea is a chronic inflammatory disorder affecting the blood vessels and pilosebaceous units of the face.[1] Rosacea is a papular or pustular eruption with an erythematous and/or telangiectatic base. Flushing is a common symptom and is often associated with the ingestion of alcohol or other foods. Hyperplasia of the affected structures often causes an enlarged, erythematous, bullous nose known as rhinophyma.[1] High-potency corticosteroids[2] (especially fluorinated corticosteroids) will induce or aggravate the condition. Treatment consists of systemic tetracycline or erythromycin. The other options presented in the question are not serious considerations in this patient.

268. D. This skin lesion should be biopsied. It is difficult, if not impossible at times, to differentiate benign from malignant skin lesions. For this reason, if you don't know what a skin lesion is, biopsy it. Using a Baker's 3 mm or 4 mm punch biopsy with local anesthesia, you can often remove the entire lesion (if it is small) or obtain a good sample for pathologic analysis.

In this patient, a basal cell carcinoma would be a primary consideration. A squamous cell carcinoma, a more aggressive tumor, is impossible to differentiate from the less malignant basal cell carcinoma without biopsy.[1]

Topical antibiotic or topical corticosteroid therapy is inappropriate when you don't know what you are treating. Cauterizing the lesion may destroy a basal cell carcinoma, but it is inappropriate without a diagnosis being made. To tell the patient not to worry but to return in 6 months is inappropriate.

269. E. Drug eruptions usually present as hives or morbilliform rashes. Patients are often on multiple medications, making the identification of the of-

fending drug more difficult. In an attempt to discover the offending medication, consider (1) the temporal relationship between the initiation of the drug and the rash and (2) the probability that a given drug is likely to cause an eruption. Drugs most likely to cause maculopapular eruptions include trimethoprim-sulfamethoxazole, penicillin G, semisynthetic penicillins, ampicillin, quinidine, and gentamicin. Diuretics, especially loop diuretics like furosemide and ethacrynic acid, are also associated with the development of fixed drug eruptions.[3]

270. E. All of the complications produced by oral glucocorticoid therapy may occur with topical therapy if the exposure is long enough, the potency of the topical glucocorticoid strong enough, and the surface area covered large enough.[4] Therefore, in addition to skin atrophy and the development of telangiectasias, topical glucocorticoid therapy may produce osteoporosis, myopathies, glaucoma, cataracts, peptic ulceration, hypertension, sodium and fluid retention, hyperglycemia, hyperlipidemia, and numerous other effects.

The lowest effective dose of topical corticosteroid should generally be used for the shortest period of time. Fluorinated corticosteroids are particularly likely to produce systemic side effects. In most cases a low potency corticosteroid like hydrocortisone or a medium potency corticosteroid like betamethasone will suffice.

SUMMARY OF THE CLASSIFICATION AND TREATMENT OF ECZEMATOID DERMATITIS AND OTHER IMPORTANT SKIN CONDITIONS

1. **Eczematoid dermatitis:**
   Contact dermatitis:
   a) allergic contact dermatitis
   b) irritant contact dermatitis
   Photodermatitis:
   a) thiazides and phenothiazines most common
   Atopic dermatitis:
   a) may continue to be a problem in adulthood
   Stasis dermatitis:
   a) usually associated with peripheral venous insufficiency
   Nummular eczematous dermatitis:

   a) coin-shaped patches predominantly on the extensor surfaces of the arms and legs
   Lichen simplex chronicus:
   a) also known as neurodermatitis
   b) characterized by an itch-scratch cycle
   Seborrheic dermatitis:
   a) characterized by an erythematous, eczematous rash with yellow, greasy scales

2. **Other important types of dermatitis seen commonly in family medicine:**
   a) rosacea
   b) drug eruptions

3. **Treatment:**
   a) remove any offending agent (as in allergic contact dermatitis and irritant contact dermatitis)
   b) topical corticosteroids form the basis of treatment for most forms of eczematoid dermatitis. Use the lowest effective strength for the shortest period of time to avoid local and systemic side effects. Be particularly cautious of the use of topical corticosteroids in children and fluorinated corticosteroids in everyone. If a dermatitis is wet, use a cream. If it is dry, use an ointment.

4. Biopsy any suspicious skin lesion.

References

1. Parker F. Skin diseases of general importance. In: Wyngaarden J, Smith L, eds. Cecil textbook of medicine. 18th Ed. Philadelphia: WB Saunders, 1988: 2300–2353.

2. Mitchell J. Dermatological therapy. In: Dunagan W, Ridner R, eds. Manual of medical therapeutics. 26th Ed. Boston: Little, Brown, 1989: 17–19.

3. Wood A, Oates J. Adverse reactions to drugs. In: Braunwald E, Isselbacher K, Petersdorf R, Wilson J, Martin J, Fauci A, eds. Harrison's principles of internal medicine. 11th Ed. New York: McGraw-Hill, 1987: 352–358.

4. Johnson G. Blue book of pharmacologic therapeutics. Philadephia: WB Saunders, 1985: 459–468.

PROBLEM 32: A 25 YEAR-OLD-MALE WITH FATIGUE, ANOREXIA, AND BLOODY URINE

A 25-year-old male presents to your office with the chief complaint of "bloody urine." He developed a sore throat 2 weeks ago. Three days ago he began having grossly bloody urine ("the color of coffee") and has been fatigued and anorexic for the past 48 hours.

On examination, his blood pressure is 150/100 mm Hg. The remainder of the physical examination is normal. A urinalysis performed reveals gross blood with clots, and a microscopic analysis is positive for red blood cell casts.

SELECT THE ONE BEST ANSWER TO THE FOLLOWING QUESTIONS:

271. The most likely diagnosis in this patient is:
    a) hemorrhagic pyelonephritis
    b) IgA nephropathy
    c) poststreptococcal glomerulonephritis
    d) hemorrhagic cystitis
    e) membranous glomerulonephritis

272. The most appropriate specific treatment(s) for the patient described above is(are):
    a) penicillin
    b) gentamicin
    c) prednisone
    d) a and b
    e) none of the above

273. Which of the following statements regarding the condition described above is(are) true?
    a) most patients eventually develop end-stage renal failure and require dialysis
    b) the prognosis depends on how aggressive the antecedent streptococcal infection is treated
    c) most patients with the acute disease recover completely within 1–2 years
    d) 5–20% of patients with the acute disease show progressive renal damage
    e) c and d

274. Which of the following is(are) complications of the condition described above?
    a) hypertensive encephalopathy
    b) congestive cardiac failure
    c) acute renal failure
    d) a and b
    e) all of the above

275. The most common cause of chronic renal failure is:
    a) glomerulonephritis
    b) chronic pyelonephritis
    c) hypertensive renal disease
    d) diabetes mellitus

    e) congenital anomalies

276. The least common cause of chronic renal failure among those causes listed below is:
    a) glomerulonephritis
    b) chronic pyelonephritis
    c) hypertensive renal disease
    d) diabetes mellitus
    e) congenital anomalies

277. Which of the following antihypertensive agents are CONTRAINDICATED in patients with chronic renal disease?
    a) hydrochlorothiazide-triamterene
    b) furosemide
    c) prazosin
    d) nifedipine
    e) alpha-methyldopa

278. The major cause of death in patients with chronic renal failure is:
    a) uremia
    b) malignant hypertension
    c) hyperkalemia-induced arrhythmias
    d) myocardial infarction
    e) subarachnoid hemorrhage

279. The anemia associated with chronic renal failure usually is:
    a) hypochromic
    b) macrocytic
    c) normochromic-normocytic
    d) microcytic
    e) hypochromic-microcytic

280. Which of the following may be indicated in the treatment of a patient with chronic renal failure?
    a) limitation of dietary protein
    b) sodium supplementation
    c) calcium supplementation
    d) a and b
    e) all of the above

ANSWERS

271. C. This patient has poststreptococcal glomerulonephritis. Poststreptococcal glomerulonephritis is the most common cause of glomerulonephritis. Nephritis may begin as early as 2 weeks after the initial streptococcal infection. In patients with mild disease, there may be no signs or symptoms. In more severe disease, malaise, headache, mild fever, flank pain, edema, hypertension, and even pulmonary edema may occur. Oliguria is common. The urine is often described as "bloody", "coffee-colored," or "smoky."[1]

A red blood cell cast found in the urinary sediment is pathognomonic for glomerulonephritis. Although other studies, including ESR and ASO titers are usually elevated, this is unnecessary for confirmation of the diagnosis.

272. E. The primary treatment of acute glomerulonephritis is symptomatic.[1] Although penicillin should be used to eradicate the B-hemolytic streptococci, this does not influence the prognosis. Prednisone is of no known value in the treatment of acute glomerulonephritis.

Symptomatic treatment should include bed rest. Protein restriction is indicated if the BUN or creatinine level is elevated. Fluid overload may be treated with loop diuretics such as furosemide. Hemodialysis is indicated if acute renal insufficiency is present and volume overload is unresponsive to more conservative measures.[1,2]

273. E. Most patients with acute glomerulonephritis recover completely within 1–2 years; 5 to 20% show progressive renal damage.[1] The treatment of the antecedent streptococcal infection has no bearing on the prognosis.

274. E. Complications of acute glomerulonephritis include hypertensive encephalopathy, congestive cardiac failure, and acute renal failure.[1]

275. A. The most common cause of chronic renal failure is glomerulonephritis.[2] Other causes include hypertensive renal disease, diabetes mellitus, congenital anomalies, and obstructive uropathies.

276. B. Chronic pyelonephritis is the least likely cause of chronic renal failure. Chronic pyelonephritis rarely leads to chronic renal failure in the absence of obstruction.[1]

277. A. Potassium-sparing diuretics such as hydrochlorothiazide-triamterene should not be administered to patients with chronic renal failure due to the worsening of hyperkalemia. All of the other agents including hydrochlorothiazide (alone), furosemide, prazosin, nifedipine and alpha-methyldopa are safe in chronic renal failure. The dosage of these agents may, however, have to be reduced.

278. D. The major causes of death in patients with chronic renal failure are myocardial infarction and cerebrovascular accidents, secondary to atherosclerosis and arteriolosclerosis. Uremia itself can usually be controlled by dialysis or renal transplantation.[1,2] Hypertension is usually controllable by step-care therapy. Arrhythmias, although they do occur in these patients, are not the major cause of death. Subarachnoid hemorrhage, as a subset of cerebrovascular accident, does occur, but is less common as a cause of death than myocardial infarction.

279. C. The anemia of chronic renal failure is usually normochromic-normocytic.[2] Hematocrit often starts to decrease when the serum creatinine reaches 200–300 μmol/L (2–3 mg/dl), or when the glomerular filtration rate has decreased to about 20–30 ms/min. The etiology of the normochromic-normocytic anemia is probably a decreased synthesis of erythropoietin by the kidney.

280. E. Treatment of chronic renal failure may include any of the following:[1]
   a) limitation of dietary protein
   b) careful control of water balance: fluid intake should be sufficient to maintain adequate urine volume, but no attempt should be made to force diuresis. If edema is present a cautious trial of furosemide or ethacrynic acid is indicated, with careful monitoring of the serum electrolytes.
   c) electrolyte supplementation/restriction: sodium supplements may be required to restore sodium losses. Potassium intake may have to be restricted or supplemented. In severe hyperkalemia, acute measures to remove potassium may be required.
   d) mineral supplementation/restriction: in the presence of bone disease (renal osteodystrophy), phosphate binders and supplemental calcium may be necessary.

e) treatment of anemia: iron is of little value unless iron deficiency exists.

f) hypertension control: blood pressure should be controlled with a combination of antihypertensive agents (see section on hypertension for detailed discussion).

g) dialysis and transplanation: hemodialysis or peritoneal dialysis may be used for long-term treatment of chronic renal failure. Although cyclosporine is associated with a decreased incidence of graft rejection, it is nephrotoxic and must be used with extreme caution.

SUMMARY OF THE DIAGNOSIS AND TREATMENT OF GLOMERULONEPHRITIS AND CHRONIC RENAL FAILURE

1. **Acute glomerulonephritis:**
   a) most common cause: poststreptococcal
   b) symptoms and signs: malaise, headache, anorexia, low-grade fever, mild generalized edema, mild hypertension, gross hematuria with red blood cell casts and proteinuria, evidence of impaired renal function
   c) treatment: symptomatic
   d) prognosis: most patients eventually recover completely

2. **Chronic renal failure:**
   a) symptoms, signs, and laboratory findings: weakness, fatigability, headaches, anorexia, nausea and vomiting, pruritis, polyuria, nocturia, hypertension, congestive cardiac failure, anemia, azotemia, acidosis, elevated serum potassium, elevated serum phosphate, decreased serum calcium, decreased serum protein
   b) treatment: protein restriction, careful fluid balance, potassium restriction or supplementation, sodium supplementation, calcium supplementation, phosphate removal, control of hypertension, hemodialysis or peritoneal dialysis, kidney transplantation

References

1. Krupp M. Disorders of the kidneys. In: Schroeder S, Krupp M, Tierney L, McPhee S, eds. Current medical diagnosis and treatment. Norwalk: Appleton and Lange, 1989: 572–581.

2. Brenner B, Lazarus M. Chronic renal failure: pathophysiologic and clinical considerations. In: Braunwald E, Isselbacher K, Petersdorf R, Wilson J, Martin J, Fauci A, eds. Harrison's principles of internal medicine. 11th Ed. New York: McGraw-Hill, 1987: 1155–1161.

Obstetrics and Gynecology

PROBLEM 33: A 25-YEAR-OLD PRIMIGRAVIDA, ACCOMPANIED BY HER HUSBAND, WHO PRESENTS TO YOUR OFFICE TO DISCUSS A BIRTH PLAN

A 25-year-old female presents to your office at 14 weeks gestation for her first prenatal visit. She is accompanied by her husband. They have come in to discuss a birth plan. She has heard that you are an excellent physician, and she would like you to look after her.

SELECT THE ONE BEST ANSWER TO THE FOLLOWING QUESTIONS:

281. When asked about birth plans you would respond:
    a) birth plans are not a good idea; most times something goes wrong and everybody ends up disappointed
    b) birth plans are not a good idea; they frequently lead to unresolved guilt
    c) birth plans should be avoided; couples who draw up a birth plan have babies with higher morbidity rates than those with no birth plans
    d) birth plans are an excellent idea; everything usually goes exactly as planned
    e) birth plans are a good idea; they involve the couple in the preparation for their baby and can be a very important part of the prenatal, intrapartum, and postpartum care.

282. The couple wish to discuss their feelings and thoughts about a number of issues. The first is electronic fetal monitoring. The couple has been told that in some hospitals, and with some physicians, routine continuous electronic fetal monitoring is standard procedure.
    Which of the following statements regarding continuous electronic fetal monitoring in low risk patients is true?
    a) the perinatal mortality rate in patients who undergo continuous fetal monitoring (CFM) is lower than in those patients who do not
    b) the perinatal morbidity rate in patients who undergo CFM is lower than in those patients who do not
    c) the incidence of cesarean section in those patients who undergo CFM is not statistically different from those who do not

    d) there is no significant difference in perinatal outcomes between those patients who undergo CFM and those patients who do not
    e) the incidence of admission to the intensive care nursery is greater in those patients who do not

283. The next question the couple wish to discuss is the use of ultrasound in pregnancy. Which of the following statements regarding the use of ultrasound in pregnancy is false?
    a) the safety of diagnostic ultrasound in pregnancy has been established
    b) no well controlled study has yet proved that routine scanning of all prenatal patients will improve the outcome of pregnancy
    c) estimation of gestational age by ultrasound for confirmation of clinical dating for patients who are to undergo elective repeat cesarean section should be performed
    d) vaginal bleeding of undetermined etiology in pregnancy should be assessed by ultrasound examination
    e) significant uterine size/clinical dates discrepancy is an absolute indication for diagnostic ultrasound

284. The routine administration of intravenous solutions is the next question that the couple asks you about. Which of the following statements regarding the use of intravenous solutions in labor is false?
    a) the use of routine intravenous solutions may limit ambulation in the first stage of labor
    b) if an epidural anesthetic is to be administered, an intravenous line must be in place
    c) there is a long first stage of labor, with ketones present in the urine

d) it is difficult to start an intravenous line in a woman who needs blood or fluid secondary to a postpartum hemorrhage; this is a rational reason for the routine use of intravenous infusions

e) none of the above statements are false

285. The conservation changes to the topic of epidural anesthesia. Regarding epidural anesthesia, which of the following statements is false?

a) before an epidural anesthetic is given, the patient should have an intravenous crystalloid solution running

b) before an epidural anesthetic is given, an internal electronic fetal monitor should be applied

c) epidural anesthesia is unlikely to prolong the second stage of labor

d) inadvertent dural puncture and spinal headache occur in 1–2% of patients receiving epidural analgesia

e) the incidence of operative vaginal delivery appears to be increased when epidural anesthesia is used

ANSWER THE FOLLOWING QUESTIONS ACCORDING TO THE CODE:

A: 1, 2, and 3 are correct
B: 1 and 3 are correct
C: 2 and 4 are correct
D: Only 4 is correct
E: All of the above are correct

286. The couple then ask you about the psychoprophylaxis of labor (Lamaze technique). Which of the following statements regarding the psychoprophylaxis of labor is(are) true?

1) patients who utilize the Lamaze technique require decreased obstetric analgesia

2) the Lamaze technique emphasizes body-building exercises, breathing techniques, and comfort aids

3) pelvic floor exercises are an important part of the Lamaze program

4) during the second stage of labor, panting alternates with pushing

287. The couple's last question is regarding episiotomy. They have been told that many of the episiotomies that are done in a modern obstetric practice are unnecessary. Which of the following statements regarding episiotomy is(are) true?

1) episiotomy pain may be more severe and long-lasting than the pain of vaginal and perineal lacerations

2) healing of episiotomy repairs is more rapid than healing of vaginal and perineal tears

3) dyspareunia is more common after episiotomy than after vaginal lacerations and perineal tears

4) episiotomy reduces the rate of subsequent pelvic relaxation problems

288. Which of the following are definite indications for the performance of an episiotomy?

1) fetal distress in the second stage of labor

2) significant maternal cardiac disease

3) prophylactic forceps

4) a prolonged second stage of labor with no other abnormalities

ANSWERS

281. E. Birth plans are an integral part of family-centered maternity care (FCMC). Family-centered maternity care enables couples to go through a labor and delivery in an informal setting, with as little intervention as necessary. Family-centered maternity care involves the husband or "significant other" as a coach in labor and allows for immediate bonding of infant to mother and father.

Breastfeeding is encouraged, and rooming-in is available. A trusting doctor-couple relationship is essential to a successful family-centered maternity care. If the couple is confident that the doctor will discuss any proposed intervention, the need for it, and the risks and benefits of the intervention, a deviation from the birth plan usually does not produce any major problem. If the couple is involved in the decision-making process throughout labor and delivery, unresolved guilt over having "failed" in any particular way does not become an issue.

282. D. A definitive prospective comparison of selective and universal continuous fetal monitoring has been completed.[1] In this study, the effects of using continuous intrapartum electronic fetal monitoring in all pregnancies, as compared to using it only in high risk pregnancies, was studied.

Universal continuous monitoring was associated with a small but significant increase in the incidence of delivery by cesarean section because of fetal distress. Perinatal outcomes as assessed by intrapartum stillbirths, low Apgar scores, need for assisted ventilation of the newborn, admission to the intensive care nursery, or neonatal seizures were not significantly different in the two groups.[1]

The conclusion from this study was that not all pregnancies, and particularly not those considered at low risk of perinatal complications, need continuous electronic fetal monitoring during labor.[1]

283. A. The safety of ultrasound in pregnancy has not been established.[2] The American College of Obstetricians and Gynecologists has urged that "only necessary or indicated diagnostic studies should be ordered."[3] No well controlled study has proved that routine scanning of all prenatal patients will improve the outcome of pregnancy. At this time, ultrasound in pregnancy should only be ordered when there is a specific indication.

284. D. The use of intravenous solutions in labor is indicated when (1) an epidural anesthetic is about to be administered and (2) there is a long first stage of labor, with ketones present in the urine.

The routine use of intravenous solutions may limit ambulation in the first stage of labor. The routine use of intravenous solutions, therefore, is not indicated in the low-risk patient.

A previous postpartum hemorrhage is not a rational reason for starting an intravenous prophylactically.[4]

285. C. Epidural anesthesia may very well prolong the second stage of labor as the mother does not have the urge to bear down and push that she would have without the epidural.[4] Operative vaginal delivery (forceps and vacuum extraction) is increased with epidural anesthesia.[5]

Epidural anesthesia should be preceded by the placement of an intravenous solution with a crystalloid running (to avoid maternal hypotension), and the placement of an internal electronic fetal monitor.[4]

One to two percent of patients receiving epidural anesthesia will experience an inadvertent dural puncture and spinal headache.[4]

286. E. Patients who utilize the Lamaze technique (psychoprophylaxis of labor) require less obstetric analgesia.

The Lamaze technique emphasizes body-building exercises, breathing techniques, and comfort aids. Pelvic floor strengthening exercises are an important part of the program. During the second stage of labor, panting alternates with pushing in patients utilizing this technique.[4]

287. B. Episiotomy is a procedure that has often been performed without justification. Although benefits including ease of repair, fewer third degree tears, prevention of fetal brain injury, and shortening of the second stage of labor have been reported,[6] most of these observations are based on subjective impressions rather than objective studies. Objectively, it would appear routine episiotomy neither decreases the risk of third degree tears nor the risk of pelvic relaxation in later life. Although it does shorten the second stage of labor, this does not appear to be detrimental in the absence of fetal distress. Objective studies have determined that (1) episiotomy pain is more severe and long-lasting than the pain of vaginal and even perineal lacerations, (2) healing of episiotomy repairs is not more rapid than healing of vaginal and perineal tears, and (3) dyspareunia is more, rather than less, common after episiotomy than after vaginal, lacerations or perineal tears.[4,7,8]

288. A. Definite indications for episiotomy include fetal distress in the second stage of labor, significant maternal cardiac disease, prophylactic forceps, premature birth, or infants in the breech presentation when vaginal delivery is anticipated.

Contraindications to episiotomy include inflammatory bowel disease, lymphogranuloma venereum, or severe perineal scarring or malformation. Complications of episiotomy include excessive blood loss and infection.

Episiotomy rates can be reduced by following these indications and contraindications and avoiding the routine use of this operative procedure. Vaginal and perineal tears can be avoided by perineal massage and stretching exercises before delivery. Communication with the patient during perineal stretching will help reduce the degree and number of tears during childbirth. Also, if professional urgency to deliver the baby rapidly is controlled, the extra time that the fetal head is on the perineum provides enough time for a great deal of stretching and the greater possibility of an intact perineum as a result.[4,9]

SUMMARY OF IMPORTANT CONSIDERATIONS IN NONINTERVENTION OBSTETRICS

1. **Birth Plans**: Involve couple in detailed preparation for birth; should foster excellent doctor-patient communication

2. **Electronic fetal monitoring**: Continous fetal monitoring not necessary for low-risk pregnancies; auscultation or intermittent fetal monitoring will provide comparable information

3. **Obstetric ultrasound**: Routine ultrasound not recommended; specific indication should be present

4. **Intravenous therapy**: Routine intravenous not necessary; specific indication should be present

5. **Anesthesia**: Epidural anesthetic is analgesic of choice; it should be offered to a patient if needed. Lamaze birth preparation classes may decrease the need for obstetric anesthesia

6. **Episiotomy**: An episiotomy does not heal any quicker and is often more painful and associated with a greater incidence of dyspareunia than vaginal and perineal lacerations. It is not associated with a decreased risk of third degree laceration, and it does not decrease the risk of pelvic relaxation in later life. It does shorten the second stage of labor, but a longer second stage does not appear to be detrimental in the absence of fetal distress.

References

1. Leveno K, et al. A prospective comparison of selective and universal fetal monitoring in 34,995 pregnancies. N Engl J Med 1986; 315: 10–16.

2. Hobbins JC, Berkowitz RL, Hohler CW. How safe is ultrasound in obstetrics? Comptemporary Ob/Gyn Special Issue, 1979; 63–74.

3. American College of Obstetricians and Gynecologists: Diagnostic ultrasound in obstetrics and gynecology. ACOG Technical Bulletin 1981: 63.

4. Klein M. Controversies in obstetrical management and maternal care. Government of Quebec, 1988.

5. Hoult IJ, MacLennan AH, Carrier LE. Lumbar epidural analgesic in labor: relation to fetal malposition and instrument delivery. Br Med J 1977; 1: 14–16.

6. Banta D, Thacker S. The risks and benefits of episiotomy: a review. BIRTH 1982; 9: 25–30.

7. Kitzinger S, ed. Episiotomy—physical and emotional aspects. London: The National Childbirth Trust. 1981.

8. Kitzinger S, Walters R. Some women's experience of episiotomy. London: The National Childbirth Trust. 1981.

9. Klein M. Rites of passage: episiotomy and the second stage of labor. Can Fam Physician 1988; 34; 2019–2025.

PROBLEM 34: A 28-YEAR-OLD PRIMIGRAVIDA IN LABOR

A 28-year-old primigravida at term is admitted to the delivery suite having 5-minute contractions. She is found to be 3 cm dilated. When examined 5 hours later she has only progressed to 4 cm and 75% effaced. The station is at station 0. Her contractions are mild to moderate and have become more irregular during the past 3 hours. She has been up walking around, but this has not helped. Her membranes are intact and bulging. The fetal heart rate tracing is reactive.

SELECT THE ONE BEST ANSWER TO THE FOLLOWING QUESTIONS:

289. The most appropriate course of action at this time would be to:
   a) perform an amniotomy
   b) begin oxytocin stimulation for hypotonic labor
   c) call the anesthesiologist to administer an epidural anesthetic
   d) reassure the patient that her contractions will eventually pick up
   e) none of the above

The appropriate action is taken for the patient described in question 288. After 4 further hours, her contractions are still mild to moderate and irregular in frequency. The cervix is now 5 cm dilated and 85% effaced. The intrapartum fetal monitor strip is reactive.

290. The most appropriate course of action at this time would be to:
    a) perform an amniotomy
    b) begin oxytocin stimulation for hypotonic labor
    c) call the anesthesiologist to administer an epidural anesthetic and prepare for cesarean section
    d) tell the patient and nursing staff to relax; everything takes time
    e) none of the above

291. The patient progresses to full cervical dilatation. After 1 1/2 hours in the second stage of labor she is exhausted. The head is at station +3 and is visible at the introitus. The occiput is straight anterior. The fetal heart rate tracing is excellent. Her contractions are strong and every 2 minutes apart.

    The most appropriate course of action at this time would be to:
    a) increase the oxytocin
    b) explain to the patient that the second stage is usually a long difficult stage and that she'll just have to try a little harder
    c) deliver the baby by outlet forceps
    d) deliver the baby with a vacuum extractor
    e) either c or d

292. Which of the following statements regarding the use of the vacuum extractor and the outlet forceps in the second stage of labor are true?
    a) the perinatal morbidity of infants delivered with outlet forceps is higher than infants delivered with the vacuum extractor
    b) the perinatal morbidity of infants delivered with the vacuum extractor is higher than infants delivered with the outlet forceps
    c) intracranial compression with the vacuum extractor is higher than with outlet forceps delivery
    d) the Apgar scores of infants delivered by the vacuum extractor is higher than infants delivered by outlet forceps
    e) the perinatal morbidity and Apgar scores of infants delivered by outlet forceps and vacuum extraction are similar

293. Which of the following criteria is essential before a forceps delivery can be referred to as outlet forceps?
    a) the scalp is or has been visible at the introitus (without the need to separate the labia)
    b) the skull has reached the pelvic floor

    c) the sagittal suture is in the anteroposterior diameter of the pelvis
    d) a and b
    e) all of the above

ANSWER THE FOLLOWING QUESTIONS ACCORDING TO THE CODE:

A: 1, 2, and 3 are correct
B: 1 and 3 are correct
C: 2 and 4 are correct
D: Only 4 is correct
E: All of the above are correct

294. Which of the following is(are) maternal indications for forceps delivery?
    1) maternal exhaustion
    2) severe cardiac or pulmonary problems accompanied by maternal dyspnea
    3) intercurrent debilitating illness
    4) second stage of labor > 45 minutes in a primigravida or 30 minutes in a multigravida

295. Which of the following is(are) fetal indications for forceps delivery if all other criteria have been met?
    1) fetal heart tones (FHT) with a persistent rate of less than 100 beats/minute or more than 160 beats/minute
    2) presence of variable decelerations on the fetal monitor strip
    3) passage of meconium-stained amniotic fluid in cephalic presentation
    4) presence of early decelerations on the fetal monitor strip

296. Which of the following conditions must be met before a forceps delivery is attempted?
    1) the cervix must be fully dilated
    2) the membranes must be ruptured
    3) the head must be engaged
    4) the bladder should be empty

ANSWERS

289. A. This patient has hypotonic labor. Once the diagnosis of active labor followed by hypotonic uterine dysfunction has been made and the head is engaged, the membranes, if intact, should probably be ruptured. Amniotomy may augment and shorten labor. The patient should be kept in the Fowler's position after amniotomy to facilitate drainage of the amniotic fluid. There is some dis-

agreement among authorities on the value of amniotomy.[1] If performed in an attempt to stimulate labor, it should be performed under aseptic conditions, and only after the head is fully engaged.

Oxytocin administration should only be considered after the membranes have been ruptured and there is still no progress in labor.

There is no indication for an epidural anesthetic at this time.

Although you could theoretically wait and see if good labor would ensue, it is reasonable to suggest that this patient has hypotonic labor that should be stimulated by amniotomy.

290. B. In this patient, amniotomy has not been of much help.

Oxytocin stimulation for hypotonic labor should now be considered. The following criteria should be adhered to before and during oxytocin administration for hypotonic labor.[1]

a) The patient must be in true labor, with cervical effacement and dilatation. It is suggested that cervical dilatation be at least 3 cm.

b) There must be no evidence of a mechanical obstruction to obstruct a safe delivery.

c) The fetus should be in a normal vertex presentation.

d) The fetus should be a singleton.

e) There should be no gross hydramnios.

f) The patient should be parity less than or equal to five.

g) The patient should not have a previous uterine scar.

h) The fetal condition should be good.

i) There should be no evidence of tetanic contractions following the initiation of oxytocin.

j) There should be continuous electronic monitoring of the fetal heart and uterine activity.

291. E. The mother is exhausted. Her contractions are strong and 2 minutes apart, and therefore not hypotonic. It would be inappropriate to increase the rate of Syntocinon infusion.

The head is at station +3 and is visible at the introitus. Therefore, delivery of the infant by either an outlet forceps or a vacuum extractor would be appropriate.

In a mother who has been pushing for 1 1/2 hours and is exhausted, it is inappropriate to advise her that she should try a little harder.

292. E. The perinatal morbidity rates and Apgar scores of infants delivered by outlet forceps and vacuum extraction are similar.

The vacuum extractor is commonly used in Europe and Canada, but uncommonly used in the United States. The Silastic vacuum extactor has the advantage over older models of being able to be immediately applied to the fetal head. The pressure can be completely released between contractions. There is lower intracranial compression with the vacuum extractor, but there is no significant difference in perinatal morbidity or Apgar scores between infants delivered by the vacuum extractor and the outlet forceps.

In the hands of experienced operators, either instrument is effective and safe.[2]

293. E. Forceps deliveries can be classified as follows:[3]

A. **Outlet forceps:** Outlet forceps is the application of forceps when the scalp is or has been visible at the introitus (without the need to separate the labia), the skull has reached the pelvic floor, and the sagittal suture is in the anteroposterior diameter of the pelvis.

B. **Low forceps:** Low forceps is the application of forceps when the skull has reached a station of +3 (at or immediately above the pelvic floor) and the sagittal suture is in the anteroposterior or an oblique diameter of the pelvis.

C. **Midforceps:** Midforceps is the application of forceps when the head is engaged but has not reached a station of +3 or the occiput has not rotated as far as the anterior oblique diameter.

D. **High forceps:** High forceps is the application of forceps at any time prior to engagement of the head. There are few, if any, indications for high forceps deliveries in present day obstetric practice.

E. **Prophylactic forceps:** Prophylactic forceps is the use of outlet forceps (not low or midforceps) and episiotomy in order to prevent injury to the fetal head and pelvic floor and to reduce maternal stress

294. A. Maternal indications for outlet forceps include maternal exhaustion, severe cardiac or pulmonary problems accompanied by dyspnea, and intercurrent debilitating illness.[3]

A second stage of labor greater than 45 minutes in a primigravida or 30 minutes in a multigravida is not an indication for forceps delivery. Maternal exhaustion, rather than the definitive length of time, is the more appropriate determinator of whether or not forceps should be employed. Obviously, if the second stage of labor is greatly prolonged (> 1 1/2 hours in a patient who has the urge to push and is not under the influence of epidural anesthesia), delivery by forceps or vacuum extraction should be considered.

295. B. The major fetal indication for termination of the second stage is fetal distress. This fetal distress may be manifested by (1) fetal heart tones (FHT) with a rate of less than 100 beats/minute or more than 160 beats/minute, (2) late deceleration patterns, (3) a grossly irregular fetal monitor pattern, (4) excessive fetal movements, or (5) the passage of meconium-stained amniotic fluid in cephalic presentation. [3]

Variable decelerations (cord compression) are not necessarily an indication for termination of the second stage of labor. This is especially true if there is quick recovery to baseline after the deceleration.

Early decelerations (head compression) are not an indication for the termination of the second stage of labor.

When faced with fetal distress, one must decide which method of delivery is preferable for the mother and baby at that time, given the condition of both. In many cases cesarean section is preferable to a forceps delivery.

296. E. The use of forceps is permissible only when ALL of the following conditions prevails, regardless of the urgent need for delivery. [1]
   a) the cervix must be fully dilated
   b) the membranes must be ruptured
   c) the head must be engaged (preferably deeply engaged to a station below +2
   d) the head must present in either vertex presentation or face presentation with chin anterior
   e) there must be no significant cephalopelvic disproportion
   f) the bladder must be empty

SUMMARY OF SOME ASPECTS OF THE ACTIVE MANAGEMENT OF THE FIRST AND SECOND STAGES OF LABOR

1. **Hypotonic labor:**
   a) establish that patient is in true labor
   b) if in true labor and not progressing, consider amniotomy
   c) if amniotomy performed or membranes have ruptured spontaneously and labor is not progressing consider oxytocin augmentation providing conditions have been fulfilled

2. **Operative vaginal delivery:**
   a) forceps and vacuum equally effective and safe if used properly
   b) follow maternal and fetal indications for operative delivery
   c) if forceps or vacuum is used, conditions for forceps delivery should all be met
   d) if considering operative vaginal delivery for fetal distress or other emergency situation, weigh carefully the risks and benefits of both vaginal and abdominal delivery before making a decision

References

1. Cunningham F, MacDonald P, Gant N. Williams obstetrics. 18th Ed. Norwalk: Appleton and Lange, 1989: 307–439.

2. Fall O, Ryden G, Finnstrom K, Finnstrom O, Leijon I. Forceps or vacuum extraction? A comparison of effects on the newborn infant. Acta Obstet Gynecol Scand 1986; 65(1): 75–80.

3. Danforth D. Operative Delivery. In: Pernoll M, Beson R, eds. Current obstetric and gynecologic diagnosis and treatment. 6th Ed. Norwalk: Appleton and Lange, 1987: 481–495.

PROBLEM 35:   A 23-YEAR-OLD PRIMIGRAVIDA WITH MANY PHYSICAL COMPLAINTS IN PREGNANCY

A 23-year-old primigravida presents for her first prenatal visit at 10-weeks gestation. She complains of nausea lasting most of the day and vomiting twice per day. These symptoms have been present for the past 2 weeks.

SELECT THE ONE BEST ANSWER TO THE FOLLOWING QUESTIONS:

297. Nausea and/or vomiting in pregnancy affects approximately 80% of pregnant women. Current theories suggest that these symptoms are most likely due to:
    a) increased levels of circulating estrogen
    b) increased levels of circulating progesterone
    c) increased levels of human chorionic gonadotrophin
    d) all of the above
    e) none of the above

298. Which of the following SHOULD NOT be part of your initial advice or treatment of this patient?
    a) reassurance that this is a self-limiting condition
    b) small frequent meals
    c) discontinuation of iron therapy if it has been previously prescribed
    d) avoidance of contact with cooking odors or brushing her teeth
    e) the prescription of an antinauseant

ANSWER THE QUESTIONS ACCORDING TO THE CODE:

A: 1, 2, and 3 are correct
B: 1 and 3 are correct
C: 2 and 4 are correct
D: Only 4 is correct
E: All of the above are correct

299. The patient's nausea clears during the following 3 weeks. However, at that time she presents with a 1-week history of constipation. She has had only 1 bowel movement during the past week. Which of the following factors have been implicated as a cause of constipation in pregnancy?
    1) reduced gut motility
    2) mechanical obstruction by the uterus
    3) increased water resorption
    4) increased estrogen levels

300. Therapy for constipation in pregnancy should include:

1) discontinuation of iron therapy if already prescribed
2) increased ingestion of fiber
3) increased fluids
4) increased exercise

301. The constipation clears on your therapeutic suggestions. She presents at 24 weeks with a 3-day history of rectal irritation and pain. You examine her and discover external hemorrhoids (not thrombosed). Your therapy at this time should include:
1) stool softeners
2) sitz baths
3) topical agents
4) mineral oil laxatives

302. The patient is well until 28 weeks. She then presents with a sensation of heartburn. She finds it difficult to sleep at night because of the associated pain. Which of the following should be recommended for relief of this symptom?
1) small frequent meals
2) calcium carbonate
3) elevation of the head of the bed
4) aluminum containing antacids

303. The patient next returns at 32-weeks gestation. Her heartburn has completely resolved but she now has significant edema of her lower extremities. Her blood pressure is 110/70 mmHg, and there is no proteinuria. She continues to work at her job as a teacher. Which of the following would you recommend for relief of this symptom?
1) a mild thiazide diuretic
2) avoidance of prolonged standing
3) complete bed rest
4) wearing support hose

304. The patient's edema improves with your treatment but she presents at 34 weeks with lumber back pain and pain in the area of the pubic symphysis and groin. Which of the following would you recommend for the treatment of this problem?
1) rest
2) acetaminophen if the pain becomes severe
3) the wearing of proper footwear
4) aspirin if the pain becomes severe

305. With your management the back pain and groin pain improve. However, at her next visit at 36 weeks she states that she has been having increased vaginal discharge. Which of the following regarding increased vaginal discharge in pregnancy is(are) TRUE?
1) in most cases the increased vaginal discharge is physiologic
2) physiologic vaginal discharge in pregnancy is caused by increased formation of mucus by cervical glands under the influence of estrogen
3) *Monilia* may be cultured in up to 25% of women approaching term
4) *Monilia* should be treated in both symptomatic and asymptomatic pregnant women

ANSWERS

297. C. and 298. E. Nausea and vomiting are common complaints in pregnancy, especially during the first trimester. Nausea, vomiting, or other gastrointestinal symptoms may occur in up to 50% of pregnant women.[1] Although the etiology has not been definitively established, increased levels of human chorionic gonadotrophin appear to be the most likely explanation.[2]

Nausea in pregnancy should be treated with conservative management if possible. Reassurance, small frequent meals, increased fluids, the avoidance of foods with a high fat content, and an intake of dry foods may be all that is necessary.[2,3] If iron therapy has been started, it should be discontinued.[2] Avoidance of contact with situations that may induce nausea (such as cooking odors) is also recommended.[2]

If persistent vomiting leading to weight loss, ketonuria, or electrolyte imbalance, hospitalization is necessary.[2]

If conservative therapy fails, antinauseants are indicated. In Canada, a combination of doxylamine and pyridoxine (Diclectin) is still available. Dimenhydrinate and meclizine may also be used. Although concern has been expressed regarding the safety of these compounds, there is no evidence suggesting that they are teratogenic or otherwise harmful to the fetus.

299. A. and 300. E. The etiology of constipation in pregnancy is multifactorial. Potential causes include hormonally mediated smooth muscle relaxation, mechanical pressure from the enlarging uterus, increased water resorption from the colon, and iron supplements.[2,4]

Treatment consists of conservative measures including discontinuing iron supplements, increasing the amount of fiber in the diet, increasing the intake of fluids, and increasing the amount of physical activity. If these measures are ineffective, a bulk-forming agent such as psyllium or methylcellulose may be added. Laxatives should be used with caution.[2]

301. A. Hemorrhoids in pregnancy can be a complication of constipation. They are also aggravated by impairment of venous return by the uterus. Treatment consists of the measures previously described to avoid constipation, softening the stools, sitz baths, and if necessary, topical agents.[3] The topical agents of choice include zinc sulfate-hydrocortisone preparations (Anusol) and Tucks (witch-hazel soaked compresses). Mineral oil is not recommended in pregnancy as a laxative as it may interfere with the absorption of lipid-soluble vitamins.

302. A. Heartburn in pregnancy is usually produced by a combination of decreased gastrointestinal motility and uterine compression.[2] This combination results in reflux of gastric contents into the esophagus.

Conservative treatment is similar to nausea in pregnancy. Small, frequent meals and the avoidance of fatty or spicy foods are usually effective.[2] Sleeping with the head of the bed elevated will decrease reflux into the esophagus. If antacids are required, calcium carbonate is the agent of choice. Aluminum-containing preparations, which interfere with the absorption of phosphate and interact with trace minerals are not recommended.[5]

303. C. Edema, a common complication of late pregnancy, occurs because of occlusion of the pelvic veins and inferior vena cava as a result of pressure from the enlarged uterus.[2] Treatment consists of avoiding prolonged standing, elevating her lower extremities, and wearing support hose.[2] In this case, the patient should probably quit her job. Because thiazide diuretics reduce intravascular volume and impede blood flow to the placenta, they are CONTRAINDICATED in pregnancy. Complete bed rest in not necessary, but the patient should try and put her feet up for at least 1 hour three times per day.

304. A. Lumbar back pain in pregnancy is often secondary to a lumbar lordosis created by the weight of

the gravid uterus. This problem should be managed by back education, the wearing of proper footwear, and rest.[2] If the back pain becomes severe and requires analgesia, acetaminophen is the drug of choice. There is no contraindication to the use of this drug in pregnancy. Aspirin may lead to coagulation abnormalities and bleeding problems in the newborn if given close to term; it may also impede labor from starting. Thus, it should be avoided.

Pain in the area of the pubic symphysis and sacroiliac joints is caused by loosening of the ligaments in preparation for birth.[2] Ligamentous laxity facilitates vaginal delivery, but frequently leads to pelvic discomfort and groin ache late in pregnancy. Treatment includes rest, heat, and acetaminophen.

305. A. The most common vaginal discharge in pregnancy is a physiologic discharge. The discharge is caused by increased formation of mucus by the cervical glands under the influence of estrogen.[4]

Monilia may be cultured from the vagina in 25% of women in late pregnancy; *Trichomonas vaginalis* may be cultured in up to 20%.[4] If symptomatic with either of these organisms, the patient should be treated; if she is not symptomatic, she does not require treatment. If treatment is required for *Trichomonas*, metronidazole should be avoided, particularly in the first trimester. The drugs of choice in pregnancy include clotrimazole for trichomoniasis and clotrimazole or miconazole for moniliasis.[6]

Once infection has been excluded, reassurance is usually the only treatment that is required for physiologic discharge. Good hygiene should be encouraged; douching should be discouraged.

SUMMARY OF THE TREATMENT OF COMMON PHYSICAL COMPLAINTS OF PREGNANCY

1. **Nausea/vomiting:**
   a) reassurance
   b) small frequent meals/dry foods
   c) discontinuation of iron therapy
   d) antinauseants if severe

2. **Constipation:**
   a) increased ingestion of fiber
   b) increased fluids
   c) increased exercise

   d) bulk-forming agents—psyllium

3. **Hemorrhoids:**
   a) stool softeners
   b) sitz baths
   c) topical preparations—zinc sulfate/hydrocortisone

4. **Heartburn:**
   a) small frequent meals/avoid fatty, greasy foods
   b) elevation of head of bed
   c) calcium carbonate antacid

5. **Edema:**
   a) avoidance of prolonged standing
   b) elevation of lower extremeties
   c) wearing of support hose
   d) avoidance of diuretics

6. **Back/pelvic/groin pain:**
   a) back education
   b) wearing of proper footwear
   c) rest
   d) acetaminophen for severe discomfort

7. **Vaginal discharge:**
   a) reassurance that increased discharge normal
   b) culture may be indicated

References

1. Biringer A. Antinauseants in pregnancy: teratogens or not? Can Fam Physician 1984; 30: 2123–2125.

2. Biringer A. Common physical discomforts of pregnancy. Can Fam Physician 1988; 34: 1965–1968.

3. Rubin P, Janowitz H. The digestive tract and pregnancy. In: Cheery S, Berkowitz R, Kase N, eds. Medical, surgical, and gynecologic complications of pregnancy. 3rd Ed. Baltimore: Williams & Wilkins, 1985: 196–206.

4. Cunningham FG, MacDonald P, Gant N, eds. Williams obstetrics. 18th Ed. Norwalk: Appleton-Century-Crofts, 1989: 135, 273.

5. Canada. Health and Welfare Canada. The Federal-Provincial Subcommittee on Nutrition, 1986. Nutrition in pregnancy national guidelines. Ottawa: Minister of Supply and Services, 1987: 81.

6. Treatment of sexually transmitted diseases. Med Let 1988; 30(757):5–10.

PROBLEM 36: A 24-YEAR-OLD PRIMIGRAVIDA WHO IS 9 CM DILATED IN THE FIRST STAGE OF LABOR

A 24-year-old female, admitted to the delivery suite 8 hours ago in active labor, in now 9 cm dilated. She is having strong, regular contractions, 2–3 minutes apart, lasting 45–60 seconds. She progressed well to 9 cm but has now been stuck at 9 cm for the past 2 1/2 hours. The station is 0. The intrapartum fetal monitor shows a reactive fetal heart with no decelerations. The membranes ruptured spontaneously 4 hours ago. The fetal position is left occiput anterior. There appears to be significant caput formation. The ischial spines appear prominent.

Her prenatal course was uneventful. The fetal head engaged at 36 weeks gestation. Obstetric ultrasound done at 36 weeks had suggested a baby of 3700 g.

SELECT THE ONE BEST ANSWER TO THE FOLLOWING QUESTIONS:

306. The most likely diagnosis in this patient is:
    a) uterine inertia
    b) inlet contraction
    c) midpelvic contraction
    d) uterine hypotonia
    e) none of the above

307. The treatment of choice in this patient at this time is:
    a) close observation for a further 1–1 1/2 hours
    b) epidural anesthesia and reassessment in 2 hours
    c) oxytocin augmentation of labor
    d) cesarean section
    e) none of the above

308. Cesarean section is most commonly performed in North America today for which of the following reasons?
    a) cephalopelvic disproportion
    b) fetal distress
    c) malpresentation
    d) previous cesarean section
    e) preeclampsia

309. Which one of the following statements regarding the risks and benefits of vaginal delivery after cesarean section (VBAC) is true?
    a) the risk of uterine rupture in VBAC is 5% in low-transverse uterine incisions
    b) the risk of uterine rupture in VBAC is the same as in scheduled repeat cesarean delivery
    c) in symptomatic uterine rupture the fetus usually dies
    d) the maternal mortality rate is higher in repeat cesarean section than in VBAC
    e) maternal morbidity, including febrile morbidity and anemia secondary to blood loss is higher in VBAC

310. In which of the following situations (reason for previous cesarean section) is a trial of labor after cesarean section contraindicated?
    a) cephalopelvic disproportion
    b) failure to progress
    c) fetal distress
    d) breech delivery
    e) none of the above

ANSWER THE FOLLOWING QUESTIONS ACCORDING TO THE CODE:

A: 1, 2, and 3 are correct
B: 1 and 3 are correct
C: 2 and 4 are correct
D: Only 4 is correct
E: All of the above are correct

311. Which of the following are(is) exclusion criteria for a trial of labor after previous cesarean section?
    1) classic cesarean incision
    2) prior incision of unknown type
    3) inadequate hospital facilities
    4) contracted pelvis

312. Which of the following guidelines should be followed in the management of VBAC delivery?
    1) frequent or continuous electronic fetal monitoring should be performed
    2) an experienced physician should remain in attendance throughout labor and delivery
    3) the patient should be typed and screened for two units of packed red blood cells
    4) the patient should be maintained on intravenous fluids throughout labor

ANSWERS

306. C. This patient most likely has a midpelvic contraction. Uterine inertia (uterine hypotonia) is unlikely because of the presence of strong, regular

contractions lasting 45–60 seconds. Inlet disproportion is unlikely because the fetal head was engaged at 36 weeks and is station 0 on examination.

Midpelvic contraction should be suspected if the AP diameter of the pelvis is short, the ischial spines are prominent (as in this patient), and the baby is large (3600 g at 36 weeks in this patient.)[1]

307. D. As this patient has a midpelvic contraction, the treatment of choice at this time is cesarean section. Nothing would be gained by waiting, and the possibility of fetal morbidity would be increased. An epidural anesthetic could certainly be given in preparation for the cesarean section. Oxytocin stimulation at this time would not be indicated; it would simply increase the risk of tetanic contractions and subsequent fetal distress.

Indications for cesarean section include pelvic contraction (inlet, midpelvic, and outlet); uterine inertia that does not respond to oxytocin or in which oxytocin is contraindicated; placenta previa; placenta abruption; malposition and malpresentation (posterior chin, transverse lie, and brow presentation), preeclampsia when induction not feasible or when induction failed; fetal distress; cord prolapse; some cases of diabetes mellitus and erythroblastosis; cervical dystocia; and previous uterine incision.[2]

308. D. The most common reason for cesarean section in North America today is previous cesarean section. It was previously thought that "once a section, always a section." This has been the primary reason for the rapid increase in incidence of cesarean section in the United States, rising from 4.5% of all deliveries in 1965 to 23% of all deliveries in 1985.[1] Repeat cesarean section accounts for nearly 40% of all cesarean sections performed today in the United States. Despite the American College of Obstetricians and Gynecologists (ACOG) guidelines on repeat cesarean section (to be discussed in a subsequent question), the incidence of vaginal delivery after cesarean section is still less than 7%.[3]

309. B. The potential for uterine rupture through the prior cesarean scar during labor is the primary risk in VBAC delivery.[4]

The incidence of uterine rupture is approximately 4% for the classical vertical cesarean incision and less than 0.5% for the low-transverse uterine incision.[4] Uterine rupture through a prior

cesarean scar may occur before or during labor. The risk of rupture through a prior low-segment transverse uterine incision is no greater in VBAC delivery following a trial of labor than in scheduled repeat cesarean delivery.[4]

Rupture may be symptomatic or asymptomatic. Surprisingly, the fetus usually fares well in both symptomatic and asymptomatic rupture. Studies done also revealed no significantly increased incidence of fetal distress during VBAC delivery. The current risk to the fetus from a ruptured uterus during VBAC delivery is lower than the fetal risk in a routine vaginal delivery.[4]

Maternal morbidity, including febrile morbidity and anemia secondary to blood loss, is reduced.[4] The incidence of iatrogenic premature delivery and the risks associated with maternal anesthesia are also reduced. With VBAC delivery, hospital stays are shorter, as are postpartum recovery periods. The maternal mortality rate is 27 times lower with VBAC delivery than with repeat cesarean.[4]

310. E. None of the above. Cephalopelvic disproportion, failure to progress, breech delivery, and fetal distress are not contraindications to a trial of labor after previous cesarean section.[5]

In a recent multicenter trial, 74% of women who had had a previous cesarean section delivered vaginally.[5]

311. E. All of the above are exclusion criteria for a trial of labor. A trial of labor is contraindicated in patients who have had a classic cesarean incision, a low-segment vertical incision or T-shaped extension of low-segment transverse incision, a prior incision of unknown type, a contracted pelvis or recurrent obstetric indication for cesarean delivery, inadequate hospital facilities or personnel for emergency delivery, and the patient's refusal to consent.[4]

312. E. The following are guidelines for the management of VBAC delivery:[4]

1. "Early in the prenatal course, the physician and the patient should discuss the option of a trial of labor.
2. "The patient should be admitted in early labor, typed and screened for 2 units of packed red blood cells, maintained without oral food, and given maintenance intravenous fluids.

3. "Frequent or continuous electronic fetal monitoring should be performed.
4. "Consent should be obtained for a vaginal delivery with possible emergency cesarean delivery.
5. "An experienced physician remains in attendance throughout labor and delivery.
6. "A surgeon, anesthesiologist, and operating room personnel are notified and remain available for emergency cesarean delivery in case of uterine rupture."

SUMMARY OF VBAC DELIVERY

1. **Current incidence**: 7%; if ACOG guidelines followed, this could theoretically be increased to 70%

2. Uterine rupture no more common in VBAC delivery than in scheduled repeat cesarean delivery (0.5%)

3. **Benefits of VBAC**: reduced maternal morbidity and maternal mortality, decreased incidence of iatrogenic premature delivery, reduced costs

4. A trial of labor may be reasonable in patients who have had up to three previous cesarean sections;[5] oxytocin induction of labor is not contraindicated with trial of labor

References

1. Cunningham FG, MacDonald P, Gant N, eds. Williams obstetrics. 18th Ed. Norwalk: Appleton and Lange, 1989: 341–392, 441–459.

2. Danforth D. Operative delivery. In: Pernoll M, Benson R, eds. Current obstetrics and gynecologic diagnosis and treatment. 6th Ed. Norwalk: Appleton and Lange, 1987: 498–500.

3. Placek PJ, Taffel SM, Moien M. Cesarean rate increases in 1985. Am J Public Health 1987; 77: 241–242.

4. Haq C. Vaginal birth after cesarean delivery. Am Fam Physician 1988; 37(6): 167–171.

5. Flamm B, et al. Vaginal birth after cesarean section: results of a multicenter study. Am J Obstet Gynecol 1988; 158: 1079–1084.

PROBLEM 37: A 26-YEAR-OLD HEALTHY PRIMIGRAVIDA IN THE THIRD TRIMESTER OF PREGNANCY

A 26-year-old primigravida, a new patient to your practice, presents at 28-weeks gestation. She has just moved to your community and you have been recommended as a physician. As part of the first visit, you take time to discuss fetal assessment in the third trimester of pregnancy. You begin your discussion with prenatal testing which is usually recommended in the latter part of the second trimester. Your first concern is whether or not this patient has been screened for gestational diabetes.

SELECT THE ONE BEST ANSWER TO THE FOLLOWING QUESTIONS:

313. Screening for gestational diabetes is recommended by some authorities. Which of the following statements regarding screening for gestational diabetes is false?
    a) a 50-g glucose load should be administered to all pregnant women between 24 and 28 weeks to screen for gestational diabetes
    b) a value greater than or equal to 7.8 mmol/L (140 mg%) should be followed by a 100-g glucose tolerance test
    c) patients with gestational diabetes mellitus are at risk for fetal macrosomia
    d) patients with gestational diabetes are at increased risk for later overt diabetes mellitus
    e) the sensitivity of the test is higher in patients in the nonfasting state than in the fasting state

314. The patient discussed in the question above has a 50-g glucose screen performed. The result is 8.3 mmol/L. A 100-g glucose tolerance test is performed and the following results are obtained: fasting— 6.0 mmol/L (108 mg/dl), 1 hour— 10.8 mmol/L (195 mg%), 2 hours— 9.6 mmol/L (163 mg%), and 3 hours— 8.0 mmol/L (144 mg%).
    Which of the following statements about this patient is correct?

a) this patient has gestational diabetes; however, no treatment is required
b) this patient does not have gestational diabetes
c) this patient has gestational diabetes; treatment should be begun with diet and insulin therapy
d) this patient has gestational diabetes; treatment should be begun with diet alone
e) this patient has gestational diabetes; treatment should be begun with diet and an oral hypo-glycemic agent

315. The patient calls you one evening in her 35th week of pregnancy. She says that she hasn't felt her baby move for the past 24 hours. At that time, you should:
a) tell her not to worry about it; all babies stop moving for periods of time
b) tell her that everything is probably all right, but ask her to check with you in the morning
c) tell her that everything is probably all right but that a nonstress test should probably be done within the next day or two; you will arrange it and call her in the morning
d) ask her to go to the hospital for a nonstress test that night
e) ask her to go the hospital for a contraction stress test that night

316. A 36-year-old primigravida at 38-weeks gestation with essential hypertension is twice weekly non-stress testing. Up to this point, all of the nonstress tests that have been performed have been "reac-tive." A "reactive" nonstress test is:
a) a nonstress test in which there are no late decelerations
b) a nonstress test in which there are no variable decelerations
c) a nonstress test in which there are no early decelerations
d) a nonstress test in which there are 3 accelera-tions lasting at least 15 seconds in a 60-minute period
e) none of the above

ANSWER THE FOLLOWING QUESTION ACCORDING TO THE CODE:

A: 1, 2, and 3 are correct
B: 1 and 3 are correct
C: 2 and 4 are correct
D: Only 4 is correct
E: All of the above are correct

317. Which of the following statements regarding the nonstress test is(are) FALSE?
1) the nonstress test has a high false-positive rate
2) the nonstress test has a high false-negative rate
3) the nonstress test is a simple, noninvasive test that is useful in the prediction of fetal hypoxia
4) if the nonstress test is being used to monitor the condition of a fetus, once per week is sufficient

SELECT THE ONE BEST ANSWER TO THE FOLLOWING QUESTION:

318. The patient described in question 316 has just undergone another nonstress test. It is reported as nonreactive. At this time you should:
a) repeat the nonstress test in 72 hours
b) order a contraction stress test
c) repeat the nonstress test in 48 hours
d) order a biophysical profile
e) reassure the patient that nothing is amiss

ANSWER THE FOLLOWING QUESTIONS ACCORDING TO THE CODE:

A: 1, 2, and 3 are correct
B: 1 and 3 are correct
C: 2 and 4 are correct
D: Only 4 is correct
E: All of the above are correct

319. Which of the following parameters is(are) a com-ponent of biophysical profile scoring?
1) gross body movements
2) fetal breathing movements
3) fetal tone
4) amniotic fluid volume

320. In which of the following situations should fetal monitoring (nonstress tests and/or biophysical profiles) be performed?
1) postdate pregnancy
2) chronic hypertension or pregnancy-induced hypertension
3) suspected small-for-gestational-age fetuses
4) normal low-risk pregnancy

ANSWERS

313. E. Gestational diabetes mellitus is carbohydrate intolerance induced by pregnancy.[1] Patients that are diagnosed as having gestational diabetes are at

high risk for fetal macrosomia. They should be carefully evaluated and followed by some of the tests that are described later in this chapter.

The 1984 Workshop-Conference on Gestational Diabetes recommends that all women should be screened using a 50-g oral glucose tolerance test between the 24th and 28th weeks of gestation without regard to time of day or last meal and that a plasma value at 1 hour exceeding 7.8 mmol/L be used as the cutoff for performing a 100-g glucose tolerance test.[2]

The diagnosis of gestational diabetes is made when two of the following four values are met or exceeded : (1) fasting— 5.8 mmol/L (105 mg/dl), 1 hour— 10.6 mmol/L (190 mg/dl), 2 hours— 9.2 mmol/L (165 mg/dl), 3 hours— 8.1 mmol/L (145 mg/dl).

Patients with gestational diabetes are at increased risk of overt Type II diabetes mellitus developing in later life.

The American College of Obstetricians and Gynecologists, in contrast, recommends screening only for women considered at high risk: those over 30, those with a family history of diabetes, those with a previous macrosomic, malformed, or stillborn infant, and those with obesity, hypertension, or glucosuria.[3]

314. D. This patient has gestational diabetes. The normal values for the 100-g glucose tolerance test are listed in question 1. If two values (out of four) are abnormal, the patient has gestational diabetes. The patient discussed in the question has three values that are abnormal. If only one value is abnormal, the diagnosis is impaired glucose tolerance.

Once the diagnosis of gestational diabetes is made, the patient should be referred to a diabetic education center, begun on a diabetic diet, and taught how to check her blood pressure on a q.i.d. basis. Eighty-five percent of gestational diabetics can be controlled on diet alone; 15 percent require diet plus insulin. Oral hypoglycemic agents should not be used to treat gestational diabetes mellitus.[1]

315. D. Absent or significantly decreased fetal movement demands further evaluation.

It is inappropriate to tell the patient not to worry or to wait until morning to be evaluated. The potential urgency of the situation demands further assessment that evening. The contraction stress test has essentially been replaced by the biophysical profile score.

Routine counting of fetal movements has been previously recommended. [4] A recent randomized controlled trial with over 68,000 women, however, has not shown any significant benefit to formal routine fetal movement counting in low-risk women.[5]

316. E. A reactive nonstress test is defined as two or more accelerations of the fetal heart rate of 15 beats per minute for at least 15 seconds during a 20-minute period. [1]

317. C. The nonstress test is a simple noninvasive test that is useful in the prediction of fetal hypoxia. If it is being used to monitor a chronic condition, it should be performed twice a week. In one study, there was a significantly lower stillbirth rate when the test was performed twice a week. The nonstress test has a high false-positive rate, and thus its specificity for the detection of fetal hypoxia is low. However, it has a high sensitivity (low false-negative rate). Thus, a reactive nonstress test[*] is reassuring.[6]

318. D. and 319 E. A nonreactive nonstress test should be followed by evaluation by biophysical profile. The biophysical profile has five components; they are (1) the nonstress test, (2) fetal breathing movements, (3) gross body movement, (4) fetal tone, and (5) qualitative analysis of amniotic fluid volume. Each one of the five parameters is assigned a maximum value of 2 points. Thus, a perfect biophysical profile is 10/10. Scores of 8/10 and 10/10 suggest normal fetuses or fetuses at low risk for chronic asphyxia. Scores of less than 8 suggest the possibility of chronic asphyxia and should be reevaluated in a short period of time (maximum— hours). If the biophysical profile continues to be low, fetal asphyxia should be strongly suspected and very careful monitoring or

---

[*] Some authorities question the reassuring nature of the nonstress test and feel that antepartum electronic fetal heart rate monitoring is not done to predict continuing fetal health but rather to identify fetal jeopardy. They feel that "This distinction is extremely important. Specifically, it is our contention that fetal heart rate accelerations do not predict fetal well-being for a definable time period, and this renders outpatient monitoring impractical since the fetus may deteriorate rapidly in women not evaluated clinically on a daily basis."[1]

delivery of the fetus (depending on the circumstances) should be undertaken.[1]

320. A. The diagnostic indications for assessment of fetal health by nonstress testing or biophysical profile scoring include among others (1) postdate pregnancy, (2) chronic hypertension or pregnancy-induced hypertension, (3) suspected small-for-gestational-age fetus, (4) diabetes (all classes), (5) history of previous stillbirth, (6) decreased fetal movement, (7) premature rupture of membranes, (8) antepartum hemorrhage, (9) major maternal medical problem, and (10) suspected abnormalities of amniotic fluid volume.[1]

A normal low-risk pregnancy is not an indication for electronic fetal monitoring or biophysical profile scoring.

SUMMARY OF THIRD TRIMESTER ASSESSMENT

1. 50-g glucose screen at 24–28 weeks (recommended routinely by 1984 Second Workshop Conference on Gestational Diabetes, but not by the American Society of Obstetricians and Gynecologists). If plasma glucose > or equal to 7.8 mmol/L (140 mg%), 100-g glucose tolerance test should be ordered.

2. Routine formal fetal movement counting can only be recommended for high-risk pregnancies. Patients should be made aware that significantly

decreased fetal activity should be reported. Significantly decreased fetal activity should be evaluated by nonstress testing or by a biophysical profile.

3. Nonstress testing and biophysical profile testing are the preferred tests for monitoring continued fetal well being.

References

1. Cunningham FG, MacDonald P, Gant N. Williams obstetrics. 18th Ed. Norwalk: Appleton and Lange, 1989: 818–819.

2. Second International Workshop-Conference on Gestational Diabetes. Diabetes 1985; 34s: 1.

3. American College of Obstetricians and Gynecologists: Management of diabetes mellitus in pregnancy. Tech Bull No 92, May 1986.

4. Swanson R. Maternal counting of fetal movements as an antenatal screening test: Part I: A review. Can Fam Physician 1988; 34: 561–565.

5. Grant A, Valentin L, Elbourne D, Alexander S. Routine formal fetal movement counting and risk of antepartum late death in normally formed singletons. Lancet 1989; II: 345–349.

6. Schneider E, et al. An assessment of the first decade's experience with antepartum fetal heart rate testing. Am J Perinatol 1988; 5(2): 134–145.

PROBLEM 38:   A 35-YEAR-OLD PRIMIGRAVIDA WITH HYPERTENSION

A 35-year-old primigravida presents to your office at 16-weeks gestation. She is a new patient. Her medical history is unremarkable. She has not had any serious illnesses. She is excited about her pregnancy and wants you to provide her prenatal care. Her blood pressure measured after 5 minutes of rest is 160/100 mm Hg. A repeat measurement 1 week later is 154/98 mm Hg.

SELECT THE ONE BEST ANSWER TO THE FOLLOWING QUESTIONS:

321. The most likely diagnosis in this patient is:
    a) preeclampsia
    b) chronic hypertension
    c) chronic hypertension with superimposed preeclampsia
    d) transient hypertension
    e) labile hypertension

322. The patient described is followed on a weekly basis. Her blood pressure remains at or around 155/98 until the 26th week of gestation. At that time, her blood pressure increases to 170/106 mm Hg. She begins to spill a small amount of protein (approximately 300 mg/day) in her urine. At this time, the most likely diagnosis is:
    a) preeclampsia
    b) an exacerbation of chronic hypertension with glomerular damage

c) chronic hypertension with superimposed preeclampsia
d) transient hypertension
e) labile hypertension

323. The treatment of choice in this patient at this time is:
a) increase rest at home; increase visits to twice weekly
b) admit to hospital for bed rest and further evaluation
c) admit to hospital and begin pharmacologic therapy
d) institute pharmacologic therapy as an outpatient; see in the office twice a week
e) admit to hospital for bed rest and pharmacologic therapy

324. This patient's blood pressure settles to a level of 140/90 mm Hg on strict bed rest and stays at that level for 8 weeks (34-weeks gestation). At that time, in spite of bed rest it rises to 170/110 mm Hg, proteinuria increases to 2 g/day, and biophysical profile testing reveals evidence of oligohydramnios. The treatment of choice at this time is:
a) begin pharmacologic therapy with a thiazide diuretic
b) begin pharmacologic therapy with a beta blocker
c) begin pharmacologic therapy with a calcium-channel blocker
d) begin pharmacologic therapy with a direct vasodilator
e) none of the above

325. A 25-year-old primigravida, a known hypertensive, who is presently on a thiazide diuretic, becomes pregnant. On examination at 8-weeks gestation her blood pressure is 120/85 mm Hg. At this time, you should:
a) discontinue the thiazide diuretic and substitute atenolol
b) discontinue the thiazide diuretic and substitute methyldopa
c) discontinue the thiazide diuretic and substitute nothing
d) continue the thiazide diuretic and see the patient every 2 weeks
e) none of the above

326. The patient described in question 325 has her blood pressure well controlled until 18-weeks ges-

tation. At that time her blood pressure rises to 160/102 mm Hg. At that time you should:
a) reinstitute the thiazide diuretic if you had stopped it or increase the dosage if you had not
b) start the patient on an angiotensin converting enzyme inhibitor
c) start the patient on a calcium-channel blocker
d) start the patient on a beta-adrenergic blocker
e) start the patient on a loop diuretic

ANSWER THE FOLLOWING QUESTION ACCORDING TO THE CODE:

A: 1,2, and 3 are correct
B: 1 and 3 are correct
C: 2 and 4 are correct
D: Only 4 is correct
E: All of the above are correct

327. Which of the following drugs are recommended for outpatient use in patients with established chronic hypertension in pregnancy?
1) atenolol
2) hydrochlorothiazide
3) methyldopa
4) nifedipine

ANSWERS

321. B. This patient most likely has chronic hypertension. Chronic hypertension in pregnancy is defined as a blood pressure of ≥ 140/90 mm Hg either predating pregnancy or occurring before the 20th gestational week.[1]

Pregnancy-induced hypertension or preeclampsia is defined as a sustained rise in arterial pressure after the 20th week to ≥ 140/90 or an increase of 30 mm Hg in systolic pressure or a 15 mm Hg increase in diastolic pressure, associated with proteinuria of >300 mg in 24 hours. Weight gain and edema are frequently present; they are not, however, necessary to make the diagnosis. Eclampsia and the presence of generalized or grand mal seizures is the major complication of preeclampsia.[1]

A patient who has chronic hypertension with superimposed preeclampsia is defined as a patient who, having preexisting hypertension, has a further increase in blood pressure or worsening of proteinuria after 20-weeks gestation.[1]

Late or transient hypertension is defined as an elevation of arterial pressure to a level ≥ 140/90 mm Hg in the immediate puerperium, with a rapid return to normal no later than the tenth postpartum day.[1]

322. C. At this time the patient has developed chronic hypertension with superimposed preeclampsia. This condition is associated with significant fetal mortality, and the fetus should be monitored closely for the duration of pregnancy.

323. B. Since this patient has developed chronic hypertension with superimposed preeclampsia, she should be admitted to hospital for bed rest and further evaluation.

Bed rest and reduced activity are essential.

The patient should be placed in the left lateral position. This position results in (1) lower blood pressure readings, (2) mobilization of extravascular fluid, (3) decreased endogenous excretion of catecholamines, (4) increased renal perfusion and diuresis, and (5) improvement in uterine blood flow.[2]

Further evaluation should include evaluation of renal function (including 24-hour urine for protein and creatinine clearance), clotting parameters (including platelets, PT, PTT, fibrinogen, fibrin degradation products, liver function tests, and uric acid levels.[3]

Pharmacologic therapy should not be instituted unless blood pressure remains significantly elevated (diastolic pressure 100—110 depending on the authority) in spite of bed rest.[1]

Rest at home or institution of outpatient pharmacologic therapy would not be appropriate in this case.

324. E. None of the above. The treatment of choice for this patient at this time is delivery. This patient now has severe preeclampsia superimposed on chronic hypertension. When blood pressure reaches a MAP of ≥ 130 mm Hg or a diastolic pressure ≥ 110 mm Hg, intravenous hypertensives should be instituted to avoid end-organ injury, particularly cerebral hemorrhage.[1] At this time, the patient's MAP is 130 mm Hg. Intravenous methyldopa, intravenous hydralazine, intravenous nitroglycerin, intravenous labetalol, or intravenous sodium nitroprusside could be used to lower blood pressure.

This fetus is in trouble. In general, lung maturity should be assured before delivery is contemplated. In the presence of intrauterine growth retardation, fetal distress, or further clinical deterioration in the maternal condition, however, delivery should take place as quickly as possible.

325. C. Patients who become pregnant while on antihypertensives and are well controlled should probably have their medications discontinued.[3] Therapy should be reinstituted if the MAP ≥ 117 mm Hg or the diastolic pressure is ≥ 100 mm Hg during the second trimester, or the MAP is ≥ 127 mm Hg or the diastolic blood pressure is ≥ 110 mm Hg during the third trimester.[1]

326. D. The best option, of those listed, is to start the patient on a beta-adrenergic receptor blocker. Examples of drugs that could be used are atenolol and metoprolol. Propranolol has been associated with many adverse fetal and neonatal effects and should not be used.[1]

Thiazide or loop diuretics should not be used as they may further decrease the intravascular volume, leading to decreased uteroplacental perfusion.[1,3]

Calcium-channel blockers may be useful in the treatment of hypertension in pregnancy, but experience with their use is lacking.

Angiotensin converting enzyme inhibitors should not be used, as congenital malformations have been associated with their use.

327. B. Atenolol and methyldopa are two of the most common drugs used to treat chronic hypertension in pregnancy. A useful substitute for atenolol is metoprolol.[1] Thiazide diuretics should not be used (see question 326). There is not enough experience with nifedipine to recommend its use at this time.

SUMMARY OF THE DIAGNOSIS AND TREATMENT OF HYPERTENSION IN PREGNANCY

1. **Classification of hypertension in pregnancy:**
   a) preeclampsia/eclampsia
   b) chronic hypertension
   c) chronic hypertension with superimposed preeclampsia
   d) late or transient hypertension

2. **Definitions of hypertension in pregnancy:**
   a) preeclampsia: blood pressure ≥ 140/90 mm Hg or increase of 30 mm Hg systolic or 15 mm Hg diastolic after 20th week of pregnancy

b) chronic hypertension: A blood pressure of ≥ 140/90 mm Hg either predating pregnancy or occurring before the 20th gestational week.

c) chronic hypertension with superimposed preclampsia: a further increase in blood pressure or a worsening of proteinuria after 20 weeks gestation in a patient with established hypertension

d) transient or late hypertension: an elevation of arterial pressure ≥ 140/90 mm Hg in the immediate puerperium, with a rapid return to normal no later than the tenth postpartum day

3. **Treatment of hypertension in pregnancy:**
   1) Patient with established chronic hypertension on medication who becomes pregnant: discontinue all antihypertensive agents in early pregnancy if arterial pressure is normal since perinatal outcome and incidence of superimposed preeclampsia is not altered by drug therapy. Reinstitute therapy if MAP ≥ 117 mm Hg or diastolic blood pressure ≥ 100 mm Hg during second trimester, or MAP ≥ 127 mm Hg or diastolic blood pressure ≥ 110 mm Hg during third trimester
   2) Drugs of choice in the treatment of hypertension in pregnancy:

Chronic hypertension:
   i)   beta blockers: atenolol, metoprolol
   ii) alpha and beta blockers: latetalol
   iii) centrally acting agent: methyldopa
Pregnancy-induced hypertension:
   a) mild–moderate: no drug therapy
   b) severe: intravenous antihypertensives to keep MAP <130 and diastolic blood pressure <110 mm Hg to avoid end-organ injury, particularly cerebral hemorrhage. Deliver once fetal lung maturity is established, or in the presence of intrauterine growth retardation, fetal distress, or further clinical deterioration in maternal condition.

References

1. Doany W, Brinkman C. Antihypertensive drugs in pregnancy. Clin Perinatol 1987; 14(4): 783–805.

2. Zuspan FP. Chronic hypertension in pregnancy. Clin Obstet Gynecol 1984; 27(4): 854–873.

3. Cunningham F, MacDonald P, Gant N. Williams obstetrics. 18th Ed. Norwalk: Appleton and Lange, 1989: 653–694.

PROBLEM 39: A 19-YEAR-OLD PRIMIGRAVIDA WITH A SMALL BABY

A 19-year-old nulliparous female with preeclampsia is being followed for possible small-for-gestational-age pregnancy (SGA). She is presently at 34-weeks gestation. She has noticed decreased fetal movements for the past 2 days. A biophysical profile gives her a score of 4 out of 10. In addition, deep decelerations are seen in response to an oxytocin challenge test. Her blood pressure is 170/100 mm Hg.

SELECT THE ONE BEST ANSWER TO THE FOLLOWING QUESTIONS:

328. In this patient, the most appropriate action at this time would be to:
   a) lower the diastolic blood pressure to 80 mm Hg and reassess the situation
   b) immediate cesarean section
   c) immediate induction of labor with prostaglandin gel
   d) best rest, antihypertensive agents, and reassessment in 24 hours
   e) immediate induction of labor with oxytocin

329. The leading cause of perinatal death in SGA fetuses is:
   a) intrauterine asphyxia
   b) preeclampsia in the mother
   c) diabetes in the mother
   d) meconium aspiration
   e) none of the above

330. The single most preventable cause of SGA pregnancy is:
   a) maternal alcohol abuse
   b) maternal malnutrition
   c) maternal cigarette smoking
   d) maternal hypertension
   e) maternal illicit drug abuse

331. The most common maternal complication causing SGA pregnancy is:

a) hypertension
b) anemia
c) renal disease
d) inflammatory bowel disease
e) valvular heart disease

332. The most common reason for suspecting SGA pregnancy is:
a) maternal socioeconomic status
b) inaccurate gestational age
c) adolescent age
d) chronic maternal disease
e) presentation late in pregnancy with no previous prenatal care

333. An SGA fetus is defined as:
a) a fetus weighing less than 2,500 g
b) a fetus whose birth weight falls below the 20th percentile for his gestational age
c) a fetus whose birth weight falls below the 10th percentile for his gestational age
d) a fetus weighing less than 1,850 g
e) none of the above

ANSWER THE FOLLOWING QUESTIONS ACCORDING TO THE CODE:

A: 1, 2, and 3 are correct
B: 1 and 3 are correct
C: 2 and 4 are correct
D: Only 4 is correct
E: All of the above are correct

334. Which of the following methods is(are) useful for the detection of SGA fetuses?
1) a complete and accurate history
2) sonographic measurements
3) a complete physical examination
4) uterine-fundal height measurements

335. Which of the following statements regarding the delivery of an SGA fetus remote from term is(are) correct?
1) the decision to deliver the fetus involves a balancing of the risks of leaving the fetus in utero compared to the risks of premature delivery
2) the stress associated with severe growth retardation often accelerates lung maturation
3) the presence of maternal disease that is worsening as a consequence of the pregnancy is a definite indication for delivery

4) when fetal weight is below the 10th percentile and remains static, additional time in utero decreases mortality

336. Which of the following is(are) causes of SGA pregnancies?
1) genetic disorders
2) congenital infections
3) multiple pregnancy
4) small maternal stature

ANSWERS

328. B. The only course of action that is reasonable in this situation is immediate cesarean section. The fetus has not been moving well for the past 2 days, has a poor biophysical profile score, and has a positive contraction stress test. This indicates acute fetal distress and immediate delivery is indicated.

Induction of labor will delay delivery and stress an already compromised uteroplacental blood flow. To bring the blood pressure down to 80 mm Hg is not only a waste of time but it will also further compromise uteroplacental blood flow. To observe this fetus in utero for 24 hours will quite probably result in the death of the baby.[1]

329. A. The leading cause of perinatal death in SGA fetuses is intrauterine asphyxia. About 20% of SGA infants are symmetrically small; 80% are asymmetrically small.

Diminished placental function is the most common causative factor in SGA pregnancy. This is most frequently due to abnormal function of a normal placenta (e.g., cigarette smoking, diminished perfusion, placental infarction, infection).

The SGA fetus is at risk for in utero complications, including hypoxia and metabolic acidosis, which may occur at any time, but are particularly likely to occur during labor.[1]

330. C. Cigarette smoking is the single most common preventable cause of SGA pregnancy in North America today. Cigarette smoking is much more common among women of child-bearing age than is alcoholism or illicit drug abuse. Birth weight is reduced by 200 g in infants of smoking mothers. The amount of reduction is related to the number of cigarettes smoked per day. Infants of smoking mothers are also shorter in length, and there is a greater risk of perinatal death or compromise in labor.[1]

Maternal malnutrition sometimes does produce an SGA fetus, but it is not a common cause of SGA.

Hypertension is the most common maternal complication causing SGA pregnancy. It cannot be classified as preventable.

331. A. Numerous maternal diseases are associated with suboptimal fetal growth via various mechanisms, including any that interfere with uptake or delivery of nutrients or oxygen to the fetus. Most of these diseases can be described by the HARM acronym (H= hypertension, A= anemia, R= renal, M= malabsorption).

Hypertension is the single most common maternal complication causing SGA pregnancy. Hypertension results in decreased blood flow through the spiral arteries perfusing the placenta, resulting in decreased delivery of oxygen and nutrients to the placenta and fetus. Hypertension may also be associated with placental infarction. Other maternal diseases associated with SGA fetuses include maternal anemia, renal disease, and maternal malabsorption.[1]

332. B. The most common reason for suspecting SGA pregnancy is inaccurate gestational age. In the majority of cases where a significant discrepancy is found between gestational age and symphysis-fundal height, inaccurate gestational age rather than true SGA is the reason. When a careful history is taken, it is often discovered that the last "period" was not a normal period, but rather a shortened period, or even just spotting. This, in most cases, represents a small bleed in early pregnancy.

The date of quickening should be established. The first perception of fetal movement occurs at 18–20 weeks in primigravidas and at 14–16 weeks in multigravidas.

If dates are in doubt, obstetric ultrasound should be performed, preferably prior to 20-weeks gestation. Obstetric ultrasound can also measure estimated fetal weight, and serial measurements of this parameter may be very useful.[1]

333. C. A newborn infant is classified as growth retarded, or small-for-gestational-age, if his birth weight falls below the 10th percentile for his gestational age. Mortality and severe morbidity are not significantly increased among fetuses and infants with lesser degrees of growth retardation and without serious malformations. For any gestational age, however, as weight decreases below the 10th percentile, the risk of fetal morbidity and mortality increases remarkably.

The term that was formerly used for SGA fetuses was "intrauterine growth retardation." However, because of the connotations of the word "retardation" for the parents and other family members, this has been replaced by "small-for-gestational-age" (SGA).[1]

334. E. All of the above are useful in the assessment of SGA fetuses.

A good history and physical examination will exlude certain maternal conditions that are associated with SGA. Sonographic measurements can estimate gestational age and can also provide accurate estimates of fetal weight, fetal condition, and amniotic fluid volume. Uterine-fundal height measurements are both sensitive and specific if performed by the same observer.[1]

335. A. When a SGA fetus is identified close to term, the decision to deliver is straightforward. However, when a SGA fetus is identified remote from term, the situation is more complex.

In many cases of SGA fetuses remote from term, there is no specific treatment that will improve the fetal situation and prompt delivery is therefore indicated.

Sometimes the growth-retarded fetus is in serious jeopardy irrespective of whether he remains in utero or is delivered. For the fetus who is severely SGA but remote from term, the decision to proceed with delivery becomes a matter of trying to determine the risk of further stay in utero compared to the risks of preterm delivery. Fortunately, the stress associated with severe fetal growth retardation often accelerates lung maturation.

The presence of maternal disease that is worsening as a consequence of the pregnancy and that therefore threatens the well-being of the mother as well as the fetus should imply delivery.

When the fetal weight is below the 10th percentile and remains static, additional time in utero increases, rather than decreases, perinatal mortality.[1]

336. E. All of the above. The etiology of SGA fetuses includes disorders associated with decreased growth potential such as genetic disorders, congenital infection, tobacco and drugs, and small maternal stature; and disorders associated with restricted growth potential such as placental disor-

ders, coexistent maternal diseases, and multiple pregnancy. [1]

SUMMARY OF THE DIAGNOSIS AND MANAGEMENT OF SMALL-FOR-GESTATIONAL-AGE PREGNANCY

1. **Definition:** < 10th percentile for gestational age

2. **Etiology:** cigarette smoking is single most common preventable cause. Hypertension is the most common coexisting maternal condition.

3. **Diagnosis:** good history, physical examination, obstetric ultrasound, and serial uterine-fundal heights

4. **Most common reason for suspecting SGA:** inaccurate dates

5. **Treatment:** in most cases risk of fetus remaining in utero is greater than risk of premature birth, even if fetus remote from term

Reference

1. Cunningham FG, MacDonald P, Gant N. Williams obstetrics. 18th Ed. Norwalk: Appleton and Lange, 1989: 764–773.

PROBLEM 40: A 24-YEAR-OLD PRIMIGRAVIDA WHO HAS GONE PAST HER DUE DATE

A 24-year-old primigravida presents to you as a new patient. She has just moved to your community and has been recommended to you by a friend. She states that she has "gone past her due date" and would like her baby delivered by induction of labor.

SELECT THE ONE BEST ANSWER TO THE FOLLOWING QUESTIONS:

337. A pregnancy is defined as post-term if it exceeds how may days of gestation?
    a) 280 days
    b) 287 days
    c) 294 days
    d) 273 days
    e) 301 days

338. You take a complete history from this patient and confirm the date of her last menstrual period as being 42 weeks previous to this date. Her antenatal course has been uneventful. A pelvic examination is done and reveals a fetal head that is fixed in the pelvis and well applied to the cervix. The cervix is soft, is 2 cm dilated, and is 30% effaced.
    What is the most appropriate action at this time?
    a) have the patient return for follow-up in 1 week
    b) perform a nonstress test and if reactive, review the patient in 1 week
    c) conduct an oxytocin challenge test
    d) schedule elective induction of labor
    e) none of the above

339. Which of the following parameters is the most sensitive test for the prediction of fetal asphyxia and resultant perinatal mortality in post-term pregnancy?
    a) nonstress test weekly
    b) nonstress test biweekly
    c) lack of a 3 cm vertical pocket of amniotic fluid on ultrasound
    d) lack of a 1 cm vertical pocket of amniotic fluid on ultrasound
    e) contraction stress test

ANSWER THE FOLLOWING QUESTIONS ACCORDING TO THE CODE:

A: 1, 2, and 3 are correct
B: 1 and 3 are correct
C: 2 and 4 are correct
D: Only 4 is correct
E: All of the above are correct

340. Which of the following statements regarding post-term pregnancy is(are) correct?
    1) the perinatal mortality rate is increased in patients beyond 42 weeks gestation

2) the incidence of meconium staining and meconium aspiration is increased in patients beyond 42 weeks gestation

3) the post-term fetus may continue to gain weight in utero and thus be an unusually large infant at birth

4) the intrauterine environment in a post-term pregnancy may predispose to the development of a dysmature or dystrophic infant

341. Some authorities have favored elective induction of all patients at 41–42 weeks gestation. Which of the following is(are) potential problems with this approach?

1) gestational age is not always precisely known

2) it is difficult to identify with precision those fetuses who are likely to develop serious morbidity

3) induction of labor is not always successful

4) delivery by cesarean section increases appreciably the risk of serious maternal morbidity

ANSWERS

337. C. A post-term pregnancy is one that persists for 294 days (42 weeks) or more from the onset of a menstrual period that was followed by ovulation about 2 weeks later.[1]

The incidence of post-term pregnancy was previously thought to be approximately 10% of all pregnancies.[1] With errors in dating taken into account, this figure may be closer to 5%.

338. D. This patient is 42 weeks by dates, and her dates are sure. The correct course of action is induction of labor with syntocinon. Induction of labor at 42 weeks in patients with definite dates has been shown to result in a decreased perinatal mortality rate.[1]

If a patient's dates are unsure, she should be followed by biophysical profile and/or nonstress testing twice weekly. The patient should also be instructed to monitor fetal activity.

339. C. The most sensitive test for the prediction of fetal asphyxia and resultant perinatal mortality in post-term pregnancy is the lack of a 3 cm amniotic fluid pocket on ultrasound. The finding of a 3 cm pocket is reassuring. A recent study has shown that the perinatal mortality using the lack of a 3 cm pocket as a test as a basis for intervention was associated with a lower perinatal mortality rate than using

nonstress testing, contraction stress testing, or the lack of 1 cm pocket on ultrasound.[2] Thus, the performance of a biophysical profile on a biweekly basis, with the demonstration of a 3 cm amniotic fluid pocket, is a reassuring sign that suggests that the fetus is in good condition.

340. E. The perinatal mortality rate and the incidence of meconium staining and meconium aspiration are increased when the gestational age is 42 weeks or beyond.[1,3]

The post-term fetus may continue to gain weight in utero and thus be unusually large at birth. On the other hand, the intrauterine environment may predispose to loss of fetal weight, loss of subcutaneous fat and muscle, and a "dystrophic" or "dysmature" appearance.

341. E. At least five difficult problems serve to discourage a policy of delivering all fetuses whose gestational age is suspected to be at least 42 weeks:[1]

a) gestational age is not always precisely known

b) it is sometimes difficult to identify those fetuses who would likely develop significant perinatal morbidity or mortality if left in utero

c) most fetuses of a gestational age of 42 weeks or greater do well

d) induction of labor is not always successful

e) cesarean section increases maternal morbidity in the present and in subsequent pregnancies

SUMMARY OF THE MANAGEMENT OF POST-TERM PREGNANCY

1. Document accurately by dates and previous ultrasound (if available)

2. If the dates are definite, induce labor at 42 weeks gestation

3. If dates are indefinite, follow carefully with biophysical profile testing and/or nonstress testing twice weekly. In biophysical profile testing, look for at least one 3 cm pocket of amniotic fluid.

References

1. Cunningham FG, MacDonald P, Gant N. Williams obstetrics. 18th Ed. Norwalk: Appleton and Lange, 1989: 758–763.

2. Benedetti T, Easterling T. Antepartum testing in postterm pregnancy. J Reproduct Med 1988; 33(3): 252–258.

3. Leveno KJ, Lowe TW, Cunningham FG, Wendel GD, Nelson S. Management of prolonged pregnancy at Parkland Hospital. Proceedings of the Society for Gynecologic Investigation, Abstract 290P, March 1985b.

PROBLEM 41: A 14-YEAR-OLD FEMALE WITH LOWER, MIDABDOMINAL, COLICKY PAIN RELATED TO THE MENSTRUAL CYCLE

A 14-year-old female presents to your office with a six-month history of lower midabdominal pain, colicky in nature, that radiates to the back and upper thighs. The pain usually starts within a few hours after the onset of menstrual flow and lasts from a few hours to 2 days. The patient's menarche began 1 year ago. The patient is not sexually active.

SELECT THE ONE BEST ANSWER TO THE FOLLOWING QUESTIONS:

342. The most likely diagnosis in this patient is:
    a) primary dysmenorrhea
    b) pelvic inflammatory disease
    c) secondary dysmenorrhea
    d) endometriosis
    e) psychogenic abdominal pain

343. Which of the following has been shown to be associated with the pain produced by the condition discussed in question 342?
    a) elevation of myometrial resting tone
    b) elevation of contractile myometrial pressure
    c) increased frequency of uterine contractions
    d) dysrhythmia of uterine contractions
    e) all of the above

ANSWER THE FOLLOWING QUESTION ACCORDING TO THE CODE:

A: 1, 2, and 3 are correct
B: 1 and 3 are correct
C: 2 and 4 are correct
D: Only 4 is correct
E: All of the above are correct

344. Which of the following is/are causes of secondary dysmenorrhea?
    1) the intrauterine device
    2) endometriosis
    3) pelvic inflammatory disease (PID)
    4) adenomyosis

345. Recommended treatments for the condition described in question 342 include:
    1) nonsteroidal anti-inflammatory drugs
    2) aerobic exercise
    3) the oral contraceptive pill
    4) narcotic analgesics

SELECT THE ONE BEST ANSWER TO THE FOLLOWING QUESTIONS:

346. The patient described in question 342 is placed on mefenamic acid for therapy of her condition. After 4 months, her menstrual periods are still painful. At this time, the most appropriate therapeutic maneuver would be to:
    a) start her on the oral contraceptive pill
    b) perform a laparoscopy and reevaluate the diagnosis
    c) switch her to a proprionic acid derivative
    d) continue the mefenamic acid for another 6 months
    e) none of the above

347. The appropriate therapeutic maneuver for the patient described in question 346 is instituted. Unfortunately, after 4 months, her menstrual periods are still painful. At this time, the recommended management would be to:
    a) start her on the oral contraceptive pill
    b) begin therapy with a NSAID from a different class
    c) arrange for a laparoscopy to reevaluate the diagnosis
    d) continue the therapeutic maneuver instituted in question 346
    e) begin to explore deep psychological issues in the hope that something will come to the surface

348. Which of the following statements about primary dysmenorrhea is FALSE?

a) there are two types of primary dysmenorrhea: spasmodic dysmenorrhea and congestive dysmenorrhea

b) patients with primary spasmodic dysmenorrhea respond less favorably to medication

c) congestive dysmenorrhea is often accompanied by irritability, fatigue, constipation, and weight gain

d) symptoms of dysmenorrhea are generally less when the patient is more educated about menstrual function

e) symptoms of dysmenorrhea may be increased by life stressors

ANSWERS

342. A. This patient has primary dysmenorrhea. Primary dysmenorrhea is the most common gynecologic complaint experienced by young women.[1] Fifty percent of menstruating women experience this symptom; in 10% of women it is severe.

Primary dysmenorrhea usually begins within 6–12 months of menarche. The pain is lower abdominal and often colicky. Onset is usually at the beginning or within a few hours of the beginning of the menstrual flow. Anovulatory cycles are not associated with dysmenorrhea. Other symptoms associated with primary dysmenorrhea include nausea, vomiting, diarrhea, headache, breast tenderness, and fatigue.[1] Secondary dysmenorrhea is dysmenorrhea that is associated with pelvic pathology. Pelvic inflammatory disease and endometriosis are the two primary causes of secondary dysmenorrhea.

Psychogenic factors, although thought by some to be a cause of dysmenorrhea, are unlikely to be responsible for the continuing cyclic problems.

343. E. Primary dysmenorrhea is associated with the following abnormalities: (1) an elevation of myometrial resting tone to above 10 mm Hg, (2) an elevation of contractile myometrial pressure to above 120 mm Hg, (3) an increased frequency of uterine contractions, and (4) dysrhythmia of uterine contractions.[1] These physiologic changes lead to an increased production of prostaglandins and uterine hypoxia.

344. E. Secondary dysmenorrhea is dysmenorrhea that is secondary to pelvic pathology. Endometriosis and chronic PID are the most common causes.[1] Other causes include the IUD, congenital malfor-

mations, adenomyosis, endometrial polyps, uterine fibroids, adhesions, ovarian cysts, pelvic congestion syndrome, and cervical stricture.

345. A. Treatments of choice for primary dysmenorrhea are the oral contraceptive pill, nonsteroidal anti-inflammatory agents, and aerobic exercise. Narcotic analgesics are not recommended for treatment of this or any other benign disorder.

An oral contraceptive is the treatment of choice in a patient who also wishes protection against pregnancy.[1] Oral contraceptives decrease both prostaglandin production and the amount of menstrual flow.

Nonsteroidal anti-inflammatories are the agents of choice in patients not wishing contraceptive protection.[1] They work by inhibiting the production of prostaglandins. The two most commonly used groups of anti-inflammatories are the propionic acids and the fenamates.[1] Proprionic acid agents include naproxen and ibuprofen. The most commonly used fenamate is mefenamic acid. Treatment should begin at the onset of menstruation and usually needs to be continued for 3 to 4 days. A particular agent should be tried for at least 4 cycles before concluding that it is ineffective. If one agent is ineffective, an agent of another class should be tried.

346. C. The most appropriate therapeutic maneuver would be to switch her to a proprionic acid derivative such as naproxen or naproxen sodium (see critique of question 345).

347. C. After failure of an adequate trial of two NSAIDs from different classes (the fenamates and the propionic acids), the diagnosis should be reevaluated and a laparoscopy performed. If, in fact, no pathology is found it would be appropriate to begin therapy with the oral contraceptive pill.

Although psychosocial issues are important, it is unlikely that a psychoanalytic approach to this problem would be of benefit.

348. B. There are two types of primary dysmenorrhea based on symptomatology; spasmodic dysmenorrhea and congestive dysmenorrhea. Spasmodic dysmenorrhea is associated with acute spasmodic pain in the lower abdomen, usually starting on the first day of menstruation. Nausea, vomiting, and diarrhea may accompany this pain. Symptoms usually last 48 hours. Congestive dysmenorrhea presents as a dull pain in the lower abdomen and

is associated with symptoms such as edema, weight gain, constipation, fatigue, and irritability.

The symptoms of congestive dysmenorrhea, in contradistinction to spasmodic dysmenorrhea, usually begin several days before menses begins and are rapidly relieved with the onset of menses.[1]

SUMMARY OF DIAGNOSIS AND TREATMENT OF DYSMENORRHEA

1. **Primary dysmenorrhea (spasmodic):** begins within 6–12 months of menarche and presents with midabdominal, colicky pain starting with or a few hours after the onset of menstrual flow and possibly lasting two days.

2. **Secondary dysmenorrhea:** suspect in patients who have pain with first menstruation, patients who have dysmenorrhea with irregular cycles related to anovulatory bleeding, patients with IUDs, and patients whose dysmenorrhea begins after the age of 25

3. **Treatment of primary dysmenorrhea:**
   a) in patients needing contraception as well: oral contraceptive pill
   b) in patients not needing contraception: nonsteroidal anti-inflammatory drugs (two classes: fenamates and proprionic acid derivatives)

   If one NSAID does not work after 4 cycles, try another agent from the other class. If this is not successful, or if the oral contraceptive pill does not work after 6 cycles in those patients in whom this was the first treament, reconsider the diagnosis. Laparoscopy is then recommended.

Reference

1. Avant R. Dysmenorrhea. Prim Care 1988; 15(3): 549–559.

PROBLEM 42: A COUPLE WHO HAVE BEEN UNSUCCESSFUL IN CONCEIVING AFTER 18 MONTHS OF TRYING

A 28-year-old female and her 27-year-old husband present to your office to discuss their inability to conceive. They have been married for 18 months and have been trying to conceive since the beginning of their marriage. They are extremely anxious, and during the interview the wife begins to cry.

The wife has a history of pelvic inflammatory disease. She had a pelvic infection at age 18.

SELECT THE ONE BEST ANSWER TO THE FOLLOWING QUESTIONS:

349. The next most appropriate step in the evaluation of this infertile couple is to:
   a) tell the couple that the infertility is due to pelvic inflammatory disease and refer them to an adoption agency
   b) refer the patient to a gynecologist to break the news
   c) begin the wife on clomiphene citrate
   d) refer the couple to a psychiatrist
   e) none of the above

350. The prevalence of infertility in North American couples is:
   a) < 1%
   b) 4–6%
   c) 10–15%
   d) 20–25%

   e) 30–35%

351. Which one of the following statements regarding the occurrence of ovulation is TRUE?
   a) the female partner should keep at least 6 months of basal body temperature charts before ovulation can be precisely determined
   b) a woman who has a menstrual period every 6 months may still be ovulating on a monthly basis
   c) if a woman has regular cycles associated with cyclical premenstrual sensations or symptoms (molimina), then she is almost certainly ovulating
   d) the only accurate method of determining ovulation is by endometrial biopsy
   e) if a woman has been anovulatory for a period of greater than 1 year, it is unlikely that she will ever ovulate again

ANSWER THE FOLLOWING QUESTIONS ACCORDING TO THE CODE:

A: 1, 2, and 3 are correct
B: 1 and 3 are correct
C: 2 and 4 are correct
D: Only 4 is correct
E: All of the above are correct

352. Which of the following statements regarding the physiology of fertility is(are) TRUE?
   1) normal quality and quantity of periovulatory cervical mucus is essential for fertilization to occur
   2) sufficient progesterone must be present in the luteal phase to properly prepare the endometrium for implantation
   3) the hypothalamic-pituitary-ovarian axis must be functioning properly in order to regulate normal folliculogenesis and ovulation
   4) sufficient progesterone levels must be present in the periovulatory phase in order to induce the luteinizing hormone (LH) surge

353. Which of the following statements regarding the investigation of infertility is(are) CORRECT?
   1) both male and female partners should be investigated simultaneously
   2) ovulation can be confirmed by the recording of basal body temperature
   3) the adequacy of the luteal phase is well assessed by midluteal serum progesterone determinations
   4) the postcoital test is negative unless 25 sperm are seen per high-power field (HPF)

354. The World Health Organization has issued parameters for the assessment of a normal sperm analysis. Which of the following is(are) part of the WHO's criteria for a normal sperm analysis?
   1) total count greater than 20 million sperm/ml
   2) sperm demonstrate greater than 50% motility
   3) sperm demonstrate greater than 50% normal morphology
   4) total semen volume is greater than 2.0 mls.

SELECT THE ONE BEST ANSWER TO THE FOLLOWING QUESTIONS:

355. The most common female factor responsible for infertility is:
   a) ovulatory/luteal phase dysfunction
   b) cervical factor

   c) tubal factor
   d) peritoneal (endometriosis)
   e) immune factor

356. Which of the following statements most correctly describes the manner in which a family physician should conduct an infertility investigation?
   a) the partners should be assessed one at a time; if no cause is found in the wife, the husband should then be checked
   b) the family physician should assess one factor at a time; the infertility investigation should be completed within 6 months
   c) the family physician should recommend an immediate referral to a gynecologist for the woman; if no infertility factor is found, he should refer the husband to a urologist for further evaluation
   d) the family physician should assess both husband and wife at the same time; preliminary investigations should be completed within 2 months.

ANSWERS

349. E. None of the above. The most appropriate first step is a complete history and physical examination on both partners.

   Infertility is defined as the inability of a couple to achieve a pregnancy after at least 1 year of unprotected intercourse, assuming a satisfactory frequency of intercourse.[1] Within 1 year, 95% of normal couples should achieve a pregnancy.[2]

   If conception does not occur within that time, a complete evaluation of both partners is indicated. In the female, a complete history including menstrual history, previous surgery, and previous pelvic infections should be obtained. The physical examination of the woman should evaluate any signs of endocrine disorder, and a complete pelvic examination (including rectovaginal) is essential. In the male, a history of mumps, current medications, epididymitis, or other male genitourinary infection is important. The physical examination of the male should include testicular size, location of urethral meatus, and the presence or absence of a varicocele. The prostate should be examined.[1]

350. C. The prevalence of infertility in North American couples is 10–15%.[3] This prevalence may be increasing due to an increase of sexually transmitted diseases, and a delay in the time of first conception.

351. C. If a woman has regular menstrual cycles associated with cyclical premenstrual sensations or symptoms (molimina), then she is almost certainly ovulating.[1] A woman who is menstruating regularly does not have to keep taking her basal body temperature for 6 months; to do so is both unnecessary and anxiety provoking. On the other hand, a woman who has a menstrual period only every 6 months is almost surely not ovulating.

Ovulation is most easily assessed by a history of regular cyclical menses; endometrial biopsy is rarely necessary. Many women who are anovulatory for long periods can have ovulation induced with clomiphene; therefore a one-year history of anovulation is not at all hopeless.

352. A. A successful pregnancy is dependent upon the following male and female factors:[1]
   a) successful vaginal intercourse with the deposition of motile spermatozoa in the upper vagina before ovulation
   b) a normal female hypothalamic-pituitary-ovarian axis that is capable of producing a luteinizing hormone (LH) surge, stimulating the production of normal cervical mucus, and producing sufficient progesterone during the luteal phase to maintain the corpus luteum and prepare the endometrium for implantation
   c) a normal quality and quantity of periovulatory cervical mucus and normal sperm-mucus interaction
   d) normal, patent fallopian tubes that allow ovum pickup, transport, and fertilization
   e) a normal hormonally stimulated uterus that is capable of supporting and maintaining implantation

353. A. Both male and female should be investigated simultaneously.[1]

A semen analysis should be performed.

In the male, a semen analysis should be obtained, preferably by masturbation. The World Health Organization's "normal" parameters of sperm count are >20 million sperm/ml, >50% motility, and >50% normal morphology.[4] An abnormal semen analysis should be repeated at least twice.

In the female, ovulation should be assessed by basal body temperature (BBT) charting. Normally, an increase in BBT of 0.5–1.0° F follows ovulation. Prolonged use of BBT records can become a significant source of anxiety and should be avoided. A 2- or 3-month period of charting is

recommended. Ovulation can be predicted prospectively with one of several rapid monoclonal antibody assay kits for the detection of urinary LH.[5] These kits, however, are expensive.

Luteal phase function can be assessed by the measurement of midluteal serum progesterone. A midluteal serum progesterone level above 10–15 ng/ml is considered evidence of an adequate luteal phase. Endometrial biopsy can also be used to diagnose a luteal phase defect.

The postcoital test measures the cervical factor in infertility. During the periovulatory period the cervical mucus should be thin, clear, acellular, and exhibit ferning and spinnbarkeit. The sperm-mucus interaction is assessed by counting the number of motile sperm per high-power field. If at least one motile sperm/HPF is found, the postcoital test is positive.

Tubal patency is assessed by laparoscopy plus intraoperative dye hydrotubation.

The uterine factor is best assessed by hysteroscopy.

Immune factors that may be involved in unexplained infertility can be assessed by measuring antisperm antibodies.

354. A. See critique of question 353. Semen volume is not part of The World Health Organization's "normal" parameters of semen analysis.

355. C. The most common female cause of infertility is the tubal factor.[6] This factor accounts for 30–50% of cases of infertility. Other factors are ovulatory/luteal phase defects (10–15%), cervical factors (10%), and male factors (40%).

356. D. Infertility investigations should be conducted quickly, and both husband and wife should be evaluated at the same time. The emotional impact of infertility can be very traumatic to a young couple. The longer the time taken to complete the investigations, the greater the emotional trauma. The family physician can perform baseline histories, physical examinations, semen analysis, basal body temperature charting, postcoital tests, and midluteal serum progesterone determinations in a short period of time. If no cause is found (suggesting a tubal or peritoneal factor), a referral to a gynecologist should be made as quickly as possible.

SUMMARY OF THE INITIAL CLINICAL SURVEY OF THE INFERTILE COUPLE

1. Complete history and physical examinations on both husband and wife

2. Basic tests that can be easily performed by family physician:
   Semen analysis (male factor)
   BBT (ovulatory factor)
   Postcoital test (cervical factor)
   Midluteal progesterone (luteal phase factor)

3. With a combination of history, physical examination, and these basic investigations, a tentative diagnosis can be reached. Referral to a gynecologist for assessment of tubal and peritoneal factors or to a urologist for further assessment of male factor is then recommended.

References

1. Jacobs L, Initial clinical survey of the infertile couple. Prim Care 1988; 15(3): 575–592.

2. Aral SO, Cates W. Increasing concern with infertility: why now? JAMA 1983; 250: 2327–2331.

3. Grimes EM. For infertile couples: a holistic approach. Contemp Obstet Gynecol 1984; 23: 179–188.

4. World Health Organization: Laboratory manual for the examination of human semen and semen cervical mucus interaction. New York: Cambridge University Press, 1987.

5. Rodrick-Highberg G, Sapp L, Kasper K, et al. Urinary LH test: evaluation with clinical specimens. Fertil Steril 1984; 41: 523–528.

6. Speroff L, Glass RH, Kase NF. Clinical gynecologic endocrinology and infertility. 3rd Ed. Baltimore: Williams & Wilkins, 1983.

PROBLEM 43: A 42-YEAR-OLD FEMALE WITH HEAVY MENSTRUAL PERIODS

A 42-year-old female presents to your office with a complaint of extremely heavy periods (with clots) for the last 6 months. Physical examination, including a pelvic examination, is normal. She is not obese. Basic screening blood work, including thyroid function studies, is normal. You decide that further evaluation is necessary and refer her to a gynecologist. The gynecologist performs a diagnostic curettage, a laparoscopy, and a hysteroscopy. No pathology is found.

SELECT THE ONE BEST ANSWER TO THE FOLLOWING QUESTIONS:

357. The most likely diagnosis in this patient is:
    a) uterine polyp
    b) submucous fibroma
    c) adenomatous hyperplasia
    d) adenomyosis
    e) none of the above

358. The most likely underlying cause of this patient's abnormal bleeding is:
    a) anovulation
    b) multiple ovulation
    c) a coagulation defect
    d) uterine pathology
    e) none of the above

359. The average volume of menstrual blood loss is:
    a) 10 cc
    b) 30 cc
    c) 50 cc
    d) 80 cc
    e) 100 cc

360. The most common physiologic correlate of dysfunctional uterine bleeding is:
    a) estrogen withdrawal
    b) estrogen breakthrough
    c) progesterone withdrawal
    d) progesterone breakthrough
    e) none of the above

ANSWER THE FOLLOWING QUESTIONS ACCORDING TO THE CODE:

A: 1, 2, and 3 are correct
B: 1 and 3 are correct
C: 2 and 4 are correct
D: Only 4 is correct
E: All of the above are correct

361. Which of the following has(have) been implicated in the etiology of dysfunctional uterine bleeding?
    1) hyperthyroidism
    2) hypothyroidism
    3) diabetes mellitus
    4) emotional stress

362. The treatment(s) of first choice for the patient described in this problem is(are):
    1) cyclic progestins
    2) the oral contraceptive pill
    3) nonsteroidal anti-inflammatory agents
    4) danazol

363. A 25-year-old female presents to your office with a 4-month history of midcycle spotting. She has a 28-day cycle and consistently spots between days 13 and 15. The treatment(s) of choice for the correction of this problem is(are):
    1) the oral contraceptive pill
    2) cyclic progestin
    3) ethinyl estradiol
    4) nonsteroidal anti-inflammatory drugs

364. A 28-year-old female presents with a 6-month history of postmenstrual spotting. Her menstrual cycles are regular, averaging 28 days in length. The treatment(s) of choice in this patient is(are):
    1) danazol
    2) the oral contraceptive pill (OCP)
    3) cyclic progestin
    4) nonsteroidal anti-inflammatory drugs

365. A 24-year-old obese female with a history of irregular menstrual periods presents to the emergency department with a 10-day history of heavy uterine bleeding. She is soaking through 20 pads/day. Her hemoglobin, when last measured 6 months ago, was 14 g%. Today it is 10.5 g%. You suspect acute hemorrhage caused by chronic anovulation. The treatment(s) of choice at this time in this patient is(are):
    1) oral contraceptives given four times/day for 5–7 days
    2) nonsteroidal anti-inflammatories
    3) intravenous Premarin
    4) cyclic progestins

366. A 20-year-old female presents to your office with an 8-month history of premenstrual spotting. She has regular 31-day cycles. The spotting begins 4–5 days before the onset of menstruation. The treatment(s) of choice in this patient is(are):

    1) the combination oral contraceptive pill
    2) nonsteroidal anti-inflammatories
    3) cyclic progestins
    4) dilation and curettage

ANSWERS

357. E. None of the above. The most likely diagnosis in this patient is dysfunctional uterine bleeding. Dysfunctional uterine bleeding is defined as uterine bleeding for which no specific genital tract lesion can be found.[1]

    The differential diagnosis of menorrhagia includes uterine fibroids (including submucous fibroids), endometriosis, adenomyosis, chronic pelvic inflammatory disease, endometrial polyps, coagulation defects, massive obesity, ovarian abnormalities, severe hypothyroidism, adenomatous hyperplasia, and endometrial carcinoma.[2]

    The evaluation of this patient included thyroid function tests, a diagnostic curettage, a laparoscopy, and a hysteroscopy. The results of these procedures were normal. Thus, with all major pathology excluded, a diagnosis of dysfunctional uterine bleeding can be made.

358. A. The most common cause of dysfunctional uterine bleeding is anovulation.[1] Anovulatory uterine bleeding may be associated with oligomenorrhea, menorrhagia, or menometrorrhagia.

    Dysfunctional uterine bleeding usually occurs during puberty and before the menopause; it is less common in the reproductive years. Ovulatory dysfunctional uterine bleeding (DUB) does occur during the reproductive years. It can be associated with midcycle spotting, premenstrual spotting, or postmenstrual spotting. Ovulatory DUB accounts for less than 10% of all DUB.[1]

359. B. The usual duration of menstrual flow is 4–6 days, and average blood loss during menstruation is 30 cc.[1] The duration of flow appears to be related to estrogen stimulation.

    In anovulatory dysfunctional uterine bleeding, the ability of the endometrium to synthesize prostaglandins appears to be altered. Nonsteroidal anti-inflammatory drugs, which are potent inhibitors of prostaglandin synthesis, may be beneficial in reducing the amount of blood loss in a patient with DUB.

360. B. The most common physiologic correlate of anovulatory DUB is estrogen breakthrough. An-

ovulation results in a continuous estrogen stimulation of the endometrium; this eventually leads to a buildup of the endometrial lining beyond the point of support. [1]

361. E. Dysfunctional uterine bleeding may be associated with endrocrine diseases (hypothyroidism, hyperthyroidism, diabetes mellitus, hyperprolactinemia); ovarian disorders (polycystic ovarian syndrome, premature menopause); drugs (including progesterone and estrogens); blood dyscrasias; emotional and physical stress; and nutritional disorders including morbid obesity and anorexia nervosa. [1]

In evaluating abnormal uterine bleeding, physiologic age grouping is often helpful. [1]

Menarche to age 20

Greater than 95% of abnormal uterine bleeding is dysfunctional and anovulatory. A careful history and physical examination is usually all that is necessary in evaluation. Oral contraceptives and NSAIDs are often beneficial.

Age 20–40

Anovulation is uncommon in this age group. A careful history and physical examination should precede any investigations. However, a hysteroscopy, endometrial sampling, and laparoscopy may be indicated in evaluation.

Age greater than 40

Anovulation is a major cause of abnormal uterine bleeding in this age group. However, uterine fibroids, uterine or cervical polyps, and endometrial carcinoma must be ruled out. Endometrial sampling is recommended.

362. B. As pelvic pathology has been excluded, this patient has dysfunctional uterine bleeding. This is most likely secondary to anovulation. Dilatation and curettage may, in this patient, be curative. If not, either cyclic progestins (Provera 10 mg from days 16–25 of the calendar month) or a nonsteroidal anti-inflammatory agent will reduce flow in 50% of patients.

As this patient is 42 years old, the oral contraceptive pill is not a reasonable treatment for dysfunctional uterine bleeding.

Danazol, although often an effective treatment, has significant side effects. If medical treatment is ineffective, surgical treatment should be considered. Endometrial ablation with the Nd:YAG laser may well become an important treatment option in the future. Hysterectomy is indicated when all other treatments have failed. [1]

363. B. The cause of midcycle spotting is estrogen withdrawal bleeding. The treatment should produce a buildup of the endometrium. Ethinyl estradiol, for 3 days before to 2 days after ovulation should be an effective therapy. The oral contraceptive pill may also be used. [1]

Because midcycle spotting is caused by estrogen withdrawal, neither cyclic progestins nor nonsteroidal anti-inflammatory drugs will correct the problem.

364. C. Postmenstrual spotting is caused by irregular endometrial shedding. This is an ovulatory DUB and responds to a NSAID or the OCP. [1]

Because this is ovulatory dysfunctional uterine bleeding, cyclic progestins would not be the drug of first choice. Danazol also would not be an appropriate treatment.

365. B. The treatment of choice for this type of heavy DUB is intravenous estrogen (Premarin 25 mg IV q4h for 3–4 doses) or an OCP given four times per day for 5–7 days. [1] In this patient, the remaining endometrial lining (basal layer) will be less responsive to progestin therapy. NSAIDs would be an excellent long-term choice; however, they are rarely helpful in a patient with this degree of acute hemorrhage.

366. B. Premenstrual spotting is a type of ovulatory dysfunctional bleeding caused by deficient progesterone production by the corpus luteum. [1] In this case, cyclic progestin administration of hydroxyprogesterone acetate (Provera) 10 mg/day from days 15–26 of the menstrual cycle is a treatment of choice. The oral contraceptive pill will also effectively stop premenstrual spotting. [1]

SUMMARY OF THE DIAGNOSIS AND TREATMENT OF DYSFUNCTIONAL UTERINE BLEEDING

1. **Definition**: abnormal uterine bleeding for which no specific genital tract lesion can be found

2. **Types of dysfunctional bleeding:**
   a) ovulatory: 10%
      midcycle spotting
      premenstrual spotting

postmenstrual spotting
b) anovulatory: 90%
oligomenorrhea
menorrhagia
menometrorrhagia

3. In patients over 20 years, exclude pelvic pathology before making the diagnosis of DUB. Also, consider the other etiologies that may be associated with DUB.

4. **Treatment:**
Ovulatory dysfunctional uterine bleeding:
midcycle spotting: ethinyl estradiol or OCP
premenstrual spotting: cyclic progestin
postmenstrual spotting: NSAID or OCP
Anovulatory dysfunctional bleeding:
a) consider therapeutic D & C

b) NSAIDs
c) cyclic progestins
d) OCP
e) surgical procedures if none of the above effective

Acute hemorrhage caused by DUB:
Premarin IV, OCPs 4 times/day for 5–7 days
OCP or oral Provera to follow

References

1. Field CS. Dysfunctional uterine bleeding. Prim Care 1988; 15(3): 561–573.

2. Poindexter AN, Ritter MB. Anovulatory uterine bleeding. Compr Ther 1983; 9: 65.

PROBLEM 44: A 49-YEAR-OLD FEMALE WITH HOT FLASHES

A 49-year-old female presents to your office with a 6-month history of "hot flashes." These flashes occur on a daily basis (approximately 10 times/day) and last for 2–3 minutes. The patient reports that her menstrual periods are becoming increasingly irregular. In addition to the "hot flashes," the patient describes disturbed sleep, headaches, and general irritability.

SELECT THE ONE BEST ANSWER TO THE FOLLOWING QUESTIONS:

367. Which of the following statements regarding this patient is FALSE?
a) over 75% of perimenopausal and menopausal women report the occurrence of hot flashes
b) there are two components to the vasomotor complex this patient describes; the hot flash and the hot flush
c) the hot flash occurs because of the pulsatile discharge of luteinizing hormone (LH)
d) hot flashes occur because of generalized vasodilation
e) skin temperature is raised significantly in patients with hot flashes

368. The treatment of choice for the patient described in question 367 is:
a) conjugated estrogen given cyclically
b) conjugated estrogen given continually
c) transdermal estrogen given cyclically
d) any of the above are satisfactory
e) a or c

369. The minimum daily dose of conjugated estrogen that is needed to relieve hot flushing is:
a) 0.125 mg
b) 0.3 mg
c) 0.625 mg
d) 1.25 mg
e) 2.5 mg

370. You decide to begin the patient described in question 367 on oral estrogen replacement therapy. Which of the following regimens is currently recommended for estrogen replacement in this situation?
a) conjugated estrogen 0.3 mg daily continuously
b) conjugated estrogen 0.625 mg daily continuously
c) conjugated estrogen 0.3 mg daily on days 1–25 of each calendar month
d) conjugated estrogen 0.625 mg daily on days 1–25 of each calendar month
e) conjugated estrogen 0.625 mg daily on days 1–25 of each calendar month plus medroxyprogesterone acetate 10 mg daily on days 16–25 of each calendar month

371. A 52-year-old woman presents with a 3-month history of dyspareunia, urinary frequency, urgency, and vaginal itching and burning. On examination, you find an atrophic vagina, with no evidence of infection.

    The treatment(s) of choice in this patient is(are):
    a) local estrogen cream
    b) oral conjugated estrogen
    c) transdermal estrogen
    d) a or b
    e) a, b, or c

ANSWER THE FOLLOWING QUESTION ACCORDING TO THE CODE:

A: 1, 2, and 3 are correct
B: 1 and 3 are correct
C: 2 and 4 are correct
D: Only 4 is correct
E: All of the above are correct

372. Which of the following condition(s) has (have) been shown to be increased when estrogen replacement therapy is administered in the postmenopausal period?
    1) breast cancer
    2) thromboembolic disease
    3) hypertension
    4) endometrial carcinoma

ANSWERS

367. C. The "hot flash" is the most common symptom of the menopause. The "hot flash" should be distinguished from the "hot flush." The hot flash usually precedes the hot flush and is described as a sensation of warmth; it is associated with vasodilation. The hot flush that follows is characterized by erythema and sweating. The skin temperature may increase by as much as 2.5° C during the hot flush. The hot flash and the hot flush are two parts of a complex vasomotor phenomenon. [1]

    Over 75% of women experience hot flashes; the majority of them, however, do not require treatment apart from explanation of the symptoms.

    Although it was originally felt that the hot flash occurred because of the pulsatile release of LH, the explanation appears to be more complex; a central hypothalamic mechanism is more likely. [1]

368. E., 369. C., and 370. E. Estrogen is the most specific and effective treatment for vasomotor symptoms. The dosage of estrogen needed to control hot flashes is usually 0.625 mg. [2] Occasionally, 1.25 mg may have to be used. The dosage can be tapered, and therapy may be able to be discontinued after 3 to 6 months.

    Estrogen should always be given cyclically and should be accompanied by the administration of a synthetic progesterone (medroxyprogesterone acetate) to prevent endometrial hyperplasia and endometrial carcinoma. The current recommendation is Premarin 0.625 mg on days 1–25 of the calendar month and Provera 10 mg on days 16–25 of the calendar month. [2]

    Estrogen may also be administered in the transdermal form. [3] Administration of transdermal estrogen bypasses the liver and may result in fewer side effects.

371. E. Estrogen deprivation can lead to significant urogenital tract symptoms including itching, burning, dryness, and dyspareunia. Urinary frequency, urgency, and discomfort also occur. [3]

    Urogenital symptoms will respond to oral estrogen (0.3–0.625 mg). Vaginal estrogen preparation [3] (Premarin vaginal cream 2–4 g/day for 3 out of 4 weeks) will also successfully treat atrophic changes. Transdermal estrogen can also be used on a cyclic basis. As in the treatment of vasomotor symptoms, progesterone should be used to prevent endometrial hyperplasia and endometrial carcinoma.

372. D. Endometrial carcinoma has been linked to the administration of postmenopausal estrogens. Endometrial carcinoma that develops secondary to estrogen replacement tends to be of a lower grade and have less invasive potential than an endometrial carcinoma that develops without the influence of postmenopausal estrogens. [3]

    Breast cancer, thromboembolic disease, and hypertension have not been found to be increased in patients who are prescribed exogenous estrogens. These conditions, however, still remain contraindications to estrogen replacement therapy. Breast cancer and thromboembolic disease are absolute contraindications, and hypertension is a relative contraindication.

SUMMARY OF THE DIAGNOSIS AND TREATMENT OF VASOMOTOR SYMPTOMS AND UROGENITAL SYMPTOMS IN THE PERIMENOPAUSAL AND POSTMENOPAUSAL PERIOD

1. **Vasomotor symptoms**: Hot flashes/ hot flushes
   a) develop in 75% of patients
   b) require treatment in 10–15% of patients

2. **Urogenital symptoms**: dyspareunia, vaginal itching, vaginal dryness; burning, urgency, and frequency of urination

3. **Treatment**:
   Premarin orally
   Estraderm patchs

Premarin intravaginally

All of the above to be used with medroxyprogesterone acetate (Provera) 10 mg for 10 days in each calendar month.

References

1. Collins J. Menopause. Prim Care 1988; 15(3): 593–606.

2. Phillips D, Gearhart J. The female reproductive system. In: Taylor R, ed. Family medicine: principles and practice. New York: Springer-Verlag, 1988: 318–319.

3. Huppert L. Hormone replacement therapy: benefits, risks, dosages. Med Clin North Am 1987; 71(1): 23–39.

PROBLEM 45: A 26-YEAR-OLD FEMALE WITH AN ABNORMAL PAP SMEAR

A 26-year-old female presents for her annual physical examination. Pelvic examination is normal and the cervix looks healthy. There is no vaginal or cervical discharge. However, the Pap smear comes back as CIN I (cervical intraepithelial neoplasia I).

SELECT THE ONE BEST ANSWER TO THE FOLLOWING QUESTIONS:

373. At this time, you should:
    a) repeat the Pap smear in 1 year
    b) repeat the Pap smear in 6 months
    c) repeat the Pap smear in 3 months
    d) refer the patient for colposcopy
    e) refer the patient for cone biopsy

374. A 26-year-old female presents for a routine health assessment. She is asymptomatic. A Pap smear is performed and the report comes back: Class II–Trichomonas present.

    At this time, you should:
    a) treat the infection and repeat the Pap smear in 1 year
    b) treat the infection and repeat the Pap smear in 6 months
    c) refer the patient for cone biopsy
    d) refer the patient for colposcopy
    e) treat the infection and repeat the Pap smear in 2 weeks

375. Which of the following statements regarding carcinoma of the cervix and/or the Pap smear is FALSE?

    a) carcinoma of the cervix is a sexually transmitted disease
    b) case-finding for carcinoma of the cervix can stop at age 60 providing the patient has been adequately screened before and has no new sexual partners after that time
    c) an Ayres spatula is a sufficient tool for obtaining a specimen for Pap smear analysis
    d) carcinoma of the cervix is a disease with a long lead time
    e) none of the above statements are false

376. Carcinoma of the cervix is usually associated with which of the following viruses?
    a) herpes simplex I virus
    b) herpes simplex II virus
    c) human papilloma virus
    d) parvovirus
    e) adenovirus

ANSWER THE FOLLOWING QUESTIONS ACCORDING TO THE CODE:

A: 1, 2, and 3 are correct
B: 1 and 3 are correct
C: 2 and 4 are correct
D: Only 4 is correct

E: All of the above are correct

377. Which of the following IS/ARE risk factors for carcinoma of the cervix?
    1) multiple sexual partners
    2) smoking
    3) early age of first coitus
    4) herpes simplex virus infections

378. Which of the following statements regarding colposcopy IS/ARE true?
    1) all women with evidence of cervical intraepithelial neoplasia should be referred for colposcopy
    2) areas of abnormality are identified by swabbing the cervix with an acetic acid solution
    3) colposcopically identified abnormalities can be treated with cryotherapy or the CO_2 laser
    4) a cone biopsy is still necessary in 15–20% of cases

ANSWERS

373. D. When a patient's Pap smear report indicates the presence of CIN she should be referred for colposcopy.

    The term "dysplasia" has been replaced in many centers by "cervical intraepithelial neoplasia (CIN).CIN is usually graded as I, II, or III.[1]

    When the Pap smear suggests the presence of neoplasia, it is almost always correct. There are very few false-positive smears. On the other hand, the false-negative rate can be very high. Thus, the Pap smear has a high "specificity" but a substantially lower "sensitivity." Previously, if a woman had an abnormal smear, it was common to repeat the smear and, if the second smear was negative, to do nothing. This is not recommended; the Pap smear that should be believed is the abnormal one, not the negative one.[1] In addition, the Pap smear may underestimate the severity of cellular atypia. Thus, an abnormal Pap smear demands a colposcopic examination.[1]

374. E. Infections such as *Trichomonas* may induce cell changes that may be interpreted as a "Class II" Pap smear. In this case, the infection should be treated and the Pap smear should be repeated in 2 weeks time. If normal, usual follow-up may occur. A second abnormal Pap smear, in this case, should result in referral for colposcopy.[1]

375. C. Carcinoma of the cervix is a sexually transmitted disease. Risk factors include early first intercourse, multiple sexual partners, and multiple sexual partners in the patient's partner.[1]

    Postmenopausal women may cease to have Pap smears after age 60 if they have no new sexual partners, and they have been adequately screened previously.

    The Pap smear should be obtained by obtaining an endocervical aspirate or a swab with a saline-moistened cotton-tipped applicator and a scraping of the exocervix with an Ayres spatula. An Ayres spatula by itself is not a sufficient tool for obtaining an accurate specimen, as the transformation zone may not be reached. The cervical cytologic brush is another excellent method for obtaining the same result.

    Carcinoma of the cervix is a disease with a long lead time. Lead time is the period of time between the detection of a medical condition by screening and when it ordinarily would have been diagnosed because an individual experienced symptoms and sought medical care. Diseases that have a long lead time usually lend themselves to effective screening programs.[2]

376. C. Carcinoma of the cervix is usually caused by the human papilloma virus (wart virus or HPV). The most common subtypes involved are types 16 and 18.

377. E. All of the above are risk factors for carcinoma of the cervix. Early age of first intercourse and multiple sexual partners have already been discussed. Additional risk factors are cigarette smoking and women with a history of a genital herpes simplex infection.[1] Women with any of the above risk factors should be screened yearly.

378. E. Any abnormal Pap smear (apart from that associated with infection) demands a colposcopic examination. Colposcopy is performed by examining an area of the cervix that has been magnified and treated with acetic acid.

    If the cytology, colposcopic impression, and histopathology all agree, and if the lesion identified by the colposcopist can be seen in its entirety, treatment of the lesion with cryotherapy or CO_2 laser vaporization is successful in greater than 95% of cases.[1] If the lesion extends into the endocervical canal and cannot be completely visualized, a cone biopsy is necessary. This will occur in 15–20% of cases.[1]

SUMMARY OF DIAGNOSIS AND TREATMENT OF CERVICAL INTRAEPITHELIAL NEOPLASIA

1. Assess risk factor status of patient and perform Pap smears at recommended intervals.

2. Obtain both an endocervical and exocervical specimen.

3. Consider cytopathologist's verbal report— if any evidence of CIN (or dysplasia in old terminology), refer for colposcopy.

4. Remember that Pap smear screening has a low sensitivity; therefore, believe the positive report, not the negative one.

References

1. Noller KL. Cervical cytology and the evaluation of the abnormal Papanicolaou smear. Prim Care 1988; 15(3): 461–471.

2. Fletcher R, Fletcher S, Wagner S. Clinical epidemiology: the essentials. Baltimore: Williams & Wilkins, 1988.

PROBLEM 46: A 24-YEAR-OLD FEMALE WITH ABDOMINAL PAIN, PELVIC PAIN, AND ADNEXAL TENDERNESS

A 24-year-old nulligravida female presents to the emergency department with a 2-day history of lower abdominal pain. On examination she has a bilateral lower abdominal tenderness, tenderness on cervical motion, and adnexal tenderness. She has a fever of 40° C. Her last menstrual period was 5 weeks ago, but she has had a small amount of spotting in the last few days. She has had one previous episode of these symptoms.

SELECT THE ONE BEST ANSWER TO THE FOLLOWING QUESTIONS:

379. The most likely diagnosis in this patient is:
    a) acute appendicitis
    b) chronic salpingitis
    c) acute salpingitis
    d) ectopic pregnancy
    e) endometritis

380. Which of the following statements regarding the relationship between the oral contraceptive pill and pelvic inflammatory disease (PID) is TRUE?
    a) the oral contraceptive pill protects against all forms of PID
    b) the oral contraceptive pill protects against chlamydial PID but not against PID caused by *Neisseria gonorrhoeae*
    c) the oral contraceptive pill protects against gonococcal PID but not against PID caused by chlamydial infection
    d) the oral contraceptive pill does not protect against any form of PID
    e) the evidence that the oral contraceptive pill protects against PID is very weak

381. Which of the following organisms IS NOT associated with acute pelvic inflammatory disease?
    a) N. gonorrhoeae
    b) *Chlamydia trachomatis*
    c) *Mycoplasma hominis*
    d) peptostreptococcus
    e) beta-hemolytic streptococcus

382. Which of the following is NOT a risk factor for acute pelvic inflammatory disease?
    a) age <25
    b) multiple sexual partners
    c) a barrier contraceptive method
    d) history of previous diagnosis of PID
    e) time of last menstrual period

383. The most appropriate treatment of the 24-year-old female previously described would be:
    a) hospitalize the patient and begin treatment
    b) begin treatment as an outpatient, but recheck the patient in 24 hours
    c) begin treatment as an outpatient, but recheck the patient if she becomes worse
    d) begin treatment as an outpatient and make an appointment for her to see a gynecologist tomorrow
    e) hospitalize the patient and discharge her for outpatient care if she has improved in 24 hours

384. If hospital management was chosen for a patient such as the one described in this question, which

of the following treatment regimens would be MOST appropriate?

a) ampicillin and gentamicin intravenously
b) ampicillin and tobramycin intravenously
c) ampicillin and doxycycline intravenously
d) cefoxitin and doxycycline intravenously
e) ampicillin intravenously

ANSWER THE FOLLOWING QUESTION ACCORDING TO THE CODE:

A: 1, 2, and 3 are correct
B: 1 and 3 are correct
C: 2 and 4 are correct
D: Only 4 is correct
E: All of the above are correct

385. If outpatient management is chosen for a patient with pelvic inflammatory disease, which of the following treatment regimens IS/ARE appropriate?

1) cefoxitin IM plus doxycycline orally
2) ampicillin, probenicid, and doxycycline orally
3) aqueous procaine penicillin G IM, plus oral probenicid and doxycycline
4) ampicillin 500 mg q.i.d. for 10 days

ANSWERS

379. C. This patient meets the diagnostic criteria for acute salpingitis. Acute salpingitis is diagnosed when there is a history of lower abdominal pain, lower abdominal tenderness, cervical motion tenderness, and adnexal tenderness that is accompanied by one of elevated temperature, elevated WBC or ESR, positive culdocentesis, an inflammatory mass on pelvic examination or sonography, or a positive gram stain or smear.[1]

The differential diagnosis of acute pelvic inflammatory disease includes acute appendicitis, endometriosis, corpus luteum bleeding, ectopic pregnancy, pelvic adhesions, benign ovarian tumor, and chronic salpingitis.[2] The patient described in the question, however, is more likely to have acute salpingitis than any of the diagnoses described above. Although the patient has had one previous episode of these symptoms, a diagnosis of chronic salpingitis cannot be made without laparoscopy.

An infection confined to the endometrium (endometritis) is unlikely in this patient. The adnexal tenderness is much more compatible with salpin-

gitis. Endometritis usually occurs post partum (especially with retained products of conception) or after a procedure such as a suction dilatation and curettage for therapeutic abortion.

380. C. The oral contraceptive pill protects against gonococcal PID. Genital tract infection with *Chlamydia trachomatis* may actually be increased.[3]

The protective effect against gonococcus may be associated with (1) a decreased average amount of menstrual blood flow, with menstrual blood acting as a culture medium; (2) a decreased permeability of cervical mucus to the infective organism; (3) a decreased cervical dilatation at mid cycle and at menstruation; and (4) a decrease in the strength of uterine contractions.[3]

381. E. The most common organisms associated with pelvic inflammatory disease are *Neiserria gonorrhoeae*, *Chlamydia trachomatis*, and *Mycoplasma hominis*.[4] Many episodes of PID appear to be polymicrobial and involve anaerobic organisms such as bacteroides and peptostreptococcus.[4] Beta-hemolytic streptococcus is not associated with acute pelvic inflammatory disease.

382. C. Barrier contraceptive methods (i.e., condom, diaphragm) are protective against, rather than contributory to, pelvic inflammatory disease. Risk factors for acute pelvic inflammatory disease include age <25, multiple sexual partners, nonbarrier contraceptive methods (especially the intrauterine device), time of last menstrual period (the closer the time to the last period, the greater the risk), a history of previous diagnosis of PID, and symptoms of urethritis in a sexual partner.[4]

383. A. Early treatment of acute pelvic inflammatory disease will decrease the probability of tubal scarring and subsequent infertility. Hospitalization and inpatient treatment is preferred in the following situations:[6]

a) the patient is an adolescent
b) the diagnosis is uncertain
c) surgical emergencies such as appendicitis and ectopic pregnancy must be excluded
d) a pelvic abscess is suspected
e) severe illness precludes outpatient management
f) the patient is pregnant
g) the patient is unable to follow or tolerate an outpatient regimen

h) the patient has failed to respond to outpatient therapy

i) follow-up within 72 hours of starting antibiotic treatment cannot be arranged

In the patient described in the question, two of these factors are present: (1) she has a severe illness, manifested by a temperature of 40° C and (2) ectopic pregnancy has not been excluded (last period 5 weeks ago and spotting in the last few days).

384. D. Combination chemotherapy is essential in patients with PID. For hospitalized patients the preferred regimen is cefoxitin, 2 g IV q6h and doxycycline 100 mg IV or PO b.i.d., for at least 4 days and at least 48 hours after improvement followed by doxycycline 100 mg PO b.i.d. to complete 10 days of treatment. An alternate regimen is clindamycin 600 mg IV q6h, and gentamicin 2 mg/kg IV q8h, for 4 days and at least 48 hours after improvement (gentamicin serum concentrations should be monitored), followed by clindamycin 450 mg PO q.i.d., to complete at least 10 days of treatment.[6]

385. A. The recommended treatments for acute pelvic inflammatory disease, treated by ouapatient therapy, are a single dose of cefoxitin 2.0 g IM; or amoxicillin 3.0 g PO; or ampicillin 3.5 g PO; or aqueous procaine penicillin G, 4.8 million U IM, at two sites, plus probenecid 1.0 g PO; or ceftriaxone, 250 mg IM; PLUS doxycycline, 100 mg b.i.d. for at least 10 days, or tetracycline 500 mg q.i.d. for at least 10 days.[6]

SUMMARY OF THE DIAGNOSIS AND TREATMENT OF ACUTE PELVIC INFLAMMATORY DISEASE

1. Use diagnostic criteria discussed in question 379.

2. Begin treatment immediately to prevent tubal scarring and subsequent infertility: hospitalize if any of the criteria discussed in the critique of question 383 are met.

3. Recognize polymicrobial nature of PID: always treat with more than one antibiotic.

4. Follow guidelines (questions 384 and 385) in the treatment of PID infections.

References

1. Hager WD, et al. Criteria for diagnosis and grading of salpingitis. Obstet Gynecol 1983; 61: 113–114.

2. Jacobson L. Differential diagnosis of acute pelvic inflammatory disease. Am J Obstet Gynecol 1980; 138(7): 1006–1011.

3. Hatcher R, Guest F, Stewart F, et al. In: Breedlove B, Judy B, Martin N, eds. Contraceptive technology. 14th Ed. New York: Irvington Publishers, 1988: 239–240.

4. Nesse R. Office management of sexually transmitted disease and management of pelvic inflammatory disease in the ambulatory patient. Prim Care 1988; 15(3): 507–515.

5. 1988 Canadian guidelines for the treatment of sexually transmitted diseases in neonates, children, adolescents, and adults. Canada Diseases Weekly Report Volume 14S2. Health and Welfare Canada (Government of Canada), 1988: 11.

PROBLEM 47:   A 35-YEAR-OLD FEMALE WITH FATIGUE, BREAST TENDERNESS, ABDOMINAL BLOATING, FLUID RETENTION, AND ANXIETY AND DEPRESSION IN THE PREMENSTRUAL PERIOD

A 35-year-old female presents with a 6-month history of fatigue, breast tenderness, abdominal bloating, fluid retention, anxiety, irritability, depression, difficulty concentrating, and hypersomnia in the 10 days prior to menstruation. She states that these symptoms usually continue until 2 days into the menstrual flow and rapidly diminish thereafter. During the 10-day period she is unable to function at work or home.

SELECT THE ONE BEST ANSWER TO THE FOLLOWING QUESTIONS:

386. The most likely diagnosis in this patient is:
    a) generalized anxiety disorder
    b) masked depression
    c) late luteal phase dysphoric disorder
    d) major depressive illness
    e) none of the above

387. Which of the following statements regarding the etiology of late luteal phase dysphoric disorder is TRUE?
    a) hormonal imbalance has been definitively established as the etiology of the condition
    b) prostaglandins have not been implicated in the etiology
    c) endorphins are more likely than prostaglandins or hormonal imbalance to be the primary cause of the disorder
    d) psychosocial factors have not been implicated in the etiology of the disorder
    e) none of the above statements are true

388. The most important element in establishing the above diagnosis is a good history. The most important information that can be obtained in the history is:
    a) the severity of symptoms
    b) the number of symptoms
    c) the timing of the symptoms in the menstrual cycle
    d) the presence and severity of the depression or anxiety
    e) all of the above symptoms are of equal importance

ANSWER THE FOLLOWING QUESTIONS ACCORDING TO THE CODE:

A: 1, 2, and 3 are correct
B: 1 and 3 are correct
C: 2 and 4 are correct
D: Only 4 is correct
E: All of the above are correct

389. For the above diagnosis to be made, which of the following criteria must be fulfilled?
    1) the symptoms must occur in at least two consecutive cycles
    2) the symptoms must be limited to the luteal phase

    3) there must be a complete absence of symptoms for at least one week in the postmenstrual period
    4) depression must be one of the symptoms

390. Which of the following treatments should form part of the regimen for patients suffering from the disorder discussed above?
    1) a high fiber, high complex carbohydrate diet
    2) increased aerobic exercise
    3) patient and spouse education
    4) vitamin B_6 (pyridoxine)

391. Which of the following is(are) recommended as drugs of first choice in the treatment of the above disorder?
    1) spironolactone
    2) combination oral contraceptive pills
    3) prostaglandin synthetase inhibitors
    4) natural progesterone

ANSWERS

386. C. This patient has late luteal phase dysphoric disorder. This is also known as premenstrual tension syndrome.

    This disorder is characterized by the occurrence of a combination of the following symptoms in the last part of the luteal phase, with a symptom-free interval in the follicular phase: (1) a labile affect, (2) persistent feelings of sadness, irritability, and anger, (3) significant anxiety or tension, (4) depressed mood, (5) decreased interest in daily activities, (6) fatigue, (7) impaired concentration, (8) change in appetite, (9) change in sleep pattern, (10) physical symptoms including breast tenderness or swelling, headaches, joint or muscle pain, and a sensation of "bloating," and (11) weight gain.[1] To make the diagnosis these symptoms must significantly interfere with work or usual social activities, and must not be associated with another major psychiatric disorder.[1] As well, these symptoms must be present for at least two cycles.

    Although premenstrual symptoms occur in up to 90% of women, severe symptoms that interfere with work or usual social activities occur in, at most, 10% of the population.

387. E. The etiology of late luteal phase disorder remains unknown. The theories that have been proposed[2] include:
    1) a hormonal imbalance with a progesterone deficiency

2) a prostaglandin-mediated syndrome

3) a syndrome caused by a relative lack of endorphins

4) a deficiency of Vitamin B6

5) a biopsychosocial theory where biologic, psychologic, and social factors interact in a complex manner.

388. C. The timing of the symptoms to the menstrual cycle is the most important factor in establishing a diagnosis of late luteal phase dysphoric disorder. The relationship of symptoms to the menstrual cycle is best established by a calendar that is kept for at least two consecutive menstrual cycles. Included in the calendar should be the day of the cycle, a daily rating of the menstrual flow (slight, moderate, heavy, or heavy with clots), and the symptoms experienced (rating scale of 1–3).[2]

389. A. For the diagnosis of late luteal phase dysphoric disorder to be made, the following criteria must apply: (1) the symptoms must occur in at least two consecutive cycles, (2) the symptoms must be limited to the luteal phase, and (3) there must be a complete absence of symptoms for at least 1 week in the postmenstrual period. Depression does not, however, have to be one of the symptoms.[1]

390. A. Treatment of luteal phase dysfunction can be divided into two phases:
Phase 1: nondrug treatment
Phase 2: drug treatment

This question addresses phase 1 treatment. The most important aspects of phase 1 treatment are:

1) patient and spouse education about the disorder

2) dietary manipulation

3) increased aerobic exercise

4) explanation and reassurance.

Physicians must acknowledge that this disorder is real, and be prepared to listen to, and offer advice to, their patients. Education will enable women to schedule activities that will avoid extra stresses around the time of maximal symptomatology. Relaxation exercises are frequently helpful.

Dietary manipulation should include limitation of salt, refined sugar, red meat, fat, alcohol, and caffeine. Dietary fiber and complex carbohydrates should be increased.

Regular (3 times/week) aerobic exercise is recommended.

Other nondrug treatments that have been suggested include Vitamin B6 (100 mg/day), evening primrose oil (containing linolenic acid), and vitamin E.[2]

391. B. Patients should be given a 3-month trial of phase 1 (nondrug) treatment before proceeding to phase 2 therapy. If, after a 3-month period of time, the patient is still having significant symptoms, the following treatments[2] may be tried:

1) spironolactone (100 mg/day) during the luteal phase if edema is a significant problem

2) a prostaglandin synthetase inhibitor during the luteal phase and into the first 2 days of the menstrual period if edema is not a significant problem

3) progesterone supplementation (vaginal suppository 200–400 mg o.d. to t.i.d.)

4) the combination oral contraceptive pill

5) danazol

6) bromocriptine

SUMMARY OF THE DIAGNOSIS AND TREATMENT OF LATE LUTEAL PHASE DYSPHORIC DISORDER

1. **Diagnosis:** criteria in question 386.

2. **Etiologic theories:** hormonal, prostaglandin, endorphin biopsychosocial

3. History is most important in diagnosis; diagnosis must be confirmed by charting symptoms for at least 2 months

4. **Treatment:**
Phase 1: Nonpharmacologic:
a) education for patient and spouse
b) diet: low fat, low sodium, avoidance of caffeine and alcohol, replacement of simple sugars by complex carbohydrates
c) aerobic exercise
d) relaxation techniques
e) vitamin B6, evening primrose oil
Phase 2: Pharmacologic:
a) edema or bloating symptoms predominate: spironolactone
b) nonedema or bloating symptoms predominate: prostaglandin synthetase inhibitor
c) consider progesterone if a or b fail
d) consider oral contraceptive if patient under 35 and also desires contraception
e) if all other treatments fail, consider danazol or bromocriptine

References

1. American Psychiatric Association. Diagnostic and Statistical Manual III—Revised. (DSM-III-R). Washington: APA Press, 1987: 369.

2. Wickes, S. Premenstrual syndrome. Prim Care 1988; 15(3): 473–487.

PROBLEM 48: A 25-YEAR-OLD NULLIPARA AT 11 WEEKS GESTATION WITH VAGINAL BLEEDING

A 25-year-old female para 0 gravida 3 presents to your office at 11-weeks gestation with vaginal bleeding and mild cramping. Her previous two pregnancies ended in miscarriages at 9 weeks. On examination a moderate bright red flow is seen coming from the cervical os. The cervix is closed. Clinical palpation reveals an 8-week uterus.

392. The diagnosis at this time is:
   a) threatened abortion
   b) inevitable abortion
   c) incomplete abortion
   d) habitual abortion
   e) complete abortion

393. Referring to the patient described in the problem, the flow increases slightly while the patient is in your office. She is now soaking through approximately 1 pad every 2 hours. You would now recommend:
   a) observation at home and outpatient investigation
   b) observation in hospital and inpatient investigation
   c) outpatient observation only, no further investigations
   d) inpatient observation only, no further investigations
   e) it doesn't really matter

394. The patient goes on to abort the fetus 3 days later. On examination it appears that most of the placental tissue is present. You would now recommend:
   a) no further treatment
   b) ergonovine maleate to contract the uterus
   c) prophylactic antibiotics to prevent infection
   d) dilatation and curettage
   e) b and c

395. The total rate of pregnancy loss after implantation, including clinically recognized spontaneous abortions, has recently been estimated using urinary concentrations of human chorionic gonadotrophin. What is this percentage?
   a) 5%
   b) 10%
   c) 15%
   d) 20%
   e) 30%

ANSWER THE FOLLOWING QUESTIONS ACCORDING TO THE CODE:

A: 1, 2, and 3 are correct
B: 1 and 3 are correct
C: 2 and 4 are correct
D: Only 4 is correct
E: All of the above are correct

396. Which of the following factors have been implicated in spontaneous abortion?
   1) endocrine defects
   2) smoking
   3) emotional trauma
   4) alcohol

397. Which of the following statements regarding chromosomal abnormalities in spontaneous abortions is(are) TRUE:
   1) most situations of a chromosomal abnormality in the fetus result from a chromosomal abnormality in one or both parents
   2) structural abnormalities are much more common than abnormalities in the number of chromosomes
   3) the most common chromosomal abnormality is 47 XX
   4) 50–60% of early spontaneous abortions are associated with a chromosomal anomaly of the conceptus

398. Which of the following statements is(are) TRUE regarding habitual abortion?
    1) habitual abortion is defined as three or more consecutive abortions
    2) repeated spontaneous abortions are likely to be a chance phenomena in most cases
    3) couples who have a history of habitual abortion should receive a complete chromosomal analysis
    4) the probability of having a successful pregnancy after three consecutive spontaneous abortions is 70–85%

ANSWERS

392. A. At this time, the diagnosis is threatened abortion. Threatened abortion is defined as bloody vaginal discharge or vaginal bleeding that appears during the first 20 weeks of pregnancy.[1] Mild abdominal cramping often accompanies the bleeding. The incidence of threatened abortion in pregnant women is 20–25%; of those 1/2 go on to abort the fetus.[1] Threatened abortion is associated with a higher risk of preterm labor, low birth weight, and perinatal mortality. There is, however, no increased risk of fetal malformations.[1]

Inevitable abortion is defined as vaginal bleeding during the first half of pregnancy accompanied by cervical dilatation and rupture of the gestational sac.[1]

Incomplete abortion refers to the incomplete evacuation of the products of conception during the abortion.[1] It is often difficult to be sure all of the products of conception have been expelled without doing a dilatation and curettage.

Habitual abortion refers to three or more consecutive completed abortions.[2] Complete abortion refers to the complete evacuation of the products of conception from the uterus during the first half of pregnancy.

393. B. In any patient with more than slight bleeding, hospitalization is wise. With the associated cramping there is a very good probability that she will go on to abort the fetus. Investigations in hospital should include a beta-HCG level and obstetric ultrasound, looking for a gestational sac with a fetal pole and fetal cardiac motion.

394. D. Unless all of the fetus and placenta can be positively identified, dilatation and curettage is indicated. It is often very difficult to be sure that an abortion is indeed complete. If the gestational age is less than 10 weeks, conservative management may be reasonable, as the embryo and accompanying placental tissue are often expelled as a unit.[1]

Ergonovine maleate and prophylactic antibiotics are most useful when excessive bleeding occurs in the postpartum period and is unlikely to be due to retained products of conception.

395. E. The total rate of pregnancy loss after implantation, including clinically recognized spontaneous abortions, was 31%. Most of the women with unrecognized early pregnancy losses had normal fertility, since 95% of them subsequently became clinically pregnant within 2 years.[3]

396. C. Many factors have been suggested as possible causes of spontaneous abortion. These include certain infections (*Mycoplasma*), chronic debilitating disease, endocrine defects (progesterone deficiency), nutrition, alcohol use, tobacco use, immunologic factors (antibodies against sperm), abnormalities of the reproductive organs, laparotomy, physical and emotional trauma, and paternal factors. Only alcohol use, tobacco use, and immunologic factors appear to have any relationship with spontaneous abortion.[1]

397. D. Chromosomal abnormalities account for 50–60% of early spontaneous abortions.[1] Abnormalities in the number of chromosomes are much more common than are structural abnormalities of chromosomes.[1]

Parents of fetuses with chromosomal abnormalities most often have normal chromosome complements themselves. Numerical abnormalities include monosomy, trisomy, and polyploidy. The most common abnormality is the monosomy 45X.

Pregnancies destined to abort because of a chromosomally abnormal zygote may go unrecognized because the products of conception are aborted with little or no delay in the onset of menstruation.

398. E. Habitual abortion is defined as three or more consecutive spontaneous abortions.[2] Repeated spontaneous abortions are likely to be a chance phenomenon in the majority of cases. The spontaneous pregnancy rate after as many as three consecutive spontaneous abortions may be as high as 70-85%.

After two or three spontaneous abortions, the parents should be karyotyped.

SUMMARY OF THE DIAGNOSIS AND MANAGEMENT OF SPONTANEOUS ABORTION

Definition of threatened abortion: bloody vaginal discharge or vaginal bleeding, which occurs during the first 20 weeks of pregnancy.

Investigation of threatened abortion:
a) serial beta-HCG levels
b) ultrasound (if questionable repeat in 1–2 weeks)

Management of threatened abortion:
a) rest in hospital (unless there is only a small amount of blood in which case rest at home is reasonable)
b) observation

c) conservative management if bleeding slows down or stops (document live fetus by ultrasound).
d) dilatation and curettage if heavy bleeding continues and ultrasound reveals no evidence of a live fetus

References

1. Cunningham FG, MacDonald P, Gant N. Williams obstetrics. 18th Ed. Norwalk: Appleton and Lange, 1989: 489–509.

2. Russell K. The course and conduct of normal labor and delivery. In: Benson R, ed. Current obstetric and gynecologic diagnosis and treatment. 5th Ed. Los Altos: Lange Medical Publications, 1984: 681–709.

3. Wilcox AJ. Incidence of early loss in pregnancy. N Engl J Med 1988; 319(4): 189–194.

PROBLEM 49: A 23-YEAR-OLD FEMALE WHO WISHES TO BEGIN TAKING THE ORAL CONTRACEPTIVE PILL

A 23-year-old female presents to your office for a complete physical assessment. She wishes to begin taking the oral contraceptive pill (OCP). Before giving her the oral contraceptive pill, you establish whether or not she has any contraindications to taking it.

SELECT THE ONE BEST ANSWER TO THE FOLLOWING QUESTIONS:

399. Which of the following IS NOT an absolute contraindication to taking the oral contraceptive pill?
    a) thrombophlebitis or thromboembolic disorder
    b) ischemic heart disease
    c) benign liver tumor
    d) diabetes mellitus
    e) undiagnosed abnormal genital bleeding

400. Which of the following IS NOT a strong relative contraindication to taking the oral contraceptive pill?
    a) severe headaches
    b) acute gall bladder disease
    c) acute phase mononucleosis
    d) long-leg cast or major injury to the lower leg
    e) greater than age 35

401. You determine that your patient has no contraindication to the oral contraceptive pill. Which of the

oral contraceptives listed below would be included in your first choices for therapy?
    a) Ortho Novum 1/80
    b) Ovral
    c) Demulen 1/50
    d) Micronor
    e) Ortho 7/7/7

402. An 18-year-old patient who you begin on the oral contraceptive pill (Loestrin 1/20) returns to the office 3 months later complaining of increasing acne. You suggest some local treatments including skin cleansers and topical clindamycin lotion. However, she returns 1 month later with no improvement in her acne. You assume that the acne is associated with the oral contraceptive pill. What would be the most reasonable course of action at this time?
    a) discontinue the oral contraceptive pill
    b) change the pill to one with less androgenic activity
    c) change the pill to one with less estrogenic activity

d) change the pill to one with less progestin activity

e) maintain the patient on the same oral contraceptive and reassess in 3 months

403. A 25-year-old female is begun on Demulen 1/35. She presents 2 months later complaining of almost daily nausea (except when she is off the pill every fourth week). What would be the most reasonable course of action at this time?
a) discontinue the oral contraceptive pill
b) switch the pill to one with lower estrogenic activity
c) switch the pill to one with lower progestin activity
d) switch the pill to one with higher estrogenic activity
e) switch the pill to one with higher progestin activity

404. A 29-year-old female is given a prescription for Ortho 7/7/7. She returns 3 months later complaining of breakthrough bleeding in the second half of the menstrual cycle. What would be the most reasonable course of action at this time?
a) discontinue the oral contraceptive pill
b) maintain the patient on the same pill for the next 6 months and reassess the situation at that time
c) switch the pill to one with lower progestin activity
d) switch the pill to one with higher progestin activity
e) switch the pill to one with higher estrogenic activity

405. A 31-year-old patient is placed on Brevicon. Three months later she returns complaining of breakthrough bleeding in the first 10 days of the menstrual cycle. What would be the most reasonable course of action at this time?
a) stop the oral contraceptive pill
b) switch the pill to one with higher estrogen activity
c) supplement the pill with ethinyl estradiol 20 µg for the first 2 weeks of the cycle
d) switch the pill to one with higher progestin activity
e) do nothing

406. A 24-year-old student, who is slightly overweight, presents for her first checkup since starting the OCP. She was given Triphasil. On her previous

examination her blood pressure was 120/70 mm Hg. Today it is 140/95 mm Hg. Her blood pressure is rechecked on two occasions during the next 2 weeks and remains at 140/95 mm Hg after 5 minutes of rest. What would be your most reasonable course of action at this time?
a) switch to a pill with a lower progestin activity
b) switch to a pill with a lower estrogenic activity
c) switch to a pill with both lower estrogenic and lower progestin activity
d) discontinue the oral contraceptive pill
e) do nothing; recheck her blood pressure in 6 months

407. An 18-year-old female presents to your office requesting a prescription for the oral contraceptive pill. She states that she is "extremely sexually active." When you question her about the meaning of "extremely sexually active" she states that she usually has intercourse every night and sees 6–7 partners on a regular basis. Your advice in this case would be:
a) the oral contraceptive pill would be a good choice for contraception
b) she should consider an alternative method of birth control because of the risk of pelvic inflammatory disease
c) she should consider the intrauterine device
d) the oral contraceptive would be a good choice for contraception; however, she should consider the use of a condom in addition
e) none of the above

408. A 25-year-old female, 6 weeks post partum, presents to your office for her postpartum checkup. She is breast feeding her baby, and the infant is thriving. She states that she would like to begin the oral contraceptive pill. Your advice to her would be:
a) the oral contraceptive pill is contraindicated in women who are lactating
b) the oral contraceptive pill can be safely used once lactation is established
c) the oral contraceptive pill can be safely used, but may decrease the quality and quantity of breast milk
d) the oral contraceptive pill has not been studied in lactating women and therefore cannot be recommended
e) the oral contraceptive pill is not needed if a woman is lactating; lactation is an effective contraceptive by itself

409. A 19-year-old female presents to your office in a state of extreme anxiety. She had unprotected intercourse at midcycle the previous night and is worried that she may get pregnant. She has multiple sexual partners who usually wear condoms. She had a new partner last night who refused to wear one. She definitely does not want to become pregnant and states that she would have an abortion if she became pregnant.

At this time, you should:
a) perform a menstrual extraction
b) tell her to relax and come back in a month if her period has not come
c) insert an intrauterine device
d) perform a serum beta-HCG test in 10 days
e) presribe Ovral 2 tablets right away and two tablets in 12 hours

ANSWER THE FOLLOWING QUESTIONS ACCORDING TO THE CODE:

A: 1, 2, and 3 are correct
B: 1 and 3 are correct
C: 2 and 4 are correct
D: Only 4 is correct
E: All of the above are correct

410. Which of the following are noncontraceptive health benefits of the oral contraceptive pill?
1) decreased benign breast disease
2) decreased rate of ectopic pregnancy
3) decreased incidence of iron-deficiency anemia
4) decreased rate of endometrial cancer

411. Which of the following drugs may interact with the oral contraceptive pill to decrease its efficacy?
1) phenobarbitol
2) clofibrate
3) valium
4) ampicillin

ANSWERS

399. D. and 400. E. The absolute contraindications to the oral contraceptive pill include thrombophlebitis or thromboembolic disorder (or history thereof); cerebrovascular disorders (or history thereof); ischemic heart disease or coronary artery disease (or history thereof); known or suspected carcinoma of the breast (or history thereof); known or suspected estrogen-dependent neoplasia (or his-

tory thereof); pregnancy, known or suspected; benign or malignant liver tumor (or history thereof); and undiagnosed abnormal genital bleeding.[1] Diabetes mellitus is a relative contraindication. The prescription of the oral contraceptive pill, however, to a patient with insulin-dependent diabetes mellitus will have very little if any effect on the daily requirement of insulin. Practically, the risk of an unplanned pregnancy in an insulin-dependent diabetic is much greater than the risk of her taking the oral contraceptive pill.

Other relative contraindications include severe headaches, particularly vascular or migraine; hypertension with resting diastolic blood pressure ≥90 mm Hg or a resting systolic blood pressure of 140 mm Hg or greater on three or more separate visits, or an accurate measurement of greater than 110 mm Hg diastolic pressure on a single visit; active gallbladder disease; acute phase mononucleosis; sickle cell disease (SS) or sickle C disease (SC); elective major surgery planned in the next 4 weeks or major surgery requiring immobilization; a long-leg cast or major injury to the lower leg; age 40 years or older, accompanied by a second risk factor for the development of cardiovascular disease (and all patients > age 45); and age 35 years or older and currently a heavy smoker. If a patient is a nonsmoker and has no other cardiovascular risk factors, she may safely take the oral contraceptive pill to age 45.[1]

401. E. No single OCP is preferable on the basis of safety, effectiveness, or patient acceptability to any other OCP. A good first choice, however, is a pill that is low in total hormonal dosage and potency for both estrogen and progesterone.[1] The biphasic or triphasic preparations tend to have the lowest monthly total hormonal dosage; they may well be the OCPs of first choice. The following table describes relative estrogen and progesterone potency of some of the commonly used oral contraceptive agents (Table 1).

If you consider the choices in the question, the OCP with the lowest amount of progestin and estrogen (potency) is Ortho 7/7/7. Demulen 1/50 is a high potency progestin pill, and Ovral and Ortho Novum 1/80 are high potency estrogen pills. Micronor is a progestin-only pill and is rarely used.

402. B. Acne or oily skin in women on oral contraceptive pills may be improved by switching to an OCP with less androgenic activity. It is reasonable to try alternative treatments such as skin cleansers and

Table 1 Relative Estrogen and Progesterone Potency of Some Commonly Used Oral Contraceptive Agents[1]

OCP	Progesterone Potency (mg)	Estrogen Potency (mg)
Loestrin 1/20	2.0	0.7–0.8
Triphasil	3.0–7.5	1.0–1.2
Lo/Ovral	9.0	1.0–1.2
Brevicon	0.5	1.2–1.4
Ortho 10/11	0.5–1.0	1.2–1.4
Ortho 7/7/7	0.5–1.0	1.2–1.4
Ortho Novum 1/35	1.0	1.2–1.4
Demulen 1/35	15	1.2–1.4
Ovral	15	1.7–2.0
Demulen 1/50	15	1.7–2.0
Ortho Novum 1/80	1.0	1.6

Table 2 Relative Androgenic Activity of Some Commonly Prescribed Oral Contraceptive Pills[1]

Oral Contraceptive	Androgen Activity
Brevicon/Modicon	0.17
Demulen 1/35	0.21
Ortho-Novum 7/7/7	0.26
Ortho-Novum 10/11	0.26
Ortho 1/35	0.34
Lo-Ovral	0.47
Loestrin 1/20	0.79

topical antibiotics first, but the most effective treatment is a change in OCPs. Table 2 lists the relative androgenic activity of some of the commonly presribed oral contraceptive pills.

In this patient's case a switch to Brevicon, Modicon, Demulen 1/35, Ortho 7/7/7, or Ortho 10/11 would be a reasonable change and would most likely improve the acne.

403. B. The most reasonable course of action (after excluding pregnancy) would be to switch to an oral contraceptive pill with less estrogenic activity. As she is presently taking Demulen 1/35, a reasonable alternative would be one like Loestrin 1/20.[1]

404. D. Spotting and breakthrough bleeding in the second half of the menstrual cycle should be managed by switching to an OCP with the same estrogen dose but a more biologically active progestin or a larger dose of the same progestin. As she is on Ortho 7/7/7, a reasonable switch would be to a pill like Demulen 1/35.[1]

405. C. Breakthrough bleeding or spotting in the first half of the menstrual cycle is most easily managed by supplementing the estrogen in the OCP for one to three cycles with an estrogen supplement (ethinyl estradiol 20 μg). By this method you will leave the progestin activity unchanged. After 3 months you can discontinue the ethinyl estradiol. The other alternative would be to switch her to an OCP with a higher estrogen potency.[1]

406. D. Approximately 4% of women who are normotensive when not taking oral contraceptives develop hypertension when they are placed on the OCP. If a woman's diastolic blood pressure is greater than 90 mm Hg on several visits while on oral contraceptives, stop their use. For women with an initial diastolic blood pressure of 60–70 mm Hg that increases to 80–90 mm Hg diastolic, decrease the progestin, or decrease both the estrogen and the progestin. If that does not work discontinue the OCP.[1]

If the patient insists on continuing the OCP, consider using the progestin-only pill (Micronor) or lowest estrogen and progestin pill available.

Hypertension induced by the oral contraceptive pill is usually reversible within 1–3 months after discontinuing the pill. The patient should return for follow-up at that time.

Patients who become hypertensive while taking the oral contraceptive pill are more likely to develop hypertension in pregnancy or chronic hypertension in later life.

407. D. The oral contraceptive pill provides the most reliable form of contraception. Also, it provides some protection against gonococcal PID. It does not, however, protect against AIDS (Acquired Immunodeficiency Syndrome) nor *Chlamydia* PID.[1] Any patient with multiple sexual partners should be urged to use condoms in addition to using the oral contraceptive. Although only a small percentage of cases of AIDS are spread by heterosexual transmission, it is likely that this mode of spread will increase in the future.

408. B. The American Academy of Pediatrics has issued a policy statement approving the use of combined oral contraceptive pills in lactating women once lactation is well established.[2] The 6-week postpartum exam is probably a good time for a nursing mother to start taking the pill. Low-dose combined oral contraceptive pills (25–30 μg estrogen) have no demonstrable adverse effect on either

the quality or quantity of breast milk, or on the sucking infant. The progestin-only contraceptive (Micronor) may also be used; it may be started immediately after delivery.

409. E. In this patient, effective postcoital contraception should be provided. The high dose combined OCP "Ovral" is preferred.[3] If four tablets of Ovral are taken two tablets at a time 12 hours apart, the pooled failure rate is only 1.8%. Morning after IUD insertion using a Copper-T or a Copper-7 is also very effective.[2]

Menstrual extraction can be avoided by proper postcoital contraception. Ordering a serum beta-HCG or telling the patient to relax will not prevent an unplanned pregnancy.

410. E. All of the choices are noncontraceptive health benefits of oral contraceptives. In addition, there is a decreased incidence of ovarian retention cysts, PID, and ovarian cancer.[1]

411. E. The drugs that are known to interact with the oral contraceptive pill and decrease its efficacy can be divided into five groups.[1] They are:
1) the anticonvulsants—phenobarbitol, carbamazepine, primidone, phenytoin, and ethosuximide
2) some cholesterol lowering agents such as clofibrate
3) the antibiotics—rifampin, isoniazid, penicillin, ampicillin, metronidazole, tetracycline, neomycin, chloramphenicol, sulfonamides, and nitrofurantoin
4) sedatives, hypnotics, tricyclics, and antipsychotics—valium, chloral hydrate, amitriptyline, largactil, etc.
5) antacids

SUMMARY OF THE MANAGEMENT OF A PATIENT USING THE ORAL CONTRACEPTIVE PILL:

1. Take a complete history and do a complete physical examination

2. Establish whether or not the patient has any absolute or relative contraindications to the pill

3. Prescribe the oral contraceptive pill on a trial basis for 3 months, using a pill with a relatively low estrogenic or progestin potency

4. If there are no symptoms or signs of altered health in 3 months, consider prescribing the pill for 1 year without further review

5. Manage side effects by considering the estrogenic potency, progestin potency, and androgenic effect of the individual pill

6. Advise the use of condoms in addition to the use of the oral contraceptive pill in a patient who has multiple sexual partners to prevent the heterosexual spread of sexually transmitted diseases including AIDS

References

1. Hatcher R, Guest F, Stewart F, et al, eds. Contraceptive technology. New York: Irvington Publishers, 1988.

2. American Academy of Pediatrics. Breast feeding and contraception. Pediatrics 1981; 68(1): 138–140.

3. Ovral as a "morning after" contraceptive. Med Let 1989; 31(803);93–94.

PROBLEM 50: A 21-YEAR-OLD FEMALE WITH A VAGINAL DISCHARGE

A 21-year-old female presents to the office with a pruritic thick, white, vaginal discharge. This is associated with erythema of the vulva. There is no discharge present at the introitus. The consistency of the discharge is curdy, the viscosity is high, and the discharge is adherent to the vaginal walls. The pH is 4.0, and there is no amine odor.

SELECT THE ONE BEST ANSWER TO THE FOLLOWING QUESTIONS:

412. The most likely diagnosis in this patient is:
a) physiologic discharge
b) bacterial vaginosis
c) candidiasis
d) trichomoniasis
e) none of the above

413. The treatment of choice in this patient is:
    a) metronidazole cream
    b) ampicillin
    c) miconazole (local)
    d) nystatin tablets
    e) none of the above

414. Which of the following factors HAS NOT been established as a risk factor for the condition described above?
    a) pregnancy
    b) antibiotic therapy
    c) diabetes mellitus
    d) oral contraceptives
    e) all of the above are established risk factors

415. A 25-year-old female presents with a profuse, gray-green malodorous discharge with irritation and pruritus. The discharge is present at the introitus. There is vulvar edema present. The discharge is adherent to the vaginal walls. The pH is 6.0. There is an amine odor present, and the microscopic examination shows 15 WBCs/hpf.
    The most likely diagnosis in this patient is:
    a) candidiasis
    b) trichomoniasis
    c) bacterial vaginosis
    d) physiologic discharge
    e) nonspecific vaginitis

416. The treatment of choice for the patient described in question 415 is:
    a) miconazole (topical)
    b) cotrimazole
    c) metronidazole
    d) ampicillin
    e) none of the above

417. A 29-year-old female presents with a 2-week history of profuse, malodorous discharge with irritation. On examination the discharge is present at the introitus. It is gray in color. It is homogeneous and has a low viscosity. It is adherent to the vaginal walls. The pH is 6.5. An amine odor is present. On microscopic examination, "clue cells" are present, but no WBCs.
    The most likely diagnosis in this patient is:
    a) bacterial vaginosis
    b) trichomoniasis
    c) candidiasis
    d) physiologic discharge
    e) nonspecific vaginitis

418. The treatment of choice for the patient described in question 417 is:
    a) miconazole
    b) cotrimazole
    c) metronidazole
    d) ampicillin
    e) none of the above

419. A 21-year-old patient presents for a periodic health assessment. On examination you notice a moderately thick, vaginal discharge. The vulva are normal. There is no discharge present at the introitus. It is white, curdy, and its viscosity is high. It is not adherent to the vaginal walls. The pH is 4.0, and no amine odor is detected on exposure to KOH. The microscopic examination reveals epithelial cells.
    The most likely diagnosis in this patient is:
    a) physiologic discharge
    b) asymptomatic candidiasis
    c) trichomoniasis
    d) bacterial vaginosis
    e) none of the above

420. The most common form of vaginitis is:
    a) candidiasis
    b) trichomoniasis
    c) bacterial vaginosis
    d) nonspecific vaginitis
    e) none of the above

ANSWERS

412. C. This patient has candidiasis.
    Candida albicans is a commensal organism in most women. When, however, *Corynebacterium* sp. and specific fungal inhibitory factors are suppressed, it can produce an infection.
    Pruritus is the symptom of vaginal candidiasis. Discharge may be normal or increased in amount. It is usually described as a white discharge with a curdy consistency that resembles "cottage cheese." Burning, irritation, and soreness may be present. Dyspareunia and vulvar (external) dysuria are common. Erythema of the vulva is common.
    Predisposing factors for vaginal candidiasis include (1) the premenstrual phase, (2) antibiotic use, and (3) coitus.
    Physical examination often reveals vulvar erythema and edema. The discharge is often adherent to the vaginal walls. The vaginal pH is usually normal (<4.5). Amine odor is absent, and

WBCs are not increased. Mycelia and/or spores may be seen on microscopy.[1]

413. C. The treatment of choice is an imidazole cream or suppository, or clotrimazole cream or suppository. Many regimens utilizing imidazole or clotrimazole have shown high cure rates. The treatment regimens vary from 1 to 7 days. Because of the presence of both internal and external symptoms, the use of the Monistat-3 Dual Pak (miconazole vaginal ovules, one/night for three nights plus miconazole cream to be applied to the vulvar area once or twice a day), can be recommended. Loose-fitting clothing and cotton underwear will decrease colonization rates.

In recurrent candidiasis, 1% gentian violet or oral nystatin or ketoconazole can be used. In recurrent candidiasis the partner should be treated with an imidazole cream, locally applied to the foreskin and the glans.[1]

414. D. Risk factors for vaginal candidiasis[1] include:
1) physical disruption of the integument
2) pregnancy
3) antibiotic therapy
4) diabetes mellitus
5) immunologic deficiencies
6) tight-fitting clothing
7) sexual behavior (including oral-genital and anal sex)

The oral contraceptive pill does not seem to increase the incidence of symptomatic candidiasis, although it may increase the frequency of the carrier state.

415. B. This patient has trichomoniasis.

The symptoms of trichomoniasis include a malodorous, copious, grayish-green vaginal discharge that adheres to the vaginal walls. Irritation, pruritis, and vulvar edema may be present. Erythema of the vaginal mucosa is common. An amine odor is present on exposure to KOH. The pH is usually greater than 5.0. Motile trichomonads and numerous white blood cells are often seen on microscopy.[1]

416. C. The treatment of choice for trichomoniasis is metronidazole. Metronidazole can be given in a single dose of 2 g orally. For patients who fail to respond to a single dose of metronidazole 2 g, a dosage of 500 mg t.i.d. can be given for 7 days.[1]

As trichomoniasis is a sexually transmitted disease, simultaneous treatment of the male partner(s) is essential. Reinfection is a major cause of recurrence.

417. A. This patient has bacterial vaginosis.

Bacterial vaginosis is the most common form of vaginitis. It has been known as nonspecific vaginitis, *Gardnerella* vaginitis, *Haemophilus* vaginitis, *Corynebacterium* vaginitis, mixed bacterial vaginitis, and anaerobic vaginitis.[1] Bacterial vaginosis is a polymicrobial infection involving a synergistic interaction between *G. vaginalis* and anaerobic bacteria.[1]

Bacterial vaginosis is frequently asymptomatic. Symptomatic patients usually present with a malodorous, profuse discharge . The discharge is present at the introitus, is gray in color, and is homogeneous. It has a low viscosity and is adherent to the vaginal walls. The pH is > 5.0, and an amine odor is present on exposure to KOH. "Clue cells" (vaginal epithelial cells that have an obscured border resulting from the adherence of bacteria to the cell border) are often seen. WBCs are absent.

418. C. The drug of choice for bacterial vaginosis is metronidazole. The dosage is 500 mg b.i.d. for 7 days. The treatment of the patient's partner is controversial.[1]

419. A. This is a physiologic discharge. If it is asympomatic, only microscopy need to be done to confirm the diagnosis. With the characteristics given, vaginal cultures are not recommended.[1]

420. C. The most common form of vaginitis is bacterial vaginosis. It accounts for 35–50% of all cases of vaginitis. Candidiasis accounts for 20–40% and trichomoniasis for 10–20%.[1]

SUMMARY OF THE DIAGNOSIS AND TREATMENT OF VAGINITIS

1. **Bacterial vaginosis:** profuse, malodorous discharge with or without irritation. Normal vulva. Discharge present at introitus, gray in color, homogeneous in consistency, low viscosity, adherent to vaginal walls, pH >5.0, amine odor present, "clue cells" present, no WBCs seen
Treatment: metronidazole 500 mg t.i.d. for 7 days
 Treat partner in recurrent cases

2. **Candidiasis:** thick, pruritic, white discharge. Erythematous vulva with or without fissures and

pustules. No discharge present at introitus. Curdy consistency, high viscosity, adeherent to vaginal walls, pH < 5.0, amine odor absent, mycelia present on microscopic examination

Treatment: miconazole vaginal tablets or suppositories, miconazole applied externally. Alternative: clotrimazole

Treat partner in recurrent cases

3. **Trichomoniasis**: profuse, malodorous discharge, with or without irritation and pruritus. Edema may or may not be present on vulva. The discharge is present at the introitus, gray-yellow to green in color, homogeneous in consistency, low viscosity, and adherent to the vaginal walls. The pH > 5.0, and the amine odor is present. Trichomonads as well as WBCs (usually greater than 10 are seen on microscopic examination).

Treatment: metronidazole 2-g dose for patient and partner

Reference

1. Chantigian P. Vaginitis: a common malady. Prim Care 1988; 15(3): 517–547.

PROBLEM 51: A 28-YEAR-OLD FEMALE WITH PELVIC PAIN AND VAGINAL BLEEDING

A 28-year-old female presents with a 2 week-history of pelvic pain and slight vaginal bleeding. There has been no vaginal discharge. She is married, has no children, and has been trying to become pregnant for the last 18 months. Her menstrual periods have always been regular, and she states that her last period occurred at its regular time.

SELECT THE ONE BEST ANSWER TO THE FOLLOWING QUESTIONS:

421. The most important diagnosis to exclude in this patient at this time is:
    a) ruptured corpus luteum cyst
    b) acute pelvic inflammatory disease
    c) ectopic pregnancy
    d) threatened abortion
    e) incomplete abortion

422. In taking a complete history in this patient, which of the following questions would be of PARTICULAR IMPORTANCE?
    a) a history of fever in the last 24 hours
    b) a history of dysmenorrhea
    c) a history of menorrhagia
    d) a history of any irregularity in the last menstrual period
    e) a history of previous miscarriages

ANSWER THE FOLLOWING QUESTIONS ACCORDING TO THE CODE:

A: 1, 2, and 3 are correct
B: 1 and 3 are correct
C: 2 and 4 are correct
D: Only 4 is correct
E: All of the above are correct

423. You perform a physical examination on the patient discussed in the question. On examination, there is moderate abdominal tenderness, but not rebound tenderness. There is also a palpable left adnexal mass.

    Based on the history and physical examination to this point, which of the following tests should be performed at this time?
    1) serum hCG
    2) culdocentesis
    3) pelvic ultrasound
    4) laparoscopy

424. The diagnosis that you suspected is confirmed. Which of the following are common signs/symptoms of this patient's condition?
    1) abdominal pain
    2) irregular vaginal bleeding
    3) abdominal tenderness
    4) amenorrhea

425. Which of the following is/are risk factors for this patient's condition?
    1) previous pelvic inflammatory disease
    2) the intrauterine device
    3) prior tubal sterilization
    4) postcoital estrogens

426. Which of the following statements regarding this patient's condition is/are true?

1) a laparoscopy should be the next step in assessment
2) a salpingectomy may be required
3) conservative surgery is a reasonable alternative in many cases
4) conservative, nonsurgical treatment is now a recommended alternative to surgery for many patients

ANSWERS

421. C. The most important diagnosis to exclude in this patient at this time is ectopic pregnancy. In a patient of childbearing age, any of the three "A's" should suggest the possibility of ectopic pregnancy. The three "A's" are amenorrhea, abdominal pain, and abnormal vaginal bleeding.

   The differential diagnosis of ectopic pregnancy includes ruptured corpus luteum cyst, pelvic infection, disease, threatened or incomplete abortion, dysfunctional uterine bleeding, torsion of an adnexa, degenerating fibroid, endometriosis, and acute appendicitis.[1]

422. D. The important question to ask in this patient is the history of the last menstrual period. She states that it "occurred at the regular time." However, in many patients with ectopic pregnancy, the last menstrual period will be abnormal. Although it may occur at the regular time, it is often lighter in amount of flow. This corresponds to shedding of the uterine decidual tissue secondary to necrosis of trophoblastic tissue.[2]

423. B. Based on the patient's history and physical examination, the probability of ectopic pregnancy is high. Therefore, a serum hCG and a pelvic ultrasound should be performed at this time. The presence of an intrauterine gestational sac virtually excludes ectopic pregnancy. The absence of gestational sac and the presence of an high titer (> 6500 mIU/ml) of serum hCG is strong evidence of ectopic pregnancy. With values of hCG < 6000 mIU/ml, the situation is less clear. Ectopic pregnancy should still be suspected, and serial quantitative hCG levels should be performed every 2 days.

   Culdocentesis, although still sometimes useful, has been largely replaced by a combination of sonography and quantitative serum hCG. Laparoscopy should be reserved for patients that have the clinical suspicion of ectopic pregnancy raised by the tests discussed above.

If serum hCG is not initially available, one of the newer urine pregnancy tests that utilize monoclonal antibodies can be used. Generally, these tests have a high sensitivity.[1,2]

424. E. There are no pathognomonic signs or symptoms of an early ectopic pregnancy. The most common symptoms noted are "the three A's": abdominal pain, abnormal vaginal bleeding, and amenorrhea. Ninety to 100% of patients with an ectopic gestation complain of pain, even before rupture. No specific type of pain is diagnostic. With tubal rupture, the pain becomes more severe.

   Amenorrhea or a history of abnormal menses is reported by 75–95% of patients. A careful history with respect to the character and timing of the last two to three menstrual cycles (amount of flow, days of flow) is extremely important. Initially, patients will often state that they have not missed a period; however, when questioned carefully, they may describe the period as being different (lighter than usual or irregular in timing). This bleeding may in fact represent bleeding from an endometrial slough.

   Irregular vaginal bleeding is noted in 50–80% of patients with an ectopic pregnancy. Usually it is mild and intermittent, resulting from uterine decidual shedding secondary to necrosis of the trophoblastic tissue. Profuse bleeding is uncommon.

   Common symptoms of early pregnancy, such as nausea and breast tenderness, are present in only 10–25% of patients with ectopic pregnancies. Symptoms of dizziness and fainting occur in 20–35% of patients. A few patients will state that they passed tissue (a decidual cast).

   Orthostatic hypotension and tachycardia are only seen in cases of massive hemoperitoneum. Most patients are afebrile.

   Abdominal tenderness is present in most patients (80–95%). Rebound tenderness is often present.

   A mass is palpable in 50% of patients with ectopic pregnancy. If there is uterine enlargement, it is not to the degree that would be expected for the duration of amenorrhea.[1,2]

425. E. Risk factors for ectopic pregnancy include previous pelvic inflammatory disease, previous ectopic pregnancy, current IUD usage, postcoital contraception, and invitro fertilization.[1,2]

426. A. Once an ectopic pregnancy is strongly suspected on clinical and laboratory grounds, a laparoscopy should be performed. This procedure is helpful in deciding whether or not a salpingectomy is required or whether more conservative surgery (salpingotomy) may be sufficient.

Conservative, nonsurgical treatments, including the use of chemotherapeutic agents such as methotrexate are being explored; however, at this time, they cannot be recommended for treatment.[1,2]

SUMMARY OF THE DIAGNOSIS AND TREATMENT OF ECTOPIC PREGNANCY

1. **Diagnosis**: The three A's: abdominal pain, abnormal vaginal bleeding, amenorrhea

2. **Confirmation of diagnosis**: Serum hCG, pelvic ultrasound

3. **Treatment**: Laparoscopy, laparotomy with salpingectomy or salpingotomy

References

1. Cunningham FG, MacDonald P, Gant N. Williams obstetrics. 18th Ed. Norwalk, CT: Appleton & Lange, 1989: 511–532.

2. Weckstein L. Clinical diagnosis of ectopic pregnancy. Clin Obstet Gynecol 1987; 30(1): 236–244.

Psychiatry

PROBLEM 52: A 37-YEAR-OLD MALE WITH WEIGHT LOSS, FATIGUE, AND A LACK OF INTEREST IN LIFE

A 37-year-old executive presents to your office with his wife. He complains of a 4-month history of weight loss, fatigue, insomnia, inability to concentrate, and a lack of interest in life. He says that he has never felt this way before. He attributes his feelings to financial problems with his company. His general health has been good and he is taking no medications at the present time.

SELECT THE ONE BEST ANSWER TO THE FOLLOWING QUESTIONS:

427. The most likely diagnosis in this patient is:
    a) adjustment disorder (secondary to financial pressure)
    b) generalized anxiety disorder
    c) major depression
    d) organic affective disorder
    e) dsythymia

428. The treatment of choice in this patient is:
    a) a tricyclic antidepressant
    b) a monoamine oxidase inhibitor
    c) psychotherapy
    d) a and c
    e) b and c

429. A 41-year-old male presents with a 3-year history of "a depressed mood." He states that he feels "depressed most of the time," although there are periods when he feels better than others. He feels chronically tired, has some difficulty concentrating at work, and has found it difficult to remain productive and efficient as chief executive officer of a major company. He has had no other symptoms. His health is otherwise good. He is on no medications.
    The most likely diagnosis in this patient is:
    a) adjustment disorder
    b) dysthymic disorder
    c) major depression
    d) organic affective disorder
    e) none of the above

430. The treatment of choice in the patient described in question 429 is:
    a) a tricyclic antidepressant

    b) a monoamine oxidase inhibitor
    c) supportive psychotherapy
    d) a and c
    e) b and c

431. A 35-year-old female presents to your office with a 3-month history of depressed mood. She feels "stressed" at work. You discover that she moved into a managerial position at work 4 months ago and is having difficulty with two of her employees. She has no previous history of psychiatric illness. She has no other symptoms. She is on no medication.
    The most likely diagnosis in this patient is:
    a) adjustment disorder
    b) dysthymic disorder
    c) major depression
    d) organic affective disorder
    e) generalized anxiety disorder

432. The treatment of choice in the patient described in question 431 is:
    a) a tricyclic antidepressant
    b) a monoamine oxidase inhibitor
    c) supportive psychotherapy
    d) a and c
    e) b and c

433. A 42-year-old female presents to your office complaining of headaches, back pain, indigestion and malaise for the past 2 months. She has had no previous history of symptoms like this, and her past medical history is unremarkable. A careful physical examination reveals no abnormalities. She is married and has two children. She states that her husband is concerned about her and that is why she is here. She denies being depressed or having a lack of interest in life. She had an episode of

depression 5 years ago that was successfully treated with tricyclic antidepressants.

The most likely diagnosis in this patient is:
a) dysthymic disorder
b) major depression
c) masked depression
d) organic affective disorder
e) none of the above

434. A complete psychiatric history is most important in evaluating depressed patients. In taking a history from a patient with depression, which of the following questions is the MOST IMPORTANT to ask?
a) family history of psychiatric problems
b) personal history of previous episodes of depression
c) suicidal ideation
d) presence or absence of hallucinations
e) presence or absence of delusions

435. With most tricyclic antidepressants, clinical response may not appear until adequate dosage has been used for:
a) 2–4 days
b) 5–7 days
c) 7–14 days
d) 14–28 days
e) 2–4 months

436. When a favorable response to a particular antidepressant has occurred during the acute phase of treatment, therapy with that drug should be continued for a period of at least:
a) 1 month
b) 2 months
c) 4 months
d) 12 months
e) 18 months

ANSWER THE FOLLOWING QUESTION ACCORDING TO THE CODE:

A: 1, 2, and 3 are correct
B: 1 and 3 are correct
C: 2 and 4 are correct
D: Only 4 is correct
E: All of the above are correct

437. Which of the following statements regarding tricyclic antidepressants is/are CORRECT?
1) most tricyclic antidepressants are equally efficacious

2) the most common limiting side effects of tricyclic antidepressants are anticholinergic side effects
3) doxepin has a lower cardiotoxicity than amitriptyline
4) if therapy with one tricyclic antidepressant is unsuccessful, it is unlikely that another one will be of benefit

ANSWERS

427. C. This patient has a major depression. A major depression is present if at least five of the following nine symptoms are present and have been present for at least 2 weeks: (1) depressed mood, (2) lack of interest or pleasure in the activities of daily living, (3) significant weight loss or weight gain, (4) insomnia or hypersomnia, (5) psychomotor agitation or retardation, (6) fatigue or loss of energy, (7) feelings of worthlessness or guilt, (8) decreased ability to concentrate, and (9) suicidal ideation. Either a depressed mood or a lack of interest or pleasure in the activities of daily living must be present before the diagnosis can be made.[1]

Adjustment disorder with depressed mood would be a diagnostic consideration in this patient if the depression had only recently developed, and if there was a chance it would resolve quickly.[2]

Organic affective disorders including thryoid dysfunction and pharmacologically induced affective disorders should be considered in all patients. The previous good general health of this patient, however, makes this diagnosis unlikely.

The patient does not present with symptoms of anxiety; generalized anxiety disorder, therefore, is not a diagnostic consideration.

Dysthmic disorder will be discussed in a subsequent question.

428. D. The treatment of choice in this patient is a combination of a tricyclic antidepressant and psychotherapy.

Supportive psychotherapy is discussed in another section of this book.

Tricyclic antidepressants are effective in 60–70% of acutely depressed patients. The tricyclic antidepressant should be tailored to the individual patient's symptoms. If the patient's symptoms include fatigue, hypersomnia, lethargy and an inability to concentrate, for example, a drive enhancing tricyclic like desipramine or nortriptyline would be appropriate. An alternative would be the new nontricyclic agent fluoxetine. If the patient's symptoms include anxiety, insomnia, and irritability, an anxiety-reducing agent such as trimipramine or amitriptyline would be more appropriate. If the patient has symptoms that seem to require both drive enhancement and anxiety reduction, then an agent such as imipramine or maprotiline would be appropriate.

All TCA's are equally effective in treating depression. The physician should consider the presenting symptoms, the side effect profile (especially anticholinergic side effects), and the cost when deciding upon therapy. Drugs with low anticholinergic side effects include desipramine, nortriptyline, and fluoxetine. Full dosage range for relief of depression is 50–300 mg/day for most agents. Fluoxetine's dosage is 20–60 mg/day.

Monoamine oxidase inhibitors should be considered if a trial of 1 or 2 tricyclic antidepressants is not effective. Phenelzine and tranylcypromine are effective agents in many cases of resistant depression.

Lithium carbonate is also useful in the treatment of tricyclic-resistant unipolar depression.[2,3]

429. B. This patient has a dysthmic disorder. Dysthmic disorder is defined as a depressive syndrome in which the patient is bothered all or most of the time by depressive symptoms, but these symptoms are not of sufficient severity to warrant a diagnosis of major depression.[1]

430. D. Because of the long history, this patient should probably be treated with a combination of supportive psychotherapy and a tricyclic antidepressant. A patient who fails to respond to a tricyclic antidepressant should be tried on an MAO inhibitor.[2,3]

431. A. This patient has an adjustment disorder. Adjustment disorder is defined as a reaction to an identifiable psychosocial stressor(s) that occurs within 3 months of the onset of the stressor. The reaction is characterized by an impairment in occupational or social functioning.[1]

432. C. The treatment of choice for adjustment disorder is supportive psychotherapy. If possible, the stressor should be removed. If not, the patient should be helped to develop coping strategies and to set and meet specific goals towards dealing with the stressor.[4]

433. C. This patient most likely has a masked depression. Patients with masked depression often present with pains in various locations, fatigue, lethargy, and bowel symptoms. Sometimes they are not even able to localize their complaints; but complain of just "not feeling quite right."

When a complete physical examination and laboratory evaluation has ruled out other disorders, the physician should explain the condition, and explain the duality (mind-body) relationship of illness. A thoughtful, empathetic explanation is often all that is required. The physician should explore environmental stressors and suggest coping strategies. Tricyclic antidepressants may be of signficant benefit to patients with masked depression.[3]

434. C. The most important question in the psychiatric history of a patient with depression is the question of feelings or thoughts of self-harm or suicide. Patients should be questioned directly and openly about suicidal thoughts. If the patient admits to thoughts of suicide he should be questioned about his plan, previous attempts, and a family history of suicide. He should be classified then as high or low risk. Any patient thought to be at high risk of suicide should be admitted. Family history of other psychiatric problems, previous episodes of depression in the patient, and the presence or absence of hallucinations or delusions are all part of a complete psychiatric history but not as important as the immediate risk of suicide.[5]

435. D. Most tricyclic antidepressants require 14–28 days to exert their antidepressant effect. Therapy should be continued for at least 4 weeks at full antidepressant dose before you consider the drug to have failed to produce a response.[3]

436. D. When a favorable response to a particular antidepressant agent occurs, therapy with that drug should be continued for at least 4 months. A shorter period of therapy will often result in relapse.[6]

437. A. Most tricyclic antidepressants are equally efficacious on a milligram to milligram basis, but differ considerably in their side effect profile. The most common side effects of TCAs are the anticholinergic side effects including dry mouth, blurred vision, constipation, and urinary retention. An agent with fewer anticholingeric side effects is often preferrable, unless insomnia is a major symptom.

Tricyclic antidepressants also vary in their cardiotoxic potential. Orthostatic hypotension and conduction disturbances are more common with agents such as amitriptyline than with an agent like doxepin.

Individuals show great variation in their response to TCAs. Dosage may have to be increased to 300 mg/day in some individuals before a therapeutic response is attained. On the other hand, elderly patients often require considerably less, averaging 50-75 mg/day.

If one TCA has been taken to full therapeutic dose and no response has been obtained, another agent should be tried. Alternatives to this include switching to either an MAO inhibitor or lithium as second-line therapy.[3,6]

SUMMARY OF THE DIAGNOSIS AND TREATMENT OF DEPRESSION:

1. **Diagnosis:** Mnemonic = SIG: E CAPS[7]
   Depressed mood plus
   S= sleep disturbance (insomnia/hypersomnia)
   I= lack of interest in activities of daily living
   G= feelings of worthlessness or guilt
   E= decreased energy or fatigue
   C= decreased ability to concentrate
   A= appetite disturbance
   P= psychomotor retardation or agitation
   S= suicidal ideation

2. **Therapy for major depression and dsythymia:**
   Tricyclic antidepressants and supportive psycho-therapy. Individualize TCA therapy to fit the patient's symptoms.

3. If one TCA does not produce a remission (at least 4 week trial) consider the use of a second TCA.

4. If TCA therapy is not successful consider the use of a monoamine oxidase inhibitor or lithium carbonate.

References

1. American Psychiatric Association: Diagnostic and statistical manual of mental disorders. 3rd Ed. Revised (DSM-III-R). Washington: APA Press, 1987.

2. Klerman G. Depression and related disorders of mood. In: Nicholi A, ed. The new Harvard guide to psychiatry. Cambridge: Harvard (Belknap) Press, 1988: 309–336.

3. Yates W. Depression. Prim Care 1987; 14(4): 657–668.

4. Popkin M. Adjustment disorder and impulse control disorder. In: Kaplan H, Sadock B, eds. Comprehensive textbook of psychiatry, V. Baltimore: Williams & Wilkins, 1989: 1141–1145.

5. Roy A. Suicide. In: Kaplan H, Sadock B, eds. Comprehensive textbook of psychiatry, V. Baltimore: Williams & Wilkins, 1989: 1414–1427.

6. Perry P, Alexander B. Rational use of antidepressants. Prim Care 1987; 14(4): 773–783.

7. Gross, C. Unpublished, Boston, Mass.

PROBLEM 53: A 42-YEAR-OLD COMPUTER SCIENCE PROFESSOR WHO HAS JUST BEEN ANOINTED BY GOD AS THE NEW LEADER OF THE COMPUTER AGE

A 42-year-old computer science professor is brought to the emergency room by his wife, who explained that for the last 4 weeks he had become increasingly irritable, angry, and suspicious. She stated that his personality had "completely changed." He had not slept for 6 nights, and had been found at 3 AM in the middle of the street working on his computer programs. He had become preoccupied with the belief that God had anointed him as the new leader of the computer age. Fearing that his ideas will be stolen by KGB spies, he has constructed an elaborate mathematical code that allows only him and his appointed "prophets" to understand the programs.

Two weeks ago the patient purchased a trench coat, dark sun glasses, and a bright red hat. He feels this attire will allow him to elude the KGB.

During the interview the patient is extremely agitated and paces the floor. He makes sexual advances towards the nurse who is observing the interview.

The patient's wife states that the patient has been depressed on and off throughout his life and has been on medication on at least three occasions. She states that her husband's family are "all nuts." When asked to expand on this answer she states that his mother is constantly calling him at 3 o'clock in the morning to see how his work is going. His father at one time was admitted to a psychiatric institution and given " shock treatments." One of his sisters is an alcoholic and his other sister ran away from home at age 14, with her current whereabouts unknown.

According to the patient's wife, the patient has never had an alcohol or drug dependency problem, and is on no medications at the present time.

SELECT THE ONE BEST ANSWER TO THE FOLLOWING QUESTIONS:

438. Given the history above, the most likely diagnosis in this patient is:
    a) schizoaffective disorder
    b) schizophrenia, paranoid type
    c) acute mania
    d) organic brain syndrome
    e) adult onset attention-deficit disorder

439. Based on the current episode and past personal and family history this is most likely part of a:
    a) chronic schizophrenia problem
    b) chronic substance abuse problem
    c) bipolar affective disorder
    d) paranoid personality disorder
    e) unclassifiable psychotic disorder

440. At this time, you should:
    a) prescribe diazepam and tell his wife that you will review the situation tomorrow
    b) prescribe lithium carbonate on an outpatient basis and see the patient in a week
    c) prescribe fluphenazine on an outpatient basis and see the patient in a week
    d) prescribe a tricyclic antidepressant on an outpatient basis and see the patient in a week
    e) none of the above

ANSWER THE FOLLOWING QUESTIONS ACCORDING TO THE CODE:

A: 1, 2, and 3 are correct
B: 1 and 3 are correct
C: 2 and 4 are correct
D: Only 4 is correct
E: All of the above are correct

441. Which of the following is/are TRUE regarding lithium carbonate?
    1) it is the drug of choice in the treatment of bipolar affective disorder
    2) lithium prevents relapses as effectively in unipolar as in bipolar affective disorders

    3) lithium is not metabolized, and therefore problems of active or inactive metabolites do not exist
    4) the average daily dose of lithium required to treat bipolar affective disorder is 900 mg

442. Patients with refractory bipolar affective disorder can be effectively treated with:
    1) fluphenazine
    2) carbamazepine
    3) alprazolam
    4) verapamil

ANSWERS

438. C. The most likely diagnosis in this patient is acute mania. Mania is defined as a distinct period of abnormally and persistently elevated, expansive, and irratible mood. It may include inflated self-esteem or grandiosity, decreased need for sleep, loquaciousness, flight of ideas, distractibility, increase in goal-directed activity, and activities such as unrestrained buying sprees, sexual indiscretions, and foolish business investments. These symptoms cause a marked impairment in occupational functioning.[1]

With no history of drug dependency problems, an organic mood disorder is less likely.

Schizophrenia is less likely because of the good premorbid functioning and the family history of affective disorder.

Schizoaffective disorder is unlikely because the patient's delusions are associated in time with affective symptoms.

Attention deficit disorder is not a consideration in a patient of this age.

439. C. This patient most likely has a bipolar affective disorder. To make the diagnosis of bipolar affective disorder at least one episode of mania has to occur. This patient has a history that is very suggestive of major depression, and thus can now be thought to have a bipolar affective disorder.[1]

His family history is also suggestive of manic-depressive disorder. His mother, who calls at 3 AM to see how his work is going may well have a bipolar affective disorder. Also, his father has had major depressive illness treated by ECT.

440. E. None of the above are true. This patient should be admitted to hospital and treated with an antipsychotic agent such as haloperidol(IM) until the psychotic symptoms subside. He should be placed on lithium carbonate at the same time. Lithium carbonate is the drug of choice for the treatment of bipolar affective disorder.[2]

Outpatient therapy is not indicated in acute mania. Diazepam or tricyclic antidepressant drugs are not recommended in the treatment of acute mania.

441. E. Lithium carbonate is the treatment of choice in the prophylaxis of bipolar affective disorder. It is also used to prevent relapses in unipolar affective disorder. In the treatment of acute mania, it may be 10–14 days before the full therapeutic effect of lithium is realized.

The dosage of lithium required to provide full therapeutic effect is considerably lower than previously thought. The average dosage may be around 900 mg/day.

Lithium is not metabolized, and therefore the accumulation of active or inactive metabolites is not a concern.[2,3]

442. C. Although lithium is the most effective prophylactic agent in bipolar affective disorder, there are some patients, perhaps 10–20%, who do not respond to it. Carbamazepine is effective in many lithium-resistant patients. Another anticonvulsant, valproic acid, may also be effective.

Verapamil (a calcium-channel blocker), is also beginning to show promise in lithium-resistant patients.

Fluphenazine, a neuroleptic, may be useful in acute mania but has no place in long term management. Alprazolam, a benzodiazepine should not be used in the treatment of bipolar affective disorder.[2,3]

SUMMARY OF THE DIAGNOSIS AND TREATMENT OF BIPOLAR AFFECTIVE DISORDER

1. At least one episode of mania is necessary to make the diagnosis of bipolar affective disorder.

2. Family history of unipolar or bipolar disorder is common.

3. **Treatment:**
   a) acute: antipsychotic plus lithium
   b) prophylaxis: lithium plus or minus other agents (carbamazepine, valproic acid)

References

1. American Psychiatric Association. Diagnostic and statistical manual of mental disorders. 3rd Ed. Revised (DSM-III-R). Washington: APA Press, 1987.

2. Klerman G. Depression and related disorders of mood. In: Nicholi A, ed. The new Harvard guide to psychiatry. Cambridge: Harvard (Belknap) Press, 1988: 309–336.

3. Schou M. Lithium treatment of manic-depressive illness. JAMA 1988; 259(12): 1834–1836.

PROBLEM 54: A 29-YEAR-OLD FEMALE WITH A POUNDING HEART, DIFFICULTY BREATHING, DIZZINESS, AND FEELINGS OF DEPERSONALIZATION

A 29-year-old female presents to the office with recurrent attacks of a pounding heart, chest pain, difficulty breathing, and a fear that she is about to die. She also trembles and is experiencing numbness and tingling sensations in her hands and feet.

SELECT THE ONE BEST ANSWER TO THE FOLLOWING QUESTIONS:

443. The most likely diagnosis in this patient is:
   a) pheochromocytoma
   b) hyperthyroidism
   c) panic disorder
   d) agoraphobia
   e) paroxsymal atrial fibrillation

ANSWER THE FOLLOWING QUESTIONS ACCORDING TO THE CODE:

A: 1, 2, and 3 are correct
B: 1 and 3 are correct
C: 2 and 4 are correct
D: Only 4 is correct
E: All of the above are correct

444. Which of the following are characteristic of the disorder described above?
    1) smothering sensations
    2) fear of going crazy
    3) fear of not being able to control the situation
    4) feelings of depersonalization

445. Which of the following is/are characteristic of agoraphobia?
    1) an intense fear of being in public places
    2) acute bursts of terrifying levels of anxiety (panic attacks)
    3) avoidance of supermarkets, shopping malls, church services, meetings, or other places where help is unavailable or escape is difficult
    4) a loss of contact with reality, including hallucinations and delusions.

446. Which of the following is/are TRUE of the disorder described in this problem?
    1) it is more common in men
    2) it typically begins in the 20s
    3) it is rarely confused with coronary artery disease
    4) it has a documented familial nature

447. Which of the following is/are effective drugs in the treatment of patients with the disorder described above?
    1) desipramine
    2) alprazolam
    3) phenelzine
    4) imipramine

448. Which of the following is/are true regarding the treatment of panic disorder?
    1) pharmacologic therapy is effective in blocking panic attacks
    2) pharmacologic therapy is effective in the treatment of phobic avoidance
    3) behavioral therapy is the treatment of choice for phobic avoidance
    4) self-desensitization by exposure to feared situations should not be recommended

ANSWERS

443. C. The most likely diagnosis in this patient is panic disorder. Panic disorder is defined as recurrent episodes of panic attacks (discrete periods of intense fear or discomfort), associated with other symptoms including dyspnea, dizziness, trembling, palpitations, choking sensation, nausea, feelings of depersonalization, numbness, hot flushes, chest pain, a fear of dying, or a fear of going crazy, or a fear of not being able to control a situation to which you may be exposed.[1]

   Although organic disease must be considered (especially thyroid dysfunction), the constellation of symptoms is almost diagnostic of panic disorder.

   Agoraphobia is discussed in a subsequent question.

444. E. All of the above can occur with panic attacks. See critique of question 443.

445. A. Agoraphobia is characterized by the following clinical features: (1) intense fear of being alone or in a public place; (2) acute bursts of terrifying levels of anxiety (panic attacks); (3) fear of panic attacks or other calamities, leading to chronic anxiety and restriction of activities, often to the point of becoming housebound; and, (4) avoidance of supermarkets, shopping malls, church services, meetings, parties, elevators, tunnels, bridges, buses, subways, and other places where help is unavailable or escape is difficult.[1,2] Agoraphobia is not characterized by hallucinations, delusions, or any other loss of contact with reality, although patients may complain of "being in a daze" or "being in a fog" (feelings of derealization or depersonalization).[2]

446. C. Panic disorder is a common medical illness. Panic disorder typically begins in the 20s, but the age of onset varies from childhood to the eighth decade. It is twice as common in women than in men. It appears to be a familial illness.

   Chest pain is a common presenting complaint among patients with panic disorder. Many patients have even been referred for coronary angiography. Other than cardiovascular symptoms, the two other most common types of somatic symptoms are neurologic and gastrointestinal symptoms.[2]

447. E. All of the drugs listed are effective for the treatment of panic disorder. The trycyclic agents

(especially imipramine and desipramine) are agents of first choice in the treatment of panic disorder. Benzodiazepine derivatives (especially alprazolam and clonazepam) have been shown to effectively block panic attacks. Phenelzine (an MAO inhibitor) is also an effective treatment.

The usual length of medical treatment is 6–12 months. If complete resolution of symptoms occurs, tapering and discontinuation of medication can be attempted after 6 months. Recurrence of symptoms demands restarting of medication.[2]

448. B. Pharmacologic therapy is effective in blocking panic attacks, but drugs have little effect on phobic avoidance. Behavioral therapy that desensitizes a patient to feared situations is important in reducing phobic avoidance. Desensitization can be facilitated by practicing exposure to feared situations. Relaxation techniques are also utilized to reduce the free-floating anxiety that is often associated with this illness.[2]

SUMMARY OF THE DIAGNOSIS AND TREATMENT OF PANIC DISORDER

1. Panic disorder often presents with many physical symptoms. Physicians must ask a patient who presents with these symptoms of their association with panic attacks.

2. Chest pain, neurologic symptoms, and gastrointestinal symptoms are most frequent somatic symptoms.

3. Panic disorder has recently been associated with an increased risk of suicide.[3]

4. **Treatment:**
   a) panic attacks: imipramine, desipramine, alprazolam, clonazepam, and phenelzine.
   b) phobic avoidance: behavioral therapy (desensitization)

References

1. American Psychiatric Association. Diagnostic and statistical manual of mental disorders. 3rd Ed. Revised (DSM-III-R). Washington: APA Press, 1987.

2. Wesner R. Panic disorder and agoraphobia. Prim Care 1987; 14(4): 649–656.

3. Weissman M, Klerman G, Markowitz J, Ouellette R. Suicidal ideation and suicide attempts in panic disorder and attacks. N Engl J Med 1989; 321: 1209–1214.

PROBLEM 55: A 45-YEAR-OLD MALE WITH AN ENLARGED LIVER

A 45-year-old executive comes into your office for his yearly physical examination. He is found to have a liver span of 20 cm. His liver edge is tender. When questioned about alcohol intake he states that he is a "social drinker." When asked to define "social", he states that he often consumes 15–18 ounces of hard liquor when spending an afternoon with a client. He denies work or family problems associated with his consumption of alcohol. He has not increased his consumption lately and he has not noticed any lessening of the effect that the alcohol has on him. He denies withdrawal symptoms.

SELECT THE ONE BEST ANSWER TO THE FOLLOWING QUESTIONS:

449. With this history, your initial impression of his drinking problem would be:
   a) excessive social drinking
   b) alcohol abuse
   c) alcoholism
   d) heavy drinking
   e) potential alcohol abuse

450. Alcoholics have a mortality rate that is approximately:

   a) the same as nonalcoholics
   b) one and one half times that of nonalcoholics
   c) twice that of nonalcoholics
   d) two and one-half times that of nonalcoholics
   e) five times that of nonalcoholics

451. Which of the following statements regarding family history and alcoholism is CORRECT?
   a) there is no increased risk of alcoholism in siblings of alcoholics
   b) in twin studies the concordance rate of alcohol abuse and alcoholism is higher in dizygotic twins than in monozygotic twins

c) the pattern of inheritance appears to be autosomal dominant

d) daughters of alcoholic fathers appear to be particularly at risk

e) men with alcoholic fathers have a highly heritable form of alcoholism that increases their risk of alcoholism ninefold

ANSWER THE FOLLOWING QUESTIONS ACCORDING TO THE CODE:

A: 1, 2, and 3 are correct
B: 1 and 3 are correct
C: 2 and 4 are correct
D: Only 4 is correct
E: All of the above are correct

452. Which of the following are common presenting symptoms in alcoholics?
1) vomiting
2) chronic diarrhea
3) dyspepsia
4) hypertension

453. Which of the following conditions may result from the excessive ingestion of alcohol?
1) acute hepatitis
2) acute and chronic gastritis
3) skeletal and cardiac myopathy
4) esophageal and gastric carcinoma

454. Which of the following conditions is/are more common in alcoholics than in nonalcoholics?
1) cigarette smoking
2) obesity
3) diabetes
4) hypertension

455. Which of the following statements regarding laboratory abnormalities in alcoholism is/are TRUE?
1) GGT (gamma-glutamyl transferase) is a very sensitive screening test for alcoholism
2) SGOT (AST) is a more sensitive and specific marker for alcoholism than GGT
3) MCV (mean corpuscular volume) has been shown to be a sensitive screening test for alcoholism
4) alcoholism questionnaires have a higher positive predictive value than laboratory markers for alcoholism

456. A 35-year-old male presents to the emergency room with profuse sweating, shaking, anxiety, and tremor. He had been admitted to a half-way house for alcoholic rehabilitation 24 hours earlier. You diagnose acute alcohol withdrawal. Which of the following is/are useful treatments in the routine management of acute alcohol withdrawal?
1) chlordiazepoxide
2) thiamine
3) diazepam
4) haloperidol

457. With respect to rehabilitation programs, which of the following is/are TRUE?
1) no type of rehabilitation program has been clearly shown to be superior to others
2) participation in Alcoholics Anonymous is generally felt to be beneficial
3) relapse following rehabilitation is common
4) disulfiram (Antabuse) should be a routine part of rehabilitation

ANSWERS

449. C. This patient is an alcoholic. The diagnosis of alcoholism requires only one of four major criteria. These criteria are: physiologic dependence (withdrawal signs and symptoms), alcohol tolerance, major alcohol related illness (including alcoholic hepatitis), or continued drinking despite strong contraindications. This patient appears to have a marked alcohol tolerance and probably also has alcoholic hepatitis.[1–3]

450. D. Alcoholics have a mortality rate 2.5 times greater than nonalcoholics. Common causes of death include cirrhosis, motor vehicle accidents, drowning, falls, homicide, and suicide.[1]

451. E. Alcoholism appears to be an inherited disease, although the actual genetic pattern has not been determined. Concordance rate for alcohol abuse and alcoholism is higher among monozygotic than dizygotic twins. Men with alcoholic fathers have a highly heritable form of alcoholism that increases their risk of alcoholism ninefold. Women are also at increased risk, but not nearly to the degree that men are.[2]

452. E. Common presenting symptoms and signs in alcoholism include anorexia, nausea, vomiting, diarrhea, dyspepsia, hypertension, dysrhythmias,

palpitations, sleep disturbances, and sexual dysfunction.[3]

453. E. Alcoholics are at risk of developing disorders of almost any organ system in the body. Frequently seen disorders include: (1) neuropsychiatric syndromes such as acute alcohol withdrawal and delirium tremens; (2) hepatic disorders such as acute hepatitis, cirrhosis and fatty liver; (3) digestive disorders such as acute and chronic gastritis, peptic ulcer, esophageal and gastric cancer, and pancreatitis; (4) hematologic disorders including bone marrow suppression and anemia; (5) nutritional deficiencies; and (6) myopathies.[1]

454. E. Cigarette smoking, obesity, diabetes, and hypertension are much more common in alcoholics than in nonalcoholics.[1]

455. D. Biochemical markers including GGT, SPOT (AST), SGPT(ALT), MCV, and HDL have been found to be neither sensitive nor specific in the diagnosis of alcoholism.[3]

Two questionnaires, the CAGE,[4] and the SMAST[5] have been found to be more sensitive and specific than laboratory markers.[3]

The CAGE questionnaire[4] asks four questions:
1) Have you ever felt you ought to CUT down on your drinking?
2) Have people ANNOYED you by criticizing your drinking?
3) Have you ever felt bad or GUILTY about your drinking?
4) Have you ever had a drink first thing in the morning (EYE OPENER) to steady your nerves or get rid of a hangover?

Two or more affirmative answers indicate probable alcoholism.

The SMAST questionnaire (Short Michigan Alcoholism Screening Test)[5] is a shortened version of the MAST (Michigan Alcoholism Screening Test).[6]

456. E. Alcohol withdrawal is best treated with benzodiazepine therapy. Chlorodiazepoxide and diazepam are the most frequently used agents. Thiamine should be administered to prevent Wernicke-Korsakoff syndrome.[2]

Withdrawal seizures can by treated with intravenous phenytoin or diazepam.[2]

Haloperidol may also be useful in patients with acute delirium.

457. A. Most studies indicate that there is no significant difference between various forms of alcoholic rehabilitation. Although evidence is lacking, many physicians believe that an inpatient program with family participation is superior to outpatient counseling. Most therapists and physicians agree that Alcoholics Anonymous (AA) participation is helpful in rehabilitation of the alcoholic.

Disulfiram (Antabuse) should not be a routine part of rehabilitation.[2]

SUMMARY OF THE DIAGNOSIS AND TREATMENT OF ALCOHOLISM

1. Diagnosis of alcoholism requires one of the following: (a) physiologic dependence, (b) alcohol tolerance, (c) major alcohol-related illness, or (d) continued drinking despite strong contraindication(s) known to the patient.

2. Office screening questionnaires: CAGE is the shortest and easiest questionnaire to use.

3. Benzodiazepines should be used for acute withdrawal.

4. Rehabilitation should involve the family.

5. Alcoholics Anonymous should be considered following cessation of drinking.

References

1. Milhorn H. The diagnosis of alcoholism. Am Fam Physician 1988; 37(6): 175–183.

2. Cook B, Garvey M, Shukla S. Alcoholism. Prim Care 1987; 14(4): 685–697.

3. Hays J, Spickard W. Alcoholism. Early diagnosis and intervention. J Gen Intern Med 1987;2: 420–427.

4. Ewing J. Detecting alcoholism. The CAGE questionnaire. JAMA 1984; 252: 1905–1907.

5. Selzer M. Vinokur A, van Rooijen L. A self-administered Short Michigan Alcoholism Screening Test (SMAST). J Stud Alcohol 1975; 36: 117–126.

6. Selzer M. The Michigan Alcoholism Screening Test: the quest for a new diagnostic instrument. Am J Psychiatry 1971; 127: 1653–1658.

PROBLEM 56: A 36-YEAR-OLD FEMALE WITH SHORTNESS OF BREATH AND PALPITATIONS

A 36-year-old female presents to your office with an 8-month history of shortness of breath, palpitations, dizziness, trouble swallowing, restlessness, fatigue, and anxiety regarding her job and the health of her two children. On careful questioning you ascertain that she is doing well at her job and her children are healthy.

SELECT THE ONE BEST ANSWER TO THE FOLLOWING QUESTION:

458. The most likely diagnosis is:
    a) panic disorder
    b) depression
    c) generalized anxiety disorder
    d) thyrotoxicosis
    e) hypochondriasis

ANSWER THE FOLLOWING QUESTIONS ACCORDING TO THE CODE:

A: 1, 2, and 3 are correct
B: 1 and 3 are correct
C: 2 and 4 are correct
D: Only 4 is correct
E: All of the above are correct

459. Which of the following are characteristic of the disorder described above?
    1) trembling
    2) nausea
    3) diarrhea
    4) dry mouth

460. Which of the following is(are) effective in the treatment of the condition described above?
    1) alprazolam
    2) lorazepam
    3) oxazepam
    4) diazepam

461. Which of the following statements regarding the use of buspirone in the treatment of the condition described above is(are) true?
    1) buspirone is a nonbenzodiazepine drug
    2) buspirone has anxiolytic efficacy similar to diazepam
    3) buspirone lacks addictive or abuse potential
    4) buspirone has signficant sedative properties

462. Which of the following has/have been shown to be beneficial in the treatment of the described disorder?
    1) supportive psychotherapy

2) family therapy
3) buspirone
4) sole treatment with biofeedback and mediation

ANSWERS

458. C.

459. E. This patient has generalized anxiety disorder (GAD).

Generalized anxiety disorder is defined as unrealistic or excessive anxiety or worry about two or more life circumstances, for a period of 6 months or longer, during which the patient has been bothered more days than not by these concerns.[1] Symptoms associated with GAD include motor tension symptoms (trembling, muscle tension, aches, restlessness, fatigibility); autonomic hyperactivity symptoms (shortness of breath, palpitations, sweating, dry mouth, dizziness, nausea, diarrhea); and other symptoms including irratibility, difficulty concentrating, and difficulty falling or staying asleep.[1]

GAD is twice as common in women as in men.[2] Symptoms usually begin in the late teens or the early twenties.

GAD must be distinguished from panic disorder and major depression. Although there is an overlap of symptoms between GAD and panic disorder, panic disorder is distinguished by the occurrence of discrete panic attacks, which are not part of GAD.[2] In GAD, anxiety symptoms are continually present and the onset of symptoms is usually earlier in life and more gradual.[2] Patients with GAD often develop a secondary depression. This can usually be distinguished from major depressive disorder by the predominance of vegetative symptoms in the latter.

Primary organic disorders such as hyperthyroidism, mitral valve prolapse, and excessive caffeine intake can result in significant anxiety and must be considered in the differential diagnosis of GAD.

Hypochondriasis is discussed in another chapter of this book.

460. E. Generalized anxiety disorder is appropriately treated pharmacologically with one of the benzodiazepines. These include alprazolam, lorazepam, oxazepam, and diazepam. These drugs will alleviate symptoms in approximately 75% of patients with GAD.[2] In elderly patients, a shorter acting agent such as lorazepam or alprazolam is preferred to avoid accumulation of drug and resulting side effects.

Imipramine, a tricyclic antidepressant, may be as good as or superior to benzodiazepines in the treatment of GAD. Also, imipramine does not have the abuse potential that benzodiazepines do, and may be preferrable for that reason.[2]

461. A. Buspirone is a nonbenzodiazepine derivative. It has anxiolytic activity as good as diazepam, but lacks the sedative side effect. It also lacks addictive or abuse potential, even when given for long-term periods. It may become the pharmacologic treatment of choice for GAD.[2]

462. A. Supportive psychotherapy is very beneficial in treating patients with GAD. In this disorder, supportive psychotherapy (and cognitive therapy) attempt to break the anxiety-physical symptom-anxiety cycle that often perpetuate GAD.

Family therapy is often helpful in treating patients with GAD. With family therapy, a better understanding of the condition by family members often facilitates greater support for the patient.

Behavioral approaches including biofeedback, relaxation training, mediation, and self-hypnosis may form a part of therapy but are seldom sufficient by themselves.

Buspirone has already been discussed.[2]

SUMMARY OF THE DIAGNOSIS AND TREATMENT OF GENERALIZED ANXIETY DISORDER

1. **GAD**: Excessive anxiety or worry with accompanying physical symptoms

2. **Major differential diagnoses**: Major depressive disorder, panic disorder

3. **Treatment:**
   a) pharmacotherapy:
      1) benzodiazepines
      2) imipramine
      3) buspirone
   b) psychotherapy:
      1) supportive and cognitive therapy
      2) family therapy
   c) behavioral therapies may be useful adjuncts

References

1. American Psychiatric Association. Diagnostic and statistical manual of mental disorders. 3rd Ed. Revised (DSM-III-R). Washington: APA Press, 1987.

2. Appenheimer T, Noyes R. Generalized anxiety disorder. Prim Care 1987; 14(4): 635–648.

PROBLEM 57: A 25-YEAR-OLD FEMALE WITH PELVIC DISCOMFORT, LOW BACK PAIN, INSOMNIA AND FATIGUE

A 25-year-old female presents to the emergency room with a 6-month history of pelvic discomfort, low back pain, lethargy, fatigue, and weight gain. She states that these problems have been getting progressively worse over the 6 month period.

She is accompanied to the emergency room by her husband.

She states that she is not depressed and that everything at home is fine. She does not look directly at you as you question her, but rather stares at the floor.

SELECT THE ONE BEST ANSWER TO THE FOLLOWING QUESTIONS:

463. Which of the following should be considered in the differential diagnosis of this patient's condition?

a) hypothyroidism
b) depression
c) spousal abuse
d) a and b only
e) all of the above

464. The estimated prevalence of spousal abuse in North America is:
    a) 1/100
    b) 1/50
    c) 1/25
    d) 1/10
    e) 1/2

465. All of the following are characteristics of spousal abuse EXCEPT:
    a) the association of violence with alcohol intake by the batterer
    b) violent behavior in the family of origin in both victim and batterer
    c) high risk of suicide attempt or gesture in the victim
    d) high incidence of neurotropic drug use in the victim
    e) a syndrome associated with lower socio-economic class

466. The main goal of psychotherapy for victims of spousal abuse is:
    a) to establish a framework by which the couple can work out their problems
    b) to establish a cause for the violence
    c) to overcome fear and reverse the concept of "learned helplessness" in the victim
    d) to find some common ground whereby the victim and batterer can begin a new relationship
    e) to convince the victim that to stay in the present relationship is an exercise in futility

467. The main goal of psychotherapy for batterers is:
    a) to establish a framework by which the couple can work out their problems
    b) to establish a cause for the violence
    c) to find some common ground whereby the victim and batterer can begin a new relationship
    d) to encourage the batterer to accept responsiblity for the violence to and facilitate his expression of anger in different ways
    e) to help the batterer deal with alcoholism and other concurrent problems

ANSWER THE FOLLOWING QUESTIONS ACCORDING TO THE CODE:

A: 1, 2, and 3 are correct
B: 1 and 3 are correct
C: 2 and 4 are correct
D: Only 4 is correct
E: All of the above are correct

468. A woman with battered wife syndrome often presents with:
    1) chronic pelvic pain
    2) dyspareunia
    3) chronic back pain
    4) chronic abdominal pain

469. Women stay in abusive relationships because of fear. Which of the following are common fears of victims of spousal abuse?
    1) fear of escalation of violence if they leave the relationship
    2) fear of being unable to function independently
    3) fear of not being believed by the person in which they confide
    4) fear of being unable to support themselves and their children

470. The purpose of an interval or transition house is to:
    1) provide an environment in which the woman and her children can feel safe
    2) provide an atmosphere where supportive counseling of both victim and batterer can take place
    3) provide education for the woman about spousal abuse
    4) facilitate the wife in seeking a divorce from her husband

ANSWERS

463. E. All of the following are diagnostic considerations in this patient. The patient may have organic disease (hypothyroidism manifested by lethargy, fatigue, and weight gain). Second, the symptoms may be a manifestation of a masked depression. Third, these symptoms may be psychophysiologic in response to spousal abuse.

The inability to diagnose spousal abuse may be explained by the fact that the profile presented to the clinician is vague. Women who are victims of spousal abuse visit their physicians often, usually with somatic or conversion symptoms or psychophysiologic reactions. Their most frequent complaints are headache, insomnia, a choking sensation, hyperventilation, gastrointestinal pain, chest pain, pelvic pain, and back pain. They may show signs of anxiety neurosis, depression, suicidal behavior, drug abuse, and noncompliance with medication.[1,2]

Unless the physician considers the possibility of spousal abuse the diagnosis will be missed.

464. D. The estimated prevalence of spousal abuse in North America is 1/10. There is some suggestion that the prevalence has been increasing in recent years due to economic recession and unemployment.[1]

465. E. Alcohol intake by the batterer is associated with spousal abuse. The majority of men who beat their spouses have an alcohol abuse problem. Sometimes, the batterer uses alcohol to disavow his behavior and convince others that he was not responsible for his actions at the time of the assault. However, alcohol doesn't cause spousal abuse. The two problems must be dealt with seperately.[1]

A nuclear family in which violence occurred is common in both victims and batterers.

Neurotropic drug use, suicide attempts, or gestures by the victim are common.[1]

Although spousal abuse may occur more commonly in the lower socioeconomic class because of chronic unemployment, it is not per se associated with the lower socioeconomic class. It occurs in ALL classes of society.[1]

466. C. The main goal of psychotherapy in spousal abuse is to overcome fear and reverse the concept of " learned helplessness" (I can't do anything to prevent this) and self-blame in the victim. This is accomplished by encouraging an increase in the victim's self-confidence and the development of a new self-concept, from "victim" and "failure" to competence and autonomy.[1]

467. D. The purpose of psychotherapy for batterers (either individual or group) is to help the batterer accept responsiblity for the abuse and to help him facilitate the expression of anger in different ways. Before marriage counseling can begin, the batterer must be prepared to follow this course. In addition, the batterer must be prepared to take steps to deal with concurrent problems, such as alcoholism.

468. E. See critique of question 463.

469. E. All of the fears listed are reasons for victims choosing to stay in the relationship. Fear of escalation of the violence and even murder are common reasons for staying. Fear of being unable to function independently and support themselves and their children are almost universal. In addition, a fear of not being believed when they finally tell their story is very common.[1]

470. B. The primary purpose of an interval or transition house is to provide a safe environment for the woman and her children. The continuation of threats and violence by the husband and the absence of provisions for safety are universally identified as deterrents to action.[1] In addition, once this barrier of fear is removed, education about the syndrome and supportive counseling can take place. The batterer has no place in an interval or transition house. The purpose of psychotherapy is not to steer the woman in the direction of divorce, but rather to develop a new self-concept in which she is capable of making her own decisions.[1]

SUMMARY OF THE DIAGNOSIS AND MANAGEMENT OF SPOUSAL ABUSE

Definition: Wife abuse is defined as the physical or psychologic abuse directed by a man against his female partner, in an attempt to control her behavior or intimidate her.

Prevalence: Current prevalence estimated at 10% of all relationships

Presenting symptoms: Usually vague somatic or psychophysiologic symptoms

Diagnosis: First, think of the diagnosis. Proceed from open-ended nonthreatening questions such as " How does your spouse express anger?" to more direct questions such as "Does your husband beat you?"

Treatment:
Victim:
1) Removal to an interval or transition house
2) Psychotherapy to reverse "learned helplessness"

Abuser:
1) Psychotherapy to help abuser accept responsibility for the abuse and to facilitate the expression of anger in other ways.

References

1. Swanson R. Battered wife syndrome. Can Med Assoc J 1984; 130: 709–713.

2. Swanson R. Recognizing battered wife syndrome. Can Fam Physician 1985; 31:823–825.

PROBLEM 58: A 25-YEAR-OLD WOMAN WHO HAS JUST LOST A BABY

A-25-year old woman presents to your office 10 months after having delivered a fetus at 18 weeks gestation. She has just been told by her physician to "get on" with her life. She is crying and tearful, and wonders if life is worth living. She feels overwhelmed and states that she is pacing the floor most of the day and night. She is having continual nightmares of the abortion process and is suffering constant abdominal pain and cramping. She is also certain that the abortion was caused by her lifting a number of heavy boxes two days before the event. She has come to see if you can help her.

SELECT THE ONE BEST ANSWER TO EACH OF THE FOLLOWING QUESTIONS:

471. The most likely diagnosis in this case is:
    a) agitated depression
    b) acute stress reaction
    c) bipolar affective disorder
    d) postpartum depression
    e) pathologic grief reaction

472. In counseling the patient regarding her lifting of the heavy boxes 2 days prior to the abortion you should explain that:
    a) yes, carrying the heavy boxes did probably cause the abortion, but not to worry; she can always get pregnant again
    b) yes, carrying the heavy boxes may have contributed to the abortion, but it probably won't happen again
    c) guilt is a universal response to grief and that is why she is wondering about carrying the boxes. However, there is no reason to believe that carrying the boxes had anything to do with the abortion.
    d) abortion is nature's way of dealing with bad chromosomes and if carrying the boxes had anything to do with the abortion then it probably was for the best
    e) boxes or no boxes, the pregnancy was doomed to failure from the start

ANSWER THE FOLLOWING QUESTIONS ACCORDING TO THE CODE:

A: 1, 2, and 3 are correct
B: 1 and 3 are correct
C: 2 and 4 are correct
D: Only 4 is correct
E: All of the above are correct

473. The family physician's role in managing perinatal loss can best be defined as that of:
    1) an empathetic listener
    2) an intensive psychotherapist
    3) a compassionate informer
    4) a source of referral to psychiatrists skilled in the management of perinatal loss

474. Which of the following are symptoms of a NORMAL grief reaction?
    1) sleeplessness
    2) preoccupation with feelings of guilt
    3) hostile reactions toward physicians and others associated with the care of the deceased
    4) loss in the pattern of activities of daily living

475. A baby dies at 32 weeks gestation after spending 4 weeks in the neonatal intensive care unit. The mother and father seem calm and do not seem very upset when their baby finally passes away. Which of the following statements are TRUE regarding this situation?
    1) this is a pathologic grief reaction
    2) this is not an uncommon occurrence
    3) a psychiatrist should be called "stat"
    4) this is an example of anticipatory grieving

ANSWERS

471. E. This patient has a pathologic grief reaction. A pathologic grief reaction is defined as the intensification of grief to the level where the person is overwhelmed, resorts to maladaptive behavior, or remains interminably in a state of grief without completing the grieving process.[1] Characteristics of pathologic grief reactions among women who have suffered an abortion include (1) nightmares, (2) recurrent abdominal pains and cramping, (3) frequent headaches and backaches, (4) vivid recollections and memories of the event, (5) recurrent anniversary effects of the loss, (6) difficulty in resuming normal activities, and (7) persistent depression.[1] The prevalence of pathologic grief reactions among women who suffer spontaneous abortions or stillbirths is estimated to be 25%.

472. C. Guilt is a universal response to a spontaneous abortion. Women often go back over their preg-

nancies and find something to "blame" the event on. The physician must ensure that the patient understands that there is NOTHING that she could have done to alter the outcome. This concept may have to be discussed repeatedly before it is finally accepted.

Although it is true that 50–60% of early spontaneous abortions may be associated with chromosomal abnormality, it is inappropriate to dismiss a miscarriage as "nature's way of dealing with bad chromosomes." The situation discussed calls for explanation about guilt feelings, time, and most of all empathy, on the part of the physician.[1,2]

473. B. The family physician's role in managing perinatal loss can best be described as that of an empathetic listener and a compassionate informer. Intensive psychotherapy is rarely required. The necessary psychotherapy can be performed by the family physician (with the help of a perinatal support team if available). See the chapter on psychotherapy for further details.

474. E. Before grief counseling can be undertaken, the physician must have a thorough knowledge of the components of a grief reaction. These are best described as:
   1) sensations of somatic distress such as sighing respirations, fatigue, sleeplessness, and digestive symptoms
   2) preoccupation with the image of the deceased
   3) preoccupation with feelings of guilt
   4) hostile reactions toward physicians and others associated with the care of the deceased
   5) loss in the pattern of activities of daily living
   These behaviors, known as "acute grief work" facilitate a separation from the deceased and the initiation of new relationships. By understanding the process of normal grieving, and their role in the tasks of grieving, family physicians can substantially decrease the incidence of pathologic grief reactions.[2,3]

475. C. This is an example of anticipatory grieving, and is common in the neonatal intense care unit setting. In this case the couple has completed a significant proportion of their "grief work" before the infant actually dies. They have "anticipated" the death of the infant and often feel relief when the event actually occurs. If we do not inform them that this is normal they will often feel intense guilt, and this itself can lead to a pathologic grief reaction. Once again, all that is required is a physician who is an "empathetic listener" and a "compassionate informer." There is no need to call a psychiatrist "stat."[2,3]

SUMMARY OF THE MANAGEMENT FOR HELPING PARENTS COPE WITH ABORTION AND STILLBIRTH

1. Keep the parents informed; be honest and forthright.

2. Recognize and facilitate anticipatory grieving.

3. Encourage the person supporting the mother to remain with her throughout the abortion or stillbirth.

4. Support the couple in seeing and spending time with the fetus or stillborn child.

5. Describe the fetus or infant in detail, particularly for couples who choose not to see it.

6. Encourage the mother to make as many choices about her care as possible.

7. Teach the couple about the grieving process.

8. If a stillbirth, allow photographs.

9. Prepare couples for hospital paperwork such as autopsy requests, death certificates, and disposal of the fetus or stillbirth.

10. Help the couple think about informing siblings.

11. Assist the couple in deciding how to tell friends of the event.

12. Discuss a subsequent pregnancy (counsel against conceiving before the grief work is complete: this may result in this child being a "replacement child").

13. Schedule frequent additional office visits (especially in the first 2 months after the event).

14. Help the couple establish contact with support groups in the community.

References

1. Hall R, Beresford T, Quinones J. Grief following spontaneous abortion. Psychiatr Clin North Am 1987; 10(3): 405–419.

2. Swanson R. Parents experiencing perinatal loss: the physician's role. Can Fam Physician 1986; 32: 599–602.

3. Worden J. Grief counseling and grief therapy. New York: Springer, 1982.

PROBLEM 59: A 29-YEAR-OLD WORKING MOTHER WITH THREE CHILDREN WHO IS UNABLE TO COPE

A 29-year-old mother who holds a full time job and has three young children at home presents to your office with complaints of fatigue and "inability to cope." She tells you that she just "can't be all things to all people anymore." You begin supportive psychotherapy.

SELECT THE ONE BEST ANSWER TO THE FOLLOWING QUESTIONS:

476. Which of the following statements regarding medical psychotherapy is FALSE?
    a) medical psychotherapy is used for patients in crisis
    b) in medical psychotherapy there is intense interaction between the patient and the therapist
    c) to be effective, medical psychotherapy must provide a rationale that can be believed by both patient and therapist
    d) all medical psychotherapy requires specialized training to be performed properly
    e) physicians can frequently use medical psychotherapy to help a patient cope with a chronic illness

ANSWER THE FOLLOWING QUESTIONS ACCORDING TO THE CODE:

A: 1, 2, and 3 are correct
B: 1 and 3 are correct
C: 2 and 4 are correct
D: Only 4 is correct
E: All of the above are correct

477. There are many reasons patients present to their family physicians for counseling or supportive psychotherapy. Which of the following is(are) common reasons for this presentation?
    1) demoralization
    2) anger
    3) depression
    4) anxiety

478. Which statement(s) BEST describes the supportive psychotherapy performed by family physicians?
    1) it provides support for the patient
    2) it attempts to provide introspective exploration of the psychic causes of the patient's problem
    3) it provides reassurance for the patient
    4) it usually requires frequent, long sessions to be successful

479. Which of the following aspects of medical psychotherapy are important in CRISIS counseling?
    1) a careful history
    2) an exploration of the previous methods of problem solving that the patient has found useful
    3) suggestions of strategies for dealing with the current problem
    4) implementation of the regimen discussed before the next visit

480. Which of the following statements regarding supportive psychotherapy in the treatment of chronic conditions is/are TRUE?
    1) goal setting is extremely important
    2) the aim of the therapist differs greatly depending on the patient
    3) the opportunity for ventilation usually provides the patient with substantial relief
    4) the therapist should assume the patient is totally helpless; this often enhances medical psychotherapy

ANSWERS

476. D. Medical psychotherapy is used in patients with crisis or in a chronic state of difficulty or illness.

Medical psychotherapy involves an intense interaction between the patient and the therapist. This interaction, however, must exist within a healing setting in which the patient feels safe.

To be effective, medical psychotherapy must provide a rationale that can be believed by both the patient and the therapist.

Family physicians provide psychotherapy even without realizing it. The support and reassurance that we provide to our patients every day is a form of medical psychotherapy. Rather than requiring extensive training, simple supportive psychotherapy simply requires an empathic physician who is prepared to spend the necessary time discussing the patient's particular problem.[1]

477. E. Demoralization, depression, anxiety, guilt, shame, and a sense of diminished self worth are all reasons for patients to present to their physicians in need of counseling or supportive psychotherapy.[2]

478. B. In performing supportive psychotherapy, the family physician provides reassurance and support for the patient. An introspective exploration of the psychic causes of the patient's problem is not a significant component of supportive psychotherapy. Medical psychotherapy for a particular problem can usually be performed in a few brief sessions.[1,2]

479. E. In crisis counseling, key elements include a careful history, an exploration of previous problem solving methods that the patient has found helpful, strategy suggestions for dealing with the current problem, and a plan for implementation of the strategies discussed before the next appointment.[2]

480. A. In patients suffering from chronic mental or physical disorders, a number of principles are important.

First, goal setting is crucial. The goals that are set should be realistic in terms of the prognosis for the condition.

Every patient is different. The aims of the therapist will depend upon the individual, the condition, previous psychologic functioning, and previous coping mechanisms.

The patient often obtains substantial relief from being able to discuss his problem and ventilate his feelings with an empathetic listener.

The patient must be an active partner in his own care. The therapist must not assume that the patient is helpless; indeed, in this situation supportive psychotherapy is doomed to failure.[1,2]

SUMMARY OF SUPPORTIVE PSYCHOTHERAPY PERFORMED BY FAMILY PHYSICIANS:

1. Establish rapport.

2. Give the patient permission to discuss his/her problem in an unhurried manner.

3. Listen to what the patient is telling you.

4. Paraphrase what the patient has just said.

5. Offer specific suggestions for the patient to work on until the next appointment (if necessary).

6. Schedule weekly visits with a view to complete resolution or major progress over 8 weeks.

References

1. Williamson P. Psychotherapy by family physicians. Prim Care 1987; 14(4): 803–815.

2. Goldberg R, Green S. Medical psychotherapy. Am Fam Physician 1985; 31(1): 173–178.

PROBLEM 60: A 19-YEAR-OLD FEMALE WITH A RAPID WEIGHT LOSS, AN INTENSE FEAR OF GAINING WEIGHT, AND AMENORRHEA

A 19-year-old female presents to the office with a 30 lb weight loss in the last 6 months. She is 5'6" tall and now weighs 90 lbs. She states that she still "feels fat" and has an intense fear of gaining weight. She also describes amenorrhea of 4 months duration.

SELECT THE ONE BEST ANSWER TO THE FOLLOWING QUESTIONS:

481. In this patient the most likely diagnosis is:
    a) bulimia
    b) anorexia nervosa
    c) personality disorder
    d) masked depression
    e) generalized anxiety disorder

482. The most serious complication of the above disorder is:
    a) muscle wasting
    b) weakness
    c) hypokalemia
    d) bradycardia
    e) hypotension

ANSWER THE FOLLOWING QUESTIONS ACCORDING TO THE CODE:

A: 1, 2, and 3 are correct
B: 1 and 3 are correct
C: 2 and 4 are correct
D: Only 4 is correct
E: All of the above are correct

483. The treatment(s) of choice for the disorder described above is(are):
    1) benzodiazepines
    2) tricyclic antidepressants
    3) psychoanalytic psychotherapy
    4) behavioral psychotherapy

484. Which of the following is/are associated with the disorder described above?
    1) personality disorder
    2) major depresssive illness
    3) substance abuse disorder
    4) panic disorder

485. A 26-year-old patient presents with recurrent episodes of binge eating (approximately 4 times/ week) after which she vomits to prevent weight gain. She states that "she has no control" over these episodes and becomes depressed because she is unable to control herself.

Which of the following statements about this patient is/are true?
    1) this patient may have an underlying personality disorder
    2) this patient may have an underlying major depression
    3) this patient may have an underlying substance abuse disorder
    4) this patient may have a normal weight

486. Complications of the disorder described in question 485 include:
    1) dental erosions and cavities
    2) callous formation on the back of the hand
    3) Mallory-Weiss tears
    4) hypokalemia

487. Treatment of the disorder described in question 485 includes:
    1) tricyclic antidepressants
    2) psychoanalytic psychotherapy
    3) behavioral psychotherapy
    4) benzodiazepines

ANSWERS

481. B. This patient has anorexia nervosa. Anorexia nervosa is defined as weight loss leading to maintenance of body weight 15% below that expected, associated with a distorted body image and an intense fear of gaining weight or becoming fat, even when underweight.[1] Many anorexic women are also amenorrheic.[1]

    Eating disorders are frequently associated with other psychiatric conditions, particularly depression, personality disorders, and substance abuse.[2]

482. C. The medical complications of anorexia include muscle wasting, weakness, fatigue, depression of cardiovascular function leading to bradycardia and hypotension, and depression of body temperature mechanisms leading to hypothermia. The most serious abnormality, however, is hypokalemia

with resultant cardiac arrhythmias and possibly sudden cardiac death.[2]

483. D. Behavioral psychotherapy forms the basis of therapy for patients with anorexia nervosa.[2] Behavioral psychotherapy is conducted with specific progress goals agreed upon by contract, and with positive reinforcement for attainment of those goals.[2]

Benzodiazepines, tricyclic antidepressants, and psychoanalytic psychotherapy have not been shown to be successful in the treatment of anorexia nervosa.[2]

484. A. Personality disorder, major depressive illness and substance abuse disorder are all associated with anorexia nervosa and bulimia. Panic disorder has not been shown to have a specific association.[2]

485. E. This patient has bulimia nervosa. Bulimia is defined as recurrent episodes of binge eating over which the patient has no control, associated with self-induced vomiting, laxative or diuretic use, strict dieting or fasting, excessive vigorous exercise, and an overconcern about body shape and image.[1] Many bulimic patients have underlying personality disorders, major depression, or substance abuse disorders.[2] Bulimics are often of normal weight, and thus are more difficult to diagnose than anorexics.[2]

486. E. Complications of bulimia include dental erosions and cavities; callous formation on the back of the hand secondary to trauma from the teeth (Russell's sign); hypokalemia from vomiting, diuretic and laxative use; and occasionally Malory-Weiss tears from repeated vomiting and wretching. Hypokalemia is the best indicator of acute risk of medical complications in bulimia and needs monitoring during treatment.[2]

487. B. As with anorexia nervosa, behavioral therapy forms the basis of treatment of bulimic patients. In addition, however, both tricyclic antidepressants and monoamine oxidase inhibitors have shown some effectiveness in decreasing binging and vomiting behaviors.[2] As in anorexia, psychoanalytic psychotherapy and benzodiazepine therapy are not appropriate.

SUMMARY OF THE DIAGNOSIS AND TREATMENT OF EATING DISORDERS

1. Anorexia nervosa and bulimia nervosa are the two most common eating disorders

2. **Major complication**: Metabolic disorders (especially hypokalemia) that may lead to cardiac arrhythmias

3. **Associated conditions**: Personality disorders, major depressive illness, substance abuse disorders

4. **Treatment**:
   a) bulimia: behavioral psychotherapy and tricyclic antidepressants
   b) anorexia nervosa: behavioral psychotherapy

References

1. American Psychiatric Association. Diagnostic and statistical manual of mental disorders. 3rd Ed. Revised. (DSM-III-R). Washington: APA Press, 1987.

2. Yates W, Sieleni B. Anorexia and bulimia. Prim Care 1987; 14(4): 737–744.

PROBLEM 61: A 27-YEAR-OLD FEMALE WITH 22 DIFFERENT SYMPTOMS

A 27-year-old female presents to your office for an initial consultation. When you ask her why she came to see you she pulls out a list of the following 22 symptoms (all of which have been present for at least 7 years): abdominal pain, nausea, bloating, intolerance to 63 different foods, back pain, generalized joint pains, shortness of breath at rest, chest pain, dizziness, amnesia, difficulty swallowing, double vision, blurred vision, trouble walking, muscle weakness, pain during intercourse, "gushing during menstruation," palpitations, painful menstruation, loss of voice, deafness, and transient blindness.

She has had 4 operations in the last 5 years to try and correct the abdominal pain; these include vagotomy and pyloroplasty, cholecystectomy, appendectomy, and hysterectomy. You are the 24th doctor she has consulted.

SELECT THE ONE BEST ANSWER TO THE FOLLOWING QUESTIONS:

488. The most likely diagnosis in this patient is:
    a) somatization disorder
    b) conversion disorder
    c) somotoform pain disorder
    d) hypochondriasis
    e) masked depression

489. After establishing the diagnosis in this patient you should:
    a) tell the patient that it was nice to meet her but you are too busy to see her again
    b) leave the office as quickly as possible
    c) prescribe a benzodiazepine and call a psychiatrist colleague for an emergency consultation
    d) prescribe an antidepressant
    e) none of the above

490. A 43-year-old woman presents to the emergency department with paralysis of both lower limbs and paraesthesias in both upper limbs beginning 2 hours ago. When first seen she is lying on a stretcher and is unble to move either lower extremity. A neurologist is consulted and states that the presentation does not fit any known neurologic disease. On further questioning you discover that the patient is being regularly beaten by her husband. Her last beating occurred 2 hours before her symptoms began. The most likely diagnosis is:
    a) complicated anxiety disorder
    b) somatization disorder
    c) conversion disorder
    d) psychogenic paralysis
    e) hypochondriasis

491. The most appropriate treatment for the patient described in question 490 is:
    a) a tricyclic antidepressant
    b) a monoamine oxidase inhibitor
    c) removal to a safe environment and supportive psychotherapy
    d) a and c
    e) b and c

492. A 45-year-old woman presents to your office in an anxious, tearful state. She states that she has chronic upper abdominal pain and is certain she has cancer of the stomach and nobody will believe her. She has attended 16 different physicians in the past year and has had a GI series performed six times; a barium enema performed three times, an ultrasound of her abdomen performed four times, and a CT scan performed twice. She is coming to you as a last resort before going to a herbal clinic in Mexico. Based on the history, the most likely diagnosis is:
    a) masked depression
    b) somatization disorder
    c) conversion disorder
    d) somatoform pain disorder
    e) hypochondriasis

493. The treatment of choice for the patient described in question 492 is:
    a) psychoanalytic psychotherapy
    b) a monoamine oxidase inhibitor
    c) a tricyclic antidepressant
    d) supportive psychotherapy
    e) electroconvulsive therapy

494. A 29-year-old female, a mother of five, initially presents to your office with a severe headache. After a complete history, physical examination, and laboratory evaluation including a lumbar puncture, you determine that she has viral meningitis. You hospitalize her. However, she remains flat in her hospital bed for 6 weeks. She is forced to leave on the verge of a nursing strike. Instead of going home, she continues to recouperate at the home of a friend, 90 miles from home. When you see her 8 weeks after discharge she walks with a cane (slowly) and complains of a constant headache. Her headache becomes chronic and she continues to need help at home 1 year later. She has had many previous health problems (mainly pain disorders) and has had a number of operations to try and diagnose and treat abdominal pain.
    The most likely diagnosis in this patient is:
    a) somatoform pain disorder
    b) hypochondriasis
    c) somatization disorder
    d) conversion disorder
    e) masked depression

ANSWER THE FOLLOWING QUESTION ACCORDING TO THE CODE:

A: 1, 2, and 3 are correct

B: 1 and 3 are correct
C: 2 and 4 are correct
D: Only 4 is correct
E: All of the above are correct

495. The patient described in question 494 may be helped by:
    1) a benzodiazepine
    2) a tricyclic antidepressant
    3) lithium carbonate
    4) supportive psychotherapy

ANSWERS

488. A. This patient has somatization disorder. Somatization disorder is defined as a history of many physical complaints or a belief that one is sick, beginning before the age of 30, and persisting for several years. Symptoms include gastrointestinal symptoms, pain symptoms, conversion symptoms, and gynecologic and sexual symptoms.[1]

   Somatization disorder is much more common in women than in men, and is familial. Twenty percent of first-degree female relatives have the condition.[2]

   Conversion disorder, somotoform pain disorder and hypochondriasis are discussed in detail in subsequent questions.

   Masked depression is discussed in another section of this book.

489. E. Treatment of somatization disorder in particular, and somatoform disorders in general should include: (1) avoiding any further inappropriate treatment (surgery, medication etc); (2) establishing a long-term empathetic relationship with the patient as the patient's sole physician; and (3) initiating frequent office consultations that center on the patient rather than on the patient's symptoms, while recognizing the importance of the symptoms to the patient.[2]

490. C. This patient has a conversion disorder secondary to spousal abuse. Conversion disorder is defined as a psychiatric disorder that results from a loss of, or alteration in physical functioning suggesting a physical disorder in which there is a temporal relationship between a psychosocial stressor and the initiation or exacerbation of the symptom(s).[1]

491. C. Therapy for this patient consists of removing the psychosocial stressor and educating the patient as to the origin of her symptoms. In this case, removal to a safe environment (an interval or transition house), supportive psychotherapy, and education regarding the origin of her symptoms are all part of the treatment.[2]

492. E. This patient has hypochondriasis. Hypochondriasis is defined as a preoccupation with the fear of having, or the belief that one has, a serious disease, based on the person's interpretation of physical signs or sensations as evidence of physical illness.[1]

   Hypochondriasis typically begins in middle or old age and is equally common in men and women.[2] The distinction between somatization disorder and hypochondriasis, which is often difficult, rests on the age of onset and the number of symptoms reported.[2]

493. D. See critique of question 489.

494. A. This patient has somatoform pain disorder. Somatoform pain disorder is defined as the preoccupation with pain in the absence of adequate physical findings to account for its occurrence or intensity.[1] In this patient, there was a strong component of secondary gain; she did not wish to go back to her role as mother and homemaker.

495. C. This patient may be helped by a combination of a tricyclic antidepressant and supportive psychotherapy. Tricyclic antidepressants have been shown to be effective in many chronic pain syndromes, including somatoform pain disorder. All tricyclic antidepressants appear to be equally efficacious; generally the dosage needed is somewhat less (50–100 mg) than the dosage needed to treat major depressive illness.[3]

SUMMARY OF THE DIAGNOSIS AND MANAGEMENT OF SOMATOFORM DISORDERS

1. **Major somatoform disorders:**
    a) somatization disorder
    b) conversion disorder
    c) hypochondriasis
    d) somatoform pain disorder

2. **Treatment:**
    a) "Do no harm," minimize medical work-ups
    b) frequent visits, concentrate on the patient, not the symptom

c) recognize the importance of the symptom to the patient
d) minimize the use of psychotropics and analgesics (except tricyclic antidepressants in somatoform pain disorder)

References

1. American Psychiatric Association. Diagnostic and statistical manual of mental disorders. 3rd Ed. Revised (DSM-III-R). Washington: APA Press, 1987.

2. Black D. Somatoform Disorders. Prim Care 1987; 14(4): 711–723.

3. Barsky A. Somatoform disorders. In: Kaplan H, Sadock B, eds. Comprehensive textbook of psychiatry, V. Baltimore: Williams & Wilkins, 1988: 1009–1027.

PROBLEM 62: A 16-YEAR-OLD MALE WITH A HISTORY OF RAPID MOOD SWINGS PRESENTING WITH TACHYCARDIA, PUPILLARY DILATION AND AN ELEVATED BLOOD PRESSURE

An 16-year-old male is brought into your office by his girl friend. She states that "he hasn't been himself lately" and seems to fluctuate from being almost "euphoric" to being depressed and irritable. The patient states that "he really is okay" and that he "just feels a little irritable occasionally." On examination his pulse is 120 beats/minute, his blood pressure is 180/110 mm Hg, his pupils are widely dilated and he is sweating.

SELECT THE ONE BEST ANSWER TO THE FOLLOWING QUESTIONS:

496. The most likely diagnosis in this patient is:
    a) acute anxiety attack
    b) pheochromocytoma
    c) thyrotoxicosis
    d) cocaine intoxication
    e) bipolar affective disorder

497. Which of the following is a complication of the disorder described above?
    a) sudden cardiac death
    b) cerebral hemorrhage
    c) respiratory arrest
    d) convulsions
    e) all of the above

498. Which of the following may be associated with the disorder described above?
    a) chronic cough
    b) hemoptysis
    c) anterior chest-wall pain
    d) lethargy
    e) all of the above

ANSWER THE FOLLOWING QUESTIONS ACCORDING TO THE CODE:

A: 1, 2, and 3 are correct
B: 1 and 3 are correct
C: 2 and 4 are correct
D: Only 4 is correct
E: All of the above are correct

499. Which of the following are characteristic of the disorder described above?
    1) no prior drug use
    2) periods of extreme self-confidence
    3) stable personality
    4) legal difficulties

500. The problem described above is often associated with which of the following disorders?
    1) conduct disorder
    2) attention deficit disorder
    3) specific developmental disorders
    4) borderline personality disorders

501. Regarding the treatment of the above condition, which of the following statements is/are TRUE?
    1) inpatient treatment programs are preferrable to outpatient treatment programs

2) adolescent patients that are currently using drugs cannot be adequately confronted in an outpatient setting

3) maintenance of sobriety is a keystone of treatment

4) outpatient treatment programs appear to be just as effective for most cocaine abusers

502. Which of the following statements regarding adolescent drug abuse is/are TRUE?

1) alcohol is still the most commonly abused drug

2) the prevalence of marijauna use has decreased in recent years

3) the prevalence of drug abuse among the very young has increased significantly

4) the prevalence of cocaine abuse has remained constant

ANSWERS

496. D. This patient shows the signs and symptoms of cocaine intoxication. Symptoms and signs of cocaine intoxication include tachycardia; pupillary dilation; elevated blood pressure; excessive perspiration or chills; nausea and vomiting; visual and tactile hallucinations; and behavioral changes including euphoria, grandiosity, rapid mood swings, psychomotor agitation, and impaired judgment and reasoning.[1]

An estimated 25 million Americans have tried cocaine at least once, 6 million use it at least once per month and 2 to 3 million persons are compulsive users.[2]

Cocaine abuse is increasing because of the availability of a less expensive form of cocaine called "crack." Snorting is still the most common method of abuse, followed by smoking (crack) and intravenous use.

Although physical disorders such as pheochromocytoma and thyrotoxicosis must be ruled out, the combination of the rapid mood shifts and the physical symptoms make cocaine abuse the most likely diagnosis. Anxiety and bipolar affective disorder would likewise be unlikely to produce the constellation of symptoms and mood swings.

497. E. Cocaine exerts many of its adverse effects by systemic vasoconstriction. Vasoconstriction leads to increased blood pressure and tachycardia. Cerebral hemorrhage, convulsions, respiratory arrest, cardiac arrhythmias, cardiac arrest, and myo-cardial infarction are potential systemic complications of cocaine abuse.[2]

498. E. Local complications of cocaine use include chronic nasal congestion, chronic cough, epistaxis, hemoptysis, and anterior chest wall pain.

Chronic cocaine use can also result in weight loss, lethargy, and impotence.[2]

499. C. The signs and symptoms of cocaine use may be nonspecific. Often a constellation of signs and symptoms will point to cocaine abuse. Diagnostic clues may include prior use of tobacco, alcohol, and marijuana; rapid mood swings (a short-lived "high" followed by an intense "low"); personality changes including acute paranoia; change in friends and peer group; chronic shortage of money; and physical signs and symptoms.[2]

500. E. Cocaine abuse is unlikely to be a sole diagnosis. Other disorders associated with cocaine abuse include conduct disorder, major depressive disorder, attention deficit disorder, intermittent explosive disorder, specific developmental disorders, and borderline personality disorder.[1,3]

501. A. Inpatient treatment programs are preferable to outpatient treatment programs. Adolescent patients who are currently using drugs cannot be adequately controlled or treated in an outpatient setting. Maintenance of sobriety is a keystone of treatment. Once inpatient treatment is completed, a follow-up outpatient service is essential for continued abstinence.[3]

502. A. Alcohol is still the most commonly abused drug in adolescents.

Marijuana use appears to be decreasing somewhat in American high schools.

There has been an alarming increase in drug use by the very young. Over fifty percent of marijuana and inhalant users report their first experience is between the sixth and ninth grade.

There has been a doubling in the prevalence of cocaine abuse in high school students (9%-17%).

From these statistics, it appears that if primary prevention of drug use is going to take place, we must begin our education programs at an earlier time. At or before the seventh grade is preferable.[3]

SUMMARY OF THE DIAGNOSIS AND TREATMENT OF COCAINE ABUSE (EMPHASIS ON ADOLESCENTS)

1. **Remember progression of abuse:** alcohol — marijuana — cocaine

2. Suspect cocaine abuse in adolescent with mood swings and evidence of sympathetic overactivity

3. Remember that drug abuse is seldom a sole diagnosis.

4. Inpatient treatment is preferable whenever possible

5. Primary prevention must begin at grade 7 or earlier

References

1. American Psychiatric Association. Diagnostic and statistical manual of mental disorders. 3rd Ed. Revised (DSM-III-R). Washington: APA Press, 1987.

2. Tarr J, Macklin M. Cocaine. Pediatr Clin North Am 1987;34(2): 319–331.

3. Semlitz L, Gold M. Adolescent drug abuse: diagnosis, treatment and prevention. Psychiatr Clin North Am 1986; 9(3): 455–473.

PROBLEM 63:   A 26-YEAR-OLD MALE WITH CHRONIC BACK PAIN

A 26-year-old male presents to your office with a chief complaint of chronic back pain. He states that he fell off a ladder 3 years ago and "broke his back." Since that time he has been unable to work and has only been able to function when taking a combination of Talwin (pentazocine) and Demerol (meperidine). He walks slowly and carefully, and is unable to flex or extend his lumbar spine because of pain. He points to the lumbar area as the point of maximum pain. He states that he doesn't like to have to take drugs, but has to, as it is the only way he can continue to function.

SELECT THE ONE BEST ANSWER TO THE FOLLOWING QUESTIONS:

503. The most likely diagnosis in this patient is:
    a) a congenital vertebral deformity with secondary lumbar fractures
    b) old lumbar fractures with chronic paravertebral muscle spasm
    c) chronic lumbar pain syndrome
    d) narcotic drug abuse
    e) somatoform pain disorder

504. After your initial history and physical examination of the patient described in question 503, your next step would be to:
    a) order a CT scan of the lumbar spine
    b) order an MRI scan of the lumbar spine
    c) refer the patient for an orthopedic consultation
    d) refer the patient for a neurosurgical consultation
    e) none of the above

505. After initiating the appropriate investigative maneuver, your next step would be to:
    a) prescibe Demerol and Talwin for 1 month and see the patient in review at that time
    b) prescribe Talwin, but not Demerol, in an effort to cut down on the amount of narcotic analgesic used
    c) prescibe Tylenol with codeine, instead of Talwin and Demerol, in an effort to decrease the addiction potential of the drug used
    d) begin to prescribe Demerol and Talwin for short periods of time (1 week) in an effort to monitor drug intake carefully
    e) none of the above

ANSWER THE FOLLOWING QUESTIONS ACCORDING TO THE CODE:

A: 1, 2, and 3 are correct
B: 1 and 3 are correct
C: 2 and 4 are correct
D: Only 4 is correct
E: All of the above are correct

506. Which of the following statements regarding drug abuse is/are correct?
    1) drug dependence is defined as the inappropriate use of a drug in terms of either its medical indications or its dose

2) drug abuse refers to physical or psychologic dependence on drugs
3) prescription drug abuse includes legal drugs that find their way into the illicit drug market
4) drug abuse may or may not lead to drug dependence

507. Which of the following prescription drugs is/are commonly abused?
1) narcotic analgesics
2) hypnosedatives
3) benzodiazepines
4) amphetamine-like substances

508. Which of the following benzodiazepines are most likely to produce rebound anxiety?
1) triazolam
2) lorazepam
3) bromazepam
4) flurazepam

509. Which of the following groups of physicians are responsible for drug diversion?
1) impaired doctors
2) "script" doctors
3) "duped" doctors
4) "dated" doctors

ANSWERS

503. D. The most likely diagnosis in this patient is narcotic drug abuse. If he himself is not a narcotic abuser, he may very well be a prescription drug trafficker.

The most common office presentations of opioid abusers are complaints of chronic pain, often related to previous trauma.[1] Chronic back pain or other orthopedic pain related to an old injury and chronic headache are the two most common complaints.

A valuable clue to narcotic abuse in this patient is his statement that his pain is ONLY relieved by taking a combination of Talwin and Demerol. A patient who names his analgesics of choice is almost certainly either a narcotic drug addict or a drug trafficker.

504. E. The ordering of either a CT scan, an NMR scan or the referral to a consultant orthopedic surgeon or neurosurgeon would not be valuable in this patient. In most cases, even if the appointment was made, the patient would not keep it. There is a significant probability that no such injury oc-

curred, and the whole episode is factitious. On the other hand, it is possible that the injury occurred and that the patient has become hooked on narcotic analgesics.

Rather, the most appropriate " investigation" would be to try and elicit a more complete history about this patient's injury, including initial emergency treatment and other physicians consulted, and to discuss with the patient your serious concerns about his use of narcotic analgesics.

His response to your concerns will, in all likelihood, further elucidate the diagnosis. The chronic pain patient may be too frightened of recurrence or too dependent upon narcotic analgesics to consider alternative forms of pain management; the prescription drug trafficker will either increase pressure, or become angry or even violent; and the patient who is going through withdrawal may admit to this at this point.

505. E. None of the above.

If the patient is a true narcotic drug addict, the most reasonable course of action is to try and convince the patient to enter an inpatient drug rehabilitation program. In programs of this type, methadone is often available for slow tapering of the narcotic dosage.[2]

Any of the other options are inappropriate. If the patient is a narcotic addict, you have simply continued to supply his habit. If he is a drug trafficker, you have just supplied him with drugs to peddle to other narcotic addicts.

506. D. Drug abuse is defined as inappropriate use of a drug in terms of either its medical indications or its dose.[3] Although drugs other than psychoactive drugs may be "abused," the definition is usually limited to this class. Drug dependence, on the other hand, refers to physical or psychologic dependence on drugs, the former being characterized by the development of chronic tolerance and a withdrawal syndrome, the latter involving a psychic drive toward periodic or continual use of the drug.[3] Drug abuse may or may not lead to drug dependence.

Prescription drug abuse refers to the abuse of drugs that are obtained by physician prescription.[3] It does not include legal drugs that find their way into the illicit drug market.

507. E. The four main classes of psychoactive drugs that tend to be chronically abused are narcotic analgesics, hypnosedatives, benzodiazepines, and am-

phetamine-like substances.[1] Some of the commonly abused prescription drugs (with their street names) include Tuinal/Seconal (Candy), Dilaudid (Ds), Fiorinal, Novahistex DH (Juice), morphine (Mojo), Percocet/Percodan (Percs), valium (Vs), and a combination of Talwin and Ritalin (Ts and Rs).[1] Some of these drugs have a street value of up to $75.00/tablet.

508. A. Rebound anxiety following discontinuation of a sedative-hypnotic can produce severe symptoms. The syndrome, however, is transient and lasts for a relatively short time.[4]

The risk of rebound anxiety is directly related to the elimination half-life after short-term use. Short acting drugs such as triazolam, lorazepam and bromazepam carry a greater risk than a longer acting agent like flurazepam.

509. E. Doctors responsible for drug diversion and the continuation of prescription drug abuse can be divided into the 4 "D's". They are: (1) the disabled or impaired doctors who prescribe medication for themselves, (2) the dishonest doctors who consciously misprescribe for profit, (3) the duped doctors who easily give into patient demands for drugs, and (4) the dated doctors who lack medical knowledge regarding the effects of their prescriptions.[5]

SUMMARY OF A RATIONAL APPROACH TO THE PRESCRIPTION OF PSYCHOACTIVE DRUGS

1. Controlled substances have legitimate clinical usefulness and the physician should not hesitate to prescribe them when they are indicated for the comfort and well-being of patients.

2. Prescribing controlled substances for legitimate medical uses requires special caution because of their potential for abuse and dependence.

3. Avoid being a physician who is one of the 4 "D's": disabled, dishonest, duped, or dated.

References

1. Goldman B. The prescription drug sting: be careful out there. Can Med Assoc J 1987; 136: 629–638.

2. Weiss K, Greenfield P. Prescription drug abuse. Psychiatr Clin North Am 1986; 9(3): 475–490.

3. Devenyi P. Prescription drug abuse. Can Med Assoc J 1985; 132: 242–243.

4. Jenike M. Drug abuse. In: Rubenstein E, Federman D, eds. Scientific American medicine. New York: Scientific American Medicine, 1987: 1–8.

5. Council on Scientific Affairs: drug abuse related to prescribing practices JAMA 1982; 247: 864–866.

PROBLEM 64: A 65-YEAR-OLD HYPERTENSIVE MALE WITH IMPOTENCE

A 65-year-old male with hypertension, congestive cardiac failure, and peptic ulcer disease presents to your office for his regular blood pressure check. You have managed to effectively control his blood pressure. Although his blood pressure is now under control, he complains of an inability to maintain an erection. He is currently taking the following medications: (1) alpha-methyldopa, (2) propranolol, (3) captopril, (4) hydrochlorothiazide, and (5) cimetidine.

SELECT THE ONE BEST ANSWER TO THE FOLLOWING QUESTIONS:

510. Which of the medications listed is the LEAST LIKELY to be the cause of this man's sexual dysfunction?
a) alpha-methyldopa
b) propranolol
c) captopril
d) hydrochlorothiazide
e) cimetidine

511. Which of the following disorders is the LEAST COMMON disorder of male sexual dysfunction?
a) hypoactive sexual desire disorder
b) male erectile disorder
c) inhibited male orgasm
d) premature ejaculation
e) postcoital headache

512. Which of the following statements regarding the etiology of male sexual dysfunction is most accurate?

a) male sexual dysfunction is almost always psychologic in origin

b) male sexual dysfunction is almost always organic in origin

c) psychologic factors seem to predominate in male sexual dysfunction, both in primary form and secondary to organic dysfunction

d) male sexual dysfunction in a younger patient has a greater probability of being organic in orgin

e) male sexual dysfunction in an older patient has a greater probability of being psychologic in origin

513. Which of the following organic disorders is the most common cause of organic male sexual dysfunction?

a) prostatism

b) hyperthyroidism

c) Parkinson's disease

d) diabetes mellitus

e) atherosclerosis of the abdominal aorta

514. The single most important aspect in the evaluation of male sexual dysfunction is:

a) the history

b) the physical examination

c) nocturnal penile tumescence measurement

d) ratio of penile/brachial blood pressure

e) serum testosterone measurement

ANSWER THE FOLLOWING QUESTIONS ACCORDING TO THE CODE:

A: 1, 2, and 3 are correct

B: 1 and 3 are correct

C: 2 and 4 are correct

D: Only 4 is correct

E: All of the above are correct

515. Which of the following investigations is/are indicated in male erectile disorder, inhibited male orgasm, and hypoactive sexual desire disorder?

1) complete blood count

2) blood urea nitrogen, creatinine

3) thyroid function studies

4) serum testosterone levels

516. Which of the following is/are important in the treatment of male sexual dysfunction?

1) reducing performance anxiety by prohibiting intercourse

2) anxiety reduction by identification and verbalization

3) introduction of the process of sensate focus

4) instruction in interpersonal communication skills

517. Which of the following is/are important in the treatment of premature ejaculation?

1) reducing performance anxiety by prohibiting intercourse

2) anxiety reduction by identification and verbalization

3) introduction of the process of sensate focus

4) teaching of the penile squeeze technique

ANSWERS

510. C. Drugs are probably the most common recognized cause of organic sexual dysfunction. Common offending drugs include the antihypertensive agents (including methyldopa, propranolol, and hydrochlorothiazide); heterocyclic antidepressants; monoamine oxidase inhibitors; major tranquilizers; abused drugs including alcohol, cannabis, and morphine; and other agents including lithium, digoxin, indomethacin, antiparkinsonian drugs, and cimetidine. Captopril has not been shown to have any adverse effect on sexual functioning. Although less common as a cause of sexual dysfunction in women than in men, drugs have been implicated in female sexual dysfunction.[1]

511. E. In men, the most common sexual dysfunctions are male erectile disorder, premature ejaculation, and inhibited male orgasm. Next most common is hypoactive sexual disorder. The least common male sexual dysfunction of the choices listed is postcoital headache.

Male erectile disorder is defined as persistent or recurrent partial or complete failure to attain or maintain erection until completion of the sexual activity. The definition includes a lack of a subjective sense of sexual excitement and pleasure.[2]

Premature ejaculation is defined as persistent or recurrent ejaculation with minimal sexual stimulation before, upon, or shortly after penetration, and before it is desired.[2]

Inhibited sexual orgasm is defined as a persistent or recurrent delay in, or absence of, orgasm in a male following a normal sexual excitement phase.[2]

Hypoactive sexual desire is defined as persistent or recurrent lack of desire for sexual activity, including lack of sexual fantasies.[2]

512. C. The etiology of male sexual dysfunction may be organic, psychologic, or a combination of both. Psychologic dysfunction probably predominates because even in cases where there is a signficant organic factor, there is also a psychologic factor. As well, male organic sexual dysfunction is complicated by the relationship with the partner.[1,3] In young men, most cases of male sexual dysfunction will be psychologic in origin. In older men, as the incidence of concurrent disease rises, so does the prevalence of organic sexual dysfunction.[1,3,4]

513. D. Diabetes mellitus is the most organic cause of impotence (other than drugs—see critique of question 501). Impotence caused by diabetes mellitus is a form of diabetic neuropathy.[4]

Other common causes of organic male sexual dysfunction include atherosclerotic vascular disease, cardiac failure, renal failure, hepatic failure, respiratory failure, genetic causes (Klinefelter's syndrome), hypothyroidism, hyperthyroidism, neurologic disorders such as multiple sclerosis and Parkinson's disease, surgical procedures such as radical prostatectomy, orchidectomy and abdominal-perineal colon resection; and radiation therapy.[1,4]

514. A. The single most important aspect in the evaluation of male (and female) sexual dysfunction is the history. For example, in a patient with an erectile disorder, if erections are achieved under certain conditions but not others, the likelihood is high that the dysfunction is psychogenic.[5] Normal erectile function during masturbation, extramarital sex, and in response to erotic material suggests a psychologic cause. Similarly, if a normal erection is lost during vaginal insertion, a psychologic cause is suspected. A complete drug history is essential.[1]

The history should include present and previous birth control, psychiatric history, family history, history of surgical procedures, marital relationship, and history of present job satisfaction and hours of work. The recurrence or persistence of the presenting sexual problem should be sought.

A complete physical examination should be done. The physical examination will determine whether there is any evidence of organic pathology that may be associated with the dysfunction.

Measurement of nocturnal penile tumescence (most simply done using a strain gauge), the ratio of penile/brachial blood pressure and the serum testosterone are investigations that have an important role to play in the overall evaluation of impotence,[5] but they do not take the place of a good history.

515. E. Based on the organic etiologies discussed in the critique of question 514, baseline screening bloodwork is indicated. This should include a complete blood count, blood urea nitrogen and creatinine, a fasting blood sugar, a fasting cholesterol level, thyroid function studies, liver function tests, and a serum testosterone level.[4]

516. E. Most cases of male sexual dysfunction have, as discussed previously, a significant psychologic component. After a complete history, a complete physical examination, screening bloodwork and the discontinuation of offending medications, sexual therapy should begin.

The treatment of male sexual (and female sexual dysfunction) has several important steps. They are (1) the reduction of performance anxiety by prohibiting intercourse, (2) anxiety reduction by identification and verbalization of the problem, (3) introduction of the process of sensate focus (semistructured touching that will permit focus on sensory awareness without any need to perform sexually), and (4) instruction in interpersonal communication skills.[1]

517. E. The initial treatment of premature ejaculation is the same as that of other male sexual dysfunctions.

In addition, an exercise known as the "squeeze technique" is used to raise the threshold of penile excitability. The penis is stimulated until impending ejaculation is perceived. At this time, the woman squeezes the coronal ridge of the glans, resulting in diminished erection and inhibited ejaculation. Eventually, with repeated practice, the threshold for ejaculatory inevitability is raised.[1]

SUMMARY OF THE DIAGNOSIS AND TREATMENT OF MALE SEXUAL DYSFUNCTION

1. **Most common male sexual dysfunctions:**
    a) male erectile disorder
    b) inhibited male orgasm
    c) premature ejaculation
    d) hypoactive sexual desire

2. Complete history especially including history of marital relationship and intake of drugs

3. Complete physical examination to help exclude organic male sexual dysfunction

4. Basic laboratory evaluation to include complete blood count, renal function, liver function, thyroid function, blood glucose, cholesterol and testosterone

5. Therapy to center on LEDO[6] approach and sensate focus:
   Lowering stress, tension, and anxiety levels through discussion, examination, and observation.
   Ensuring that both parties understand each other's desires, pleasures, and difficulties.
   Determining the partner's genuine awareness and knowledge of their own and each other's sexual anatomy and the process of intercourse.
   Outlining, drawing and explaining alternative approaches to arousal and excitation, and intercourse techniques.

6. Referral to speciality care for sexual dysfunction that cannot be handled by primary care physicians (including penile implants and injection therapy)

References

1. Kaplan HJ, Sadock B. Synopsis of psychiatry. 5th Ed. Baltimore: Williams & Wilkins, 1988: 363–376.

2. American Psychiatric Association. Diagnostic and statistical manual of mental disorders. 3rd Ed. Revised. (DSM-III-R). Washington: APA Press, 1987: 279–286.

3. Golden J. Psychiatric aspects of male sexual dysfunction. Postgrad Med 1983; 74(4): 221–229.

4. Braunstein G. Endocrine causes of impotence. Postgrad Med 1983; 74(4): 207–217.

5. Sacks S. Evaluation of impotence. Postgrad Med 1983; 74(4): 182–195.

6. Felstein I. Understanding sexual medicine: a guide for family practioners and students. Lancaster, PA: MTP Press Limited, 1986: 120.

PROBLEM 65:   A 20-YEAR-OLD FEMALE WITH VAGINISMUS

A 24-year-old female, who was married 6 months ago, presents to the office in tears. She and her husband have been unable to have sexual intercourse. She says that when he tries to penetrate her she "tenses up" and she is unable to go any farther.

She was raped at the age of 12 and still has vivid memories of the event.

You suspect vaginismus.

SELECT THE ONE BEST ANSWER TO THE FOLLOWING QUESTIONS:

518. Which of the following statements regarding vaginismus is FALSE?
   a) most women with vaginismus also have difficulty with sexual arousal
   b) there is a strong association between vaginismus and an intense childhood and adolescent exposure to religious orthodoxy
   c) there is a strong association between vaginismus and a traumatic sexual experience
   d) vaginismus is a condition of involuntary spasm or constriction of the musculature surrounding the vaginal outlet
   e) vaginismus may begin with a poorly healed episiotomy following childbirth

519. Regarding the diagnosis and treatment of vaginismus, which of the following statements is FALSE?
   a) throughout the diagnostic examination the woman must feel that she is in control, and may terminate the examination at any time
   b) the diagnosis of vaginismus can often be made without inserting a speculum
   c) the sexual partner should be involved in all aspects of the treatment process
   d) the insertion of vaginal dilators is not a recognized part of the treatment protocol
   e) sensate focus techniques are an important part of the treatment protocol

520. Which of the following statements regarding female sexual arousal disorder is FALSE?
   a) sexual arousal disorder is more common in women than in men

b) the diagnosis takes into account the focus, intensity, and duration of the sexual activity

c) if sexual stimulation is inadequate in focus, intensity, or duration, the diagnosis cannot be made

d) sexual arousal disorder in women is not associated with inadequate vaginal lubrication

e) female sexual arousal disorder is often associated with inhibited female orgasm

521. Of the following, which is the most common cause of hypoactive sexual desire disorder in women?
a) major psychiatric illness in the woman
b) major psychiatric illness in the woman's partner
c) dual-career families, with increased responsibilities on the woman both at work and in the home
d) major physical illness in the woman
e) alcoholism in the woman's partner

522. Which of the following statements regarding inhibited female orgasm is FALSE?
a) inhibited female orgasm is the least common female sexual dysfunction
b) primary anorgasmia is more common among unmarried women than among married women
c) women over the age of 35 seem to have increased orgasm potential
d) women may have more than one orgasm without a refractory period
e) fear of impregnation is a common cause of inhibited female orgasm

ANSWER THE FOLLOWING QUESTIONS ACCORDING TO THE CODE:

A: 1, 2, and 3 are correct
B: 1 and 3 are correct
C: 2 and 4 are correct
D: Only 4 is correct
E: All of the above are correct

523. Which of the following statements regarding dyspareunia is/are TRUE?
1) it may be caused by endometriosis
2) it may be caused by vaginitis or cervicitis
3) it may be caused by an episiotomy scar
4) it is usually unrelated to vaginismus

524. Which of the following methods is/are useful in the treatment of female sexual dysfunction?

1) sexual anatomy and physiology education
2) sensate focus exercises
3) treatment of underlying anxiety and depression
4) long term use of a vibrator

ANSWERS

518. A. Vaginismus is defined as recurrent or persistent involuntary spasm of the musculature of the outer third of the vagina that interferes with coitus.[1]

There is a strong association between vaginismus and an intense childhood and adolescent exposure to religious orthodoxy.[2] Vaginismus may occur when an episiotomy fails to properly heal following childbirth.[3] Most women with vaginismus have normal sexual arousal.[2]

In this patient, the etiology of vaginismus is most likely from the traumatic sexual experience that took place in her childhood.[2,3]

519. D. The evaluation and treatment of vaginismus begins with a carefully performed physical examination in which the patient is always in full control. She may terminate the examination at any time.

On inspection of the external genitalia, spasm and rigidity of the perineal muscles are often felt. In this case the diagnosis can be made even without inserting a speculum. From inspection, the examination may proceed to the insertion of one of the examiner's fingers.

The use of vaginal dilators in gradually increasing sizes has proved helpful in the treatment of vaginismus. Beginning with the smallest size, the woman inserts these herself until she becomes both comfortable and relaxed with their insertion. When the largest plastic dilator can be inserted, the couple can proceed to intercourse.

The partner must be involved in all aspects of assessment and treatment. Ideally, he should be present to observe the entire evaluation and treatment. Together with anatomy and physiology education, the couple learns the concept of sensate focus exercises, which play a major part in the therapy of any sexual dysfunction.[3]

520. D. Female sexual arousal disorder is defined as persistent or recurrent partial or complete failure to attain or maintain the lubrication-swelling response of sexual excitement until completion of the sexual activity.[1] The diagnosis includes the subjective sense of sexual excitement and

pleasure, and requires the focus, intensity, and duration of stimulation to be adequate.[1]

Sexual arousal disorder is often associated with inhibited female orgasm.[2]

521. C. Hypoactive sexual desire disorder is defined as persistent or recurrent deficient or absent desire for sexual activity.[1] The definition includes a lack of sexual fantasies. The major reasons for hypoactive sexual desire disorder are (1) major marital dysfunction, in which the lack of desire to have sexual intercourse is a symptom of the dysfunction, and (2) a change in family structure from single-career families to dual-career families. The woman, now, as well as having major work responsibilities, is still often left with the majority of the child care and home care in the evenings. By the time she gets everything done, she is just too tired for sex.

522. A. Inhibited female orgasm is defined as persistent or recurrent delay in, or absence of, orgasm in a female following a normal sexual excitement phase during sexual activity.[1] The definition takes into account the adequacy in focus, intensity, and duration of the sexual activity.[1] Inhibited female orgasm is the most common female sexual dysfunction.

Primary anorgasmia (never having had an orgasm) is more common in unmarried women than in married women. Women over the age of 35 appear to have an increased orgasmic potential.[3]

Women may have more than one orgasm without a refractory period.[3]

Causes for inhibited female orgasm include: (1) fear of impregnation, (2) rejection by the sexual partner, (3) hostility towards men, and (4) feelings of guilt regarding sexual impulses.[2]

523. A. Dyspareunia is defined as recurrent or persistent genital pain before, during, or after sexual intercourse.[1] This dyspareunia cannot be caused exclusively by lack of lubrication or by vaginismus.[1] In many cases, however, vaginismus and dyspareunia are closely associated. Other causes of dyspareunia include episiotomy scars, vaginitis and/or cervicitis, endometriosis, postmenopausal vaginal atrophy, and anxiety regarding the sexual act itself.[2,3]

524. A. In the summary of the chapter on male sexual dysfunction, the LEDO[4] approach to sexual counseling was discussed. This applies equally well to female sexual dysfunction.

In the absence of other psychiatric pathology, dual-sex therapy is the most accepted approach to the treatment of sexual dysfunction. The sexual problem often reflects other areas of disharmony or misunderstanding in the marriage. The marital relationship as a whole is treated, with emphasis on sexual functioning as a part of that relationship. Both a female and a male therapist are involved in the treatment of the couple's sexual problem. The therapy is short term and behaviorally oriented; the goal is to reestablish communication within the marital unit. Information regarding anatomy and physiology is given. Specific sensate focus exercises are prescribed. The couple proceeds from nongenital touching and sensory awareness to genital touching and finally to intercourse. The couple learns to communicate with each other through these graded exercises.[2,3]

If underlying anxiety, depression, or other psychiatric pathology is present, it must be treated separately.

The long term use of a vibrator has no place in sexual therapy.

SUMMARY OF THE DIAGNOSIS AND TREATMENT OF FEMALE SEXUAL DYSFUNCTION

1. **Diagnosis:**
   a) Inhibited female orgasm
   b) Female sexual arousal disorder
   c) Vaginismus
   d) Hypoactive sexual desire disorder
   e) Dyspareunia

2. Complete history (including complete sexual history) and physical examination (See chapter on male sexual dysfunction)

3. **Treatment:**
   a) LEDO[4] (see chapter on male sexual dysfunction)
   b) dual-sex therapy

References

1. American Psychiatric Association. Diagnostic and statistical manual of mental disorders. 3rd Ed. Revised (DSM-III-R). Washington: APA Press, 1987.

2. Kaplan HJ, Sadock B. Synopsis of psychiatry. 5th Ed. Baltimore: Williams & Wilkins, 1988: 363–376.

3. Kolodny R, Masters W, Johnson V. Textbook of sexual medicine. Boston: Little, Brown, 1979.

4. Felstein I. Understanding sexual medicine: a guide for family practioners and students. Lancaster, PA: MTP Press, 1986: 120.

PROBLEM 66: A 48-YEAR-OLD MALE WITH A 6 MONTH HISTORY OF SNORING, NOCTURNAL BREATH CESSATIONS, AND EXCESSIVE DAYTIME SLEEPINESS

A 48-year-old man presents to the office with a 6-month history of snoring and excessive daytime sleepiness. His wife states that he often stops breathing temporarily during the night. These symptoms have been occurring regularly for the past 6 months. The patient weighs 280 pounds and is 5'8" tall, and his blood pressure is 180/105 mm Hg.

SELECT THE ONE BEST ANSWER TO THE FOLLOWING QUESTIONS:

525. The most likely diagnosis in this patient is:
    a) narcolepsy
    b) obstructive sleep apnea syndrome
    c) generalized poor physical condition
    d) central sleep apnea syndrome
    e) adult onset adenoid hypertrophy

526. The condition described above may be associated with which of the following disorders?
    a) hypertension
    b) obesity
    c) polycythemia
    d) a and b
    e) all of the above

527. Which of the following investigations is indicated in patients with the condition described above?
    a) a 24-hour electrocardiographic monitor
    b) a sleep laboratory evaluation
    c) a chest x-ray
    d) b and c
    e) all of the above

ANSWER THE FOLLOWING QUESTIONS ACCORDING TO THE CODE:

A: 1, 2, and 3 are correct
B: 1 and 3 are correct
C: 2 and 4 are correct
D: Only 4 is correct
E: All of the above are correct

528. Which of the following medications is/are contraindicated in the patient with the condition described above?
    1) sedative hypnotics
    2) alcohol
    3) barbiturates
    4) tricyclic antidepressants

529. Which of the following may be indicated in the treatment of the condition described above?
    1) weight loss
    2) uvulopalatopharyngoplasty
    3) tracheostomy
    4) nasal continuous positive airway pressure

SELECT THE ONE BEST ANSWER TO THE FOLLOWING QUESTIONS:

530. A 35-year-old male presents to your office with a chief complaint of "weak muscles" especially after laughing. On further questioning you discover that the patient has excessive daytime sleepiness and "weird imaginings" just before going to sleep at night. The patient appears anxious and tense. Your tentative diagnosis is:
    a) narcolepsy
    b) hysterical conversion reaction
    c) psychosomatic symptoms secondary to chronic anxiety
    d) hypochondriasis
    e) serious psychiatric disturbance NYD

531. Which of the following is/are first line drugs to use in the treatment of the patient discussed in question 530?
    a) methylphenidate
    b) imipramine
    c) both a and b
    d) neither a nor b

ANSWERS

525. **B.** This patient has obstructive sleep apnea syndrome. Obstructive sleep apnea syndrome is characterized by a history of snoring and typical intermittent snorting and gasping sounds; nocturnal breath cessations observable by the bed partner and often perceived by the patient; excessive daytime sleepiness and sleep attacks; nocturnal body movements, excessive sweating, nocturnal enuresis, loss of libido, morning headaches, obesity, and cognitive impairment; and hypertension and other cardiovascular complications.[1] Central sleep apnea, although associated with nocturnal breath cessations and usually excessive daytime sleepiness, is not usually associated with snoring.[1] Obstructive sleep apnea is much more common than central sleep apnea.

Narcolepsy is discussed in a subsequent question.

Generalized poor physical condition is not a reasonable explanation for the presenting symptoms.

Adult onset adenoid hypertrophy does not occur.

526. **E.** Patients with sleep apnea often have coexisting hypertension and obesity. Pulmonary hypertension, with subsequent right-sided cardiac failure may occur. Hypoxia and carbon dioxide retention also occur, and polycythemia may result from the latter two.[1]

527. **E.** A thorough history should be taken from both the patient and the patient's spouse. The characteristics of the "snoring" should be elicited. The loud and abrupt snorting and choking sounds that occur after each breath cessation are quite different from ordinary snoring.[1]

A complete physical examination including a complete ENT evaluation should be performed. A chest x-ray, electrocardiogram, and complete blood count is recommended. A 24-hour electrocardiographic monitor will detect nocturnal dysrhythmias. A complete sleep laboratory evaluation with recording of respiration and monitoring of ear oxymetry is necessary to confirm the diagnosis.[1]

528. **A.** In patients with sleep apnea, drugs that depress the ventilatory drive are contraindicated. These include sedative hypnotics, barbiturates, narcotics, sedating analgesics, and alcohol. Drugs that impair respiration through other mechanisms (like the metabolic alkalosis produced by thiazide and loop diuretics, the decreased ventilatory response to carbon dioxide produced by propranolol, and the general obesity and soft tissue proliferation produced by corticosteroids) should be avoided.[1]

Tricyclic antidepressants are not contraindicated; on the contrary, they are sometimes prescribed as treatment.

529. **E.** The treatment of obstructive sleep apnea depends upon the severity of the condition. Weight reduction should be recommended in all patients. Steps to treat underlying cardiovascular abnormalities such as hypertension and congestive cardiac failure should be initiated. Severe obstructive sleep apnea may be treated by tracheostomy or uvulopalatopharyngoplasty. The latter operation surgically enlarges the pharyngeal space. Nasal continuous positive airway pressure appears to be a safe and effective treatment, although the number of patients treated so far is small.[1]

The use of medication appears to be primarily indicated in relatively mild cases of obstructive sleep apnea. Protriptyline, an activating tricyclic antidepressant, and medroxyprogesterone acetate have only limited efficacy, and long-term data on the efficacy of their use is lacking.[1]

530. **A.** The patient described in this question has narcolepsy.[1,2] Narcolepsy is characterized by excessive daytime sleepiness and sleep attacks associated with one or more of cataplexy, sleep paralysis, and hypnagogic hallucinations.[1,2]

Cataplexy, which is present in the majority of patients with narcolepsy, is a brief, sudden loss of muscle control that may cause conscious collapse of the patient.[1] Cataplexy is frequently precipitated by laughter or anger.

Sleep paralysis and hypnagogic hallucinations occur less frequently than cataplexy. Sleep paralysis and hypnagogic hallucinations usually occur in the transition period between wakefulness and sleep. Sleep paralysis is a temporary loss of muscle tone and a resulting inability to move. Hypnagogic hallucinations are vivid visual or auditory perceptions that occur while falling asleep.[1]

531. **C.** There are seperate treatments for the sleep attacks and for the cataplexy.

Methylphenidate is the preferred drug for treating the sleep attacks of narcolepsy.[1]

Imipramine is the pharmacologic agent of choice for cataplexy.[1] It also alleviates sleep paralysis, but has little effect on the sleep attacks.[1] Dosage is 10–75 mg/day, which is considerably less than the antidepressant dosage.

Although methylphenidate and imipramine can be combined, the combination may produce serious hypertension. Therefore, careful titration and frequent monitoring of blood pressure is essential.

SUMMARY OF THE DIAGNOSIS AND TREATMENT OF OBSTRUCTIVE SLEEP APNEA AND NARCOLEPSY

1. **Diagnosis:**
   a) obstructive sleep apnea-snoring, intermittent gasping, nocturnal breath cessations and excessive daytime sleepiness
   b) narcolepsy: excessive daytime sleepiness with irresistible sleep attacks with cataplexy, sleep paralysis, and hypnagogic hallucinations

c) always interview spouse to substantiate history
d) treatment:
   1) obstructive sleep apnea- weight loss, control of hypertension and cardiovascular complications, tracheostomy, uvulo-palatopharyngoplasty, possibly protrip-tyline or medroxyprogesterone
   2) narcolepsy: methylphenidate for sleep attacks; imipramine for cataplexy and sleep paralysis

References

1. Kales A, Vela-bueno A, Kales J. Sleep disorders: sleep apnea and narcolepsy. Ann Intern Med 1987; 106: 434–443.

2. Kaplan HJ, Sadock B, eds. Comprehensive textbook of psychiatry, V. Baltimore: Williams & Wilkins, 1989.

PROBLEM 67: A 26-YEAR-OLD PRIMIGRAVIDA, 4 DAYS POSTPARTUM, WHO IS TEARFUL AND DEPRESSED

A 26-year-old primigravida delivers a healthy male infant at 40 weeks gestation. She is doing well until the 4th day postpartum. At that time she develops insomnia, weepiness, depression, and fatigue. She has no previous history of psychiatric disease. She begins to improve on the 8th postpartum day and returns to her normal mental state by 2 weeks postpartum.

SELECT THE ONE BEST ANSWER TO THE FOLLOWING QUESTIONS:

532. The most likely diagnosis in this patient is:
   a) postpartum depression
   b) postpartum blues
   c) acute adjustment reaction
   d) postpartum anxiety
   e) none of the above

533. The treatment of choice in this patient is a brief course of:
   a) a tricyclic antidepressant
   b) lithium carbonate
   c) a monoamine oxidase inhibitor
   d) a benzodiazepine
   e) none of the above

534. A 28-year-old primigravida delivers a healthy female infant at 39 weeks gestation. She is well until the 4th postpartum day when she develops tearfulness, despondency, guilt, anorexia, depression, insomnia, and feelings of inadequacy in coping with the infant. She continues to have these feelings when she sees you for her 3-week postpartum check-up.

The most likely diagnosis in this patient is:
   a) postpartum depression
   b) postpartum blues
   c) acute adjustment reaction
   d) early bipolar affective illness
   e) none of the above

ANSWER THE FOLLOWING QUESTIONS ACCORDING TO THE CODE:

A: 1, 2, and 3 are correct
B: 1 and 3 are correct
C: 2 and 4 are correct
D: Only 4 is correct
E: All of the above are correct

535. The treatment of choice for the patient described in question 534 may include:
    1) a tricyclic antidepressant
    2) a monoamine oxidase inhibitor
    3) supportive psychotherapy
    4) lithium carbonate

536. A 29-year-old primigravida is found on her 4th postpartum day loudly singing hymns at 4 AM in the corridor. During the next 24 hours she causes turmoil on the maternity ward. She rushes into other patients' rooms announcing that she is about to start classes in bioenergetics and urges them to participate. She refuses meals and denies any need to sleep since she is "in touch with the source of superior power." She is hyperactive and talkative and invites the obstetrician to make love to her. When the psychiatrist is hastily summoned, she shoves him out of her room.

    Which of the following statements is/are TRUE about this patient?
    1) the patient has a postpartum psychosis
    2) the patient probably has schizophrenia
    3) this patient is likely to have a personal or a family history of bipolar or unipolar affective disorder
    4) the patient is unlikely to recover

537. Which of the following may be indicated in the treatment of the patient discussed in question 536?
    1) haloperidol
    2) chloropromazine
    3) lithium carbonate
    4) diazepam

ANSWERS

532. B. This patient has postpartum blues.

    Postpartum blues occur in about 50–80% of puerperal women. The syndrome is transitory, resolving spontaneously within a few hours to 2 weeks.[1]

    Postpartum blues usually starts with a brief period of weeping on the third or fourth day after delivery and peaks between the fifth and the tenth days. Symptoms include insomnia, weepiness, anxiety, headaches, poor concentration, and confusion. Elation may occur.[1]

    The etiology of postpartum blues is unknown, but a hormonal basis is postulated.[1]

533. E. The treatment of choice in this patient is reassurance and brief, supportive psychotherapy,

along with information about newborn care. The patient should be reassured that these symptoms are extremely common in new mothers, and that they will disappear spontaneously.[1]

Most women recover completely within 2 weeks. A few patients progress to a more serious postpartum depression. Postpartum blues is a recurrent condition, with many women experiencing symptoms in future pregnancies. As recovery is rapid in the vast majority of cases, pharmacotherapy is not necessary.[1]

534. A. This patient has a postpartum depression. Postpartum depression occurs in appoximately 10% of all childbearing women. The syndrome disables the patient for more than 2 weeks and is characterized by a depressed mood and difficulty coping, especially with the infant. Other symptoms include tearfulness, despondency, worrying about not loving their baby enough, anxiety about feeding or spoiling the baby, fears about the baby's sleep, and fears about older children's jealousy.[1] Hypochondriasis, irritability, impaired concentration, poor memory, and undue fatigue are also common in postpartum depression.

    As with postpartum blues, the origin of postpartum depression is unclear.[1]

535. A. The treatment of postpartum depression should center on supportive psychotherapy. The condition should be presented as a treatable emotional disorder. Information about newborn care, social assistance, marriage counseling, and homemaking support should be provided.

    Either a tricyclic antidepressant or a monoamine oxidase inhibitor will be effective in treating depression and restoring sleep. Tranquilizing drugs such as diazepam should be avoided as they may produce dependency. Lithium carbonate should be reserved for patients with bipolar symptoms.[1]

536. B. Postpartum psychoses occur in 1 to 2 per 1000 postpartum women; they may present as schizophrenic or affective disorders or as confusional states. Postpartum psychosis is felt to be an atypical psychosis, as most episodes do not meet the criteria for an organic mental disorder, a schizophreniform disorder, a paranoid disorder, or an affective disorder.[1]

    This patient presents with a hypomanic episode. She likely has either a personal or family history of unipolar or bipolar affective disorder. She will likely recover with proper treatment.[1]

537. A. Since this patient has a psychosis, an antipsychotic should form the first line of treatment. Chloropromazine or haloperidol usually controls the psychotic symptoms. The hypomanic presentation should be managed with lithium carbonate. It is reasonable to begin the lithium at the same time as the antipsychotic is being administered; this will allow control of the acute symptoms while the serum lithium level is being built up.[1]

This treatment regimen will likely return the patient to normal function. She should, however, be on lithium carbonate for several months. Women who have a history of a bipolar affective disorder are liable to have a recurrence after a future pregnancy; lithium carbonate should be considered for immediate administration after a subsequent birth.[1]

The use of psychotropic drugs in breast-feeding is an important consideration. It is probably wise to suggest that a woman on psychotropic medication of any kind should bottle feed rather than breast-feed.

SUMMARY OF THE DIAGNOSIS AND TREATMENT OF POSTPARTUM PSYCHIATRIC DISORDERS

Three disorders:

1. Postpartum blues — prevalence, 50–70%
    Begins 3rd–4th day, resolves by 2 weeks
    Treatment: reassurance, supportive psychotherapy

2. Postpartum depression — prevalence, 10%
    Usually begins 3rd–5th day, lasts longer than 2 weeks
    Treatment: supportive psychotherapy, tricyclic antidepressants or monoamine oxidase inhibitors

3. Postpartum psychosis — prevalence, 0.1–0.2%
    Usually begins after 3rd day postpartum
    May be associated with history of bipolar affective disorder or schizophrenia
    Treatment: antipsychotics, lithium carbonate if hypomanic or manic episode is initial presentation

Reference

1. Robinson G, Stewart D. Postpartum psychiatric disorders. Can Med Assoc J 1986; 134(1): 31–36.

PROBLEM 68: A 55-YEAR-OLD MALE WITH "NO WILL TO CARRY ON LIVING"

A 55-year-old male is brought to the emergency department by his wife at 2 AM. She says her husband has been crying for the last week. He says that he has nothing more to live for. While you begin to question her he begins to cry. Apparently, he just updated his will and bought a new handgun last night. When you begin to question the patient, he begins to sob uncontrollably and says that he is sorry to put you to all of this trouble.

SELECT THE ONE BEST ANSWER TO THE FOLLOWING QUESTIONS:

537. Given the history to this point, and assuming that no more relevant information can be obtained from the patient you should:
    a) prescribe a tricyclic antidepressant and see the patient in a week
    b) prescribe diazepam for both husband and wife and ask them to come for counseling in 2 weeks
    c) try to form a "no suicide contract" with the patient
    d) hospitalize the patient
    e) prescribe a major tranquilizer for the patient and see him in the morning

538. Which of the following is/are associated with high suicide risk?
    a) major affective disorder
    b) schizophrenia
    c) alcoholism
    d) all of the above
    e) a and b only

539. The ratio of male to female successful suicides is:
    a) 1 to 3
    b) 5 to 1
    c) 3 to 1
    d) 1 to 1
    e) 1 to 5

ANSWER THE FOLLOWING QUESTIONS ACCORDING TO THE CODE:

A: 1, 2, and 3 are correct
B: 1 and 3 are correct
C: 2 and 4 are correct
D: Only 4 is correct
D: All of the above are correct

540. Which of the following is/are suicide death risk factors in adults?
1) family history
2) psychiatric diagnosis
3) medical illness
4) unemployment

541. Which of the following is/are true regarding the emergence of an acute suicidal episode?
1) the emergence is superimposed upon the preexisting or concurrent psychiatric illness
2) feelings of hopelessness, despair, pessimism, and helplessness are more important than depression
3) the emergence is often precipitated by psychosocial life events
4) most patients are receiving treatment for psychiatric illness at the time of emergence

542. Which of the following is/are important in the clinical management of suicidal patients?
1) inquire about suicidal thoughts and plans at every visit
2) follow up missed appointment
3) prescribe adequate doses of antidepressant medication
4) form a "no-suicide" contract with the patient

ANSWERS

537. D. You should hospitalize the patient. This patient has just updated his will and bought a new handgun. This is enough evidence to conclude that the patient is a serious suicidal risk.

For patients who are acutely suicidal, inpatient evaluation and management is the safest option. It protects the patient from himself and from others, and provides a relief from environmental stressors. It also allows for continuous assessment and reassessment of response to treatment. If the patient refuses hospitalization, involuntary commitment may be necessary.[1]

538. D. Most suicidal patients suffer from a psychiatric disorder. The psychiatric disorders most closely associated with suicide risk include major affective disorder, schizophrenia, alcoholism, and panic disorder.[1,2] Patients with these conditions may face up to a 30% lifetime probability of death from suicide.[1,2]

539. C. Men commit suicide more than three times as often as women do, a rate that is stable over all ages. Women, on the other hand are three times as likely to attempt suicide than are men.[1]

540. E. The suicide death risk factors for adults are (1) a family history of suicide; (2) male sex; (3) a psychiatric diagnosis; (4) never married, divorced, widowed, or separated marital status; (5) lack of social supports; (6) medical illness; (7) unemployment; (8) fall in social and/or economic status; (9) inadequate treatment of acute suicidal episode; and (10) previous suicide attempts.[1]

541. A. The emergence of an acute suicidal episode is often superimposed upon the preexisting or concurrent psychiatric diagnosis.

Feelings of hopelessness, despair, pessimism, and helplessness tend to be more predictive of acute suicidal risk than depression.

The emergence of an acute suicidal episode is often precipitated by psychosocial life stressors.

Although most patients who are acutely suicidal have visited a physician recently, most are not receiving treatment for psychiatric illness at the time of the emergence.[1,3]

542. E. Inquiry into suicidal thoughts and plans is important in every patient who is being actively treated for major depressive disorder, schizophrenia, alcoholism, and panic disorder. If a patient misses an appointment, follow-up should be initiated immediately.

Tricyclic antidepressants, antipsychotic medications and ECT form the basis of pharmacologic management of patients who are acutely suicidal or at risk for emergence of an acute suicidal episode. In patients who are at risk for suicide and who are being treated as outpatients, antidepressant and antipsychotic medications should be issued only in a small supply. This will prevent deliberate overdose.

Physicians should form a "no-suicide" contract with a patient who is at risk for the development of an acute suicidal episode. The physician or his designate must be available on a 24-hour basis to respond to the emergence of a crisis.

Family members, social support networks, and community resources must be mobilized to help suicidal patients and those at risk for suicide.[1–3]

SUMMARY OF THE DIAGNOSIS AND MANAGEMENT OF THE SUICIDAL PATIENT

1. **Review risk factors:** Pay particular attention to history of major affective disorder, alcoholism, schizophrenia, and panic disorder

2. Establish the presence or absence of hopelessness in assessing risk of acute suicidal episode.

3. Hospitalize patient in suicidal crisis

4. Establish a "no-suicide contract" with individuals at risk but not in acute crisis. Ensure availability of 24-hour contact.

5. Treat depression in a suicidal patient with tricyclic antidepressants and ECT.

6. Enlist support of family and community in ongoing management.

References

1. Blumenthal SJ. Suicide: a guide to risk factors, assessment, and treatment of suicidal patients. Med Clin North Am 1988; 72(4): 937–971.

2. Weissman M, Klerman G, Markowitz J, Ouellette R. Suicidal ideation and suicide attempts in panic disorder and attacks. N Engl J Med 1989; 321: 1209–1214.

3. Klerman G. Clinical epidemiology of suicide. J Clin Psychiatry 1987; 48(12): 33–38.

Pediatrics

PROBLEM 69: A 5-YEAR-OLD CHILD WITH FEVER, IRRITABILITY, AND A LEFT-SIDED EARACHE

A mother presents to your office with her 5-year-old boy. The child has had a fever for the past 24 hours and developed a left-sided earache 8 hours ago. The child has had a respiratory tract infection for 1 week. The boy is extremely irritable and examination of the tympanic membrane is difficult. You are, however, able to see a bulging, red, tympanic membrane. The eardrum does not move when air is infused with a pneumatic otoscope head. The right tympanic membrane is normal and the rest of the examination of the head and neck is normal.

SELECT THE ONE BEST ANSWER TO THE FOLLOWING QUESTIONS:

543. According to standard nomenclature, this child has:
    a) acute otitis media
    b) acute suppurative otitis media
    c) purulent otitis media
    d) otitis media with effusion — acute
    e) acute serous otitis media

544. Which one of the following statements regarding otitis media is false?
    a) over 50% of children will have at least one episode of otitis media before the age of 1 year
    b) the incidence and prevalence of acute otitis media is higher among boys than among girls
    c) day-care attendance has not had any significant effect on the incidence of otitis media
    d) otitis media is more prevalent in large families
    e) the incidence of otitis media is higher in winter than in summer

545. Which of the following statements regarding otitis media is false?
    a) acute otitis media usually begins a few days after onset of a cold or other upper respiratory tract infection
    b) otitis media is usually associated with eustachian tube dysfunction
    c) environmental factors such as pollen, dusts, molds, and cigarette smoke are unlikely to be associated with an increase in the incidence of otitis media
    d) most cases of acute otitis media are considered to be bacterial in origin
    e) none of the above statements are false

546. The most common bacterial causes of acute otitis media in order of frequency are:
    a) pneumococcus, group A streptococci, *Haemophilus influenzae*
    b) pneumococcus, *Haemophilus influenzae*, staphylococci
    c) pneumococcus, *Haemophilus influenzae*, *Branhamella catarrhalis*
    d) *Haemophilus influenzae*, pneumococcus, group A streptococcus
    e) *Haemophilus influenzae*, pneumococcus, *Branhamella catarrhalis*

547. The drug of choice for acute otitis media is:
    a) penicillin
    b) erythromycin
    c) erythromycin-sulfisoxazole
    d) amoxicillin
    e) cefaclor

ANSWER THE FOLLOWING QUESTIONS ACCORDING TO THE CODE:

A: 1, 2, and 3 are correct
B: 1 and 3 are correct
C: 2 and 4 are correct
D: Only 4 is correct
E: All of the above are correct

548. Which of the following statements regarding the symptomatic treatment of children with otitis media is/are true?
    1) earache and fever should be treated with aspirin
    2) topical decongestants are useful in improving eustachian tube function

3) eardrops provide significant relief in children with acute otitis media

4) systemic antihistamine-decongestants have not been shown to affect the symptoms or course of acute otitis media

549. Which of the following statements regarding recurrent episodes of acute otitis media in children is/are true?
1) recurrent bouts of acute otitis media usually occur in the winter or early spring
2) recurrent bouts of acute otitis media should be managed by myringotomy and the insertion of ventilation tubes
3) medical management appears to be just as effective and somewhat safer than myringotomy and the insertion of ventilation tubes in children with recurrent acute otitis media
4) amoxicillin does not have a significant role to play in the management of recurrent acute otitis media

ANSWERS

543. A. This patient has acute otitis media.

Acute otitis media is defined as a clinical syndrome of otalgia, fever, and irritability (either singly or in combination) in association with a full or bulging tympanic membrane, and with pneumatoscopic evidence of effusion.[1,2] Acute otitis media usually lasts 2–6 weeks. Other otitis media syndromes include subacute otitis media (infection lasting 6 weeks to 3 months, with associated effusion), and chronic otitis media (infection lasting greater than 3 months).[1]

544. C. Otitis media is a common condition. Over 50% of children will have one episode of otitis media before the age of 1 year.

Both upper respiratory tract infection and otitis media are more common in winter in temperate climates. A viral upper respiratory tract infection is an important cause of otitis media.

The incidence and prevalence of acute otitis media is higher in boys than girls, and is higher among lower socioeconomic groups than middle and upper class children.

Otitis media is more common in large families, and in situations such as day-care centers where there is a high rate of infectivity.[1]

545. C. Acute otitis media usually begins a few days after onset of a cold or other upper respiratory tract

infection. The upper respiratory tract infection usually produces eustachian tube dysfunction and obstruction. This subsequently leads to the accumulation of fluid in the middle ear and infection.[1]

Environmental factors such as exposure to respiratory tract irritants, (e.g., pollen, dust, molds, tobacco smoke) may increase the incidence of upper respiratory tract infection and acute otitis media.[1]

Supine nursing (i.e., habitually putting the infant to bed with a bottle) may also contribute directly to risk of otitis media.[1]

Most cases of otitis media are considered to be bacterial in orgin.[1]

546. C. The bacteriology of acute otitis shows the following frequency: pneumococcus, *Haemophilus influenzae, Branhamella catarrhalis*, Group A streptococci, and *Staphylococcus aureus.*[1,2]

547. D. The drug of choice for acute otitis media remains amoxicillin or ampicillin. The usual length of treatment is 7–10 days.

A patient who does not improve on amoxicillin most likely has an infection with a beta-lactamase producing organism. In this case, second line agents including trimethoprim-sulfamethoxazole, erythromycin-sulfamethoxazole, amoxicillin-clavulinic acid, or cefaclor can be used.[1,2]

548. D. Symptoms of earache or fever should be treated with systemic analgesic/antipyretic agents. Acetaminophen is preferable to aspirin because of the reported link between some viral infections and the development of Reye's syndrome.

Ear drops do not provide any symptomatic relief in otitis media, and interfere with otoscopic examination and follow-up.

Topical decongestants (sympathomimetic nose drops and sprays), used to relieve obstruction of the eustachian tube, and systemic antihistamine-decongestant combinations have not been shown to be effective in the treatment of otitis media.[1]

549. B. Recurrent episodes of otitis media can be managed with prophylactic antibiotic therapy. Half-strength doses of sulfisoxazole or amoxicillin are appropriate. Such preventive therapy can be used episodically or continuously throughout the winter and early spring (the peak season for upper respiratory tract infection). This therapy appears to be just as effective as myringotomy and the inser-

tion of ventilation tubes in the treatment of recurrent otitis media.[1]

SUMMARY OF THE DIAGNOSIS AND MANAGEMENT OF ACUTE OTITIS MEDIA

1. **Definition:** The clinical syndrome of otalgia, fever, and irritability associated with a full or bulging tympanic membrane and with pneumatoscopic evidence of effusion

2. **Etiologic agents:** Pneumococci, *Haemophilus influenzae, Branhamella catarrhalis,* and group A streptococci

3. **Treatment:** Amoxicillin/ ampicillin are drugs of choice. Systemic decongestants-antihistamines,

topical decongestants, and ear drops are not useful in treatment. Acetaminophen is the drug of choice for pyrexia.

4. Recurrent bouts of acute otitis media appear to be safely and effectively treated with antibiotics, myringotomy and the insertion of ventilation tubes may not be necessary.

References

1. Stool S. Otitis media: update on a common, frustrating problem. Postgrad Med 1989; 85(1): 40–53.

2. Eichenwald H. Developments in diagnosing and treating otitis media. Am Fam Physician 1985; 31(3) 155–163.

PROBLEM 70:   A 7-YEAR-OLD CHILD WITH FEVER, CERVICAL LYMPHADENOPATHY AND A SORE THROAT

A 7-year-old boy presents to the office with his mother for assessment of a fever and a sore throat. The fever (which has been as high as 39° C) began 2 days ago, and his sore throat began 24 hours ago.

On examination, his throat is red. There are no exudates. There are moderately enlarged cervical lymph nodes, which are nontender.

SELECT THE ONE BEST ANSWER TO THE FOLLOWING QUESTIONS:

550. Which of the following statements regarding the etiology of this child's sore throat is true?
    a) the etiology is much more likely to be streptococcal than viral
    b) the etiology is much more likely to be viral than streptococcal
    c) the etiology is uncertain; a viral pharyngitis is often clinically indistinguishable from a streptococcal pharyngitis
    d) the causative agent is most likely the Epstein-Barr virus
    e) the etiology is uncertain; an antibiotic should be given just to be on the safe side

551. Which of the following symptoms is more likely to be associated with a viral pharyngitis than a streptococcal pharyngitis?
    a) severe sore throat
    b) oral temperature > 38° C
    c) beefy red or exudative pharyngitis
    d) tender anterior cervical lymph nodes

    e) rhinorrhea

552. Which of the following organisms is the most common bacterial pathogen in bacterial pharyngitis?
    a) group A beta-hemolytic streptococci
    b) group B streptococci
    c) group C streptococci
    d) *Streptococcus pneumoniae*
    e) group G streptococci

553. Which of the following statements regarding the diagnosis of streptococcal pharyngitis is true?
    a) the sensitivity of ELISA (enzyme linked immunosorbent assay) techniques for diagnosing streptococcal pharyngitis is as high as throat culture
    b) throat cultures should be taken on most children with sore throats
    c) the throat culture remains the gold standard for the diagnosis of streptococcal pharyngitis
    d) ELISA negative throat swabs from children with symptoms suggestive of streptococcal pharyngitis do not need to be cultured

e) a positive throat culture is definitive evidence of streptococcal pharyngitis infection

554. The antibiotic of choice for the treatment of streptococcal pharyngitis is:
    a) penicillin
    b) erythromycin
    c) tetracycline
    d) sulfamethoxazole
    e) cefaclor

555. Which of the following statements regarding standardized symptomatic treatment versus penicillin as initial therapy for streptococcal pharyngitis is (are) true?
    a) penicillin is superior to standarized symptomatic therapy (analgesics and education) for the relief of the initial symptoms of streptococcal pharyngitis
    b) standarized symptomatic therapy (analgesics and education) appear to be as effective as penicillin for the relief of the initial symptoms of streptococcal pharyngitis
    c) penicillin usually produces rapid relief of fever, malaise, odynophagia, adenitis and pharyngitis in patients with streptococcal pharyngitis
    d) a and c

ANSWER THE FOLLOWING QUESTION ACCORDING TO THE CODE:

A: 1, 2, and 3 are correct
B: 1 and 3 are correct
C: 2 and 4 are correct
D: Only 4 is correct
E: All of the above are correct

556. Which of the following is/are complications of streptococcal pharyngitis?
    1) otitis media
    2) peritonsillar abscess
    3) sinusitis
    4) glomerulonephritis

ANSWERS

550. C. Acute pharyngitis is most commonly caused by viruses. Group A beta-hemolytic streptococcus is the only common bacterial cause. It, however, accounts for fewer than 15% of cases.

Although the clinical manifestations of viral and bacterial pharyngitis differ somewhat, there is considerable overlap in signs and symptoms, and it is often impossible (as in this case) to clinically distinguish one form of pharyngitis from another.

Viral pharyngitis usually has a gradual onset with fever, malaise, anorexia, hoarseness, cough, rhinitis, and sore throat being the most common symptoms. Often the sore throat begins 24–48 hours after the pain. Pharyngeal inflammation is usually relatively slight, although small ulcers and exudates (indistinguishable from streptococcal pharyngitis) may occur. Cervical lymphadenopathy, which may be tender, is not uncommon.

The white blood cell count may be significantly elevated, and in the early stages of illness, a polymorphonuclear leukocytosis (as in streptococcal pharyngitis) may occur.

The duration of illness is usually short (1–5 days).

Streptococcal pharyngitis often initially presents with headache, abdominal pain, vomiting, and fever. The fever may be as high as 40° C (104° F). The sore throat usually follows, and tonsillar enlargement, exudation, and pharyngeal erythema are found. Pharyngeal pain may be slight to severe. Many patients have only mild erythema, with no enlargement of the tonsils and with no exudate. Tender anterior cervical lymphadenopathy usually occurs early. The course of the disease may last from a few days up to 2 weeks. The physical findings most likely to be associated with streptococcal disease include diffuse redness of the tonsils and tonsillar pillars, and petechial mottling of the soft palate.[1]

551. E. Conjunctivitis, rhinitis, cough, and hoarseness rarely occur with streptococcal pharyngitis. Two or more of these symptoms suggests viral and the presence of two or more of these symptoms suggests viral pharyngitis.

Children with all four of the following are more likely to have streptococcal pharyngitis than viral pharyngitis: (1) moderate to severe sore throat, (2) beefy red or exudative pharyngitis, (3) oral temperature > 38° C (100.4° F) and (4) anterior cervical lymph node tenderness and palpable enlargement.[1]

552. A. The most common pathogen in bacterial pharyngitis is group A beta-hemolytic streptococci. Rarely, group B, C, and G streptococci cause clinical pharyngitis.

Group B streptococci is not associated with streptococcal pharyngitis.

Streptococcal pneumoniae has occasionally been implicated in clinical pharyngitis.[1,2]

553. C. Diagnosis of streptococcal pharyngitis can be made by rapid antigen detection methods (ELISA) or by culture after pharyngeal swabbing.[1,2]

The throat culture remains the gold standard for the diagnosis of streptococcal pharyngitis.

The sensitivity of the throat culture exceeds the sensitivity of ELISA tests. ELISA tests are more specific than sensitive (there will be more false negatives ELISA tests than false positives).

Most children who present with a sore throat do not have streptococcal pharyngitis (approximately 85% have a viral pharyngitis). Culturing all or most children, therefore, will result in a very high false-positive pick-up (low positive predictive value).

554. A. The antibiotic of choice for the treatment of streptococcal pharyngitis is penicillin. The use of antibiotics should be guided by the results of antigen detection tests or cultures, unless there are strong clinical and epidemiologic grounds to suspect a streptococcal infection. If used, penicillin should be given for a full 10 days.[1-3]

Erythromycin is a satisfactory alternative if the patient is allergic to penicillin.

Tetracycline should not be given to young children (< 10 years) because of the risk of staining of tooth enamel.

Cefaclor and sulfamethoxazole are not considered to be first line drugs in the treatment of streptococcal infection.

555. B. There is no significant difference between the prescription of penicillin (while awaiting culture results) and symptomatic treatment consisting of analgesics and education, for the relief of most of the symptoms associated with streptococcal pharyngitis.[3]

556. E. The only significant complications of viral pharyngitis is purulent bacterial otitis media. With streptococcal disease, peritonsillar abscess, sinusitis, otitis media, and occasionally meningitis.

Acute glomerulonephritis and rheumatic fever may also follow streptococcal infections.

Mesenteric adenitis, which may mimic appendicitis, may be associated with both viral and bacterial pharyngitis.[1]

SUMMARY OF THE DIAGNOSIS AND TREATMENT OF PHARYNGITIS

1. Most cases (85%) of pharyngitis are viral. It is often impossible to clinically distinguish one form of pharyngitis from another. However, if any two of conjunctivitis, rhinitis, cough, and hoarseness are present, the diagnosis is almost certainly viral. If the following four signs and symptoms are present, the probability of streptococcal pharyngitis is significantly increased: (1) moderate to severe sore throat, (2) beefy red or exudative pharyngitis, (3) oral temperature > 38° C (100.4 ° F), and (4) anterior cervical lymph node tenderness and palpable enlargement.

2. **Diagnosis:** The throat culture remains the gold standard for diagnosis.

3. **Treatment:** Symptomatic treatment is just as effective as penicillin in alleviating the signs and symptoms of streptococcal pharyngitis. Symptomatic treatment can be suggested while awaiting a throat culture. Penicillin remains the antibiotic of choice for the treatment of streptococcal pharyngitis.

References

1. Boat T, Doershuk C, Stern R, Heggie A. Acute pharyngitis. In: Behrman R, Vaughan V, eds. Nelson's textbook of pediatrics. 13th Ed. Philadelphia: WB Saunders, 1987: 871–872.

2. Denny F. Current problems in managing streptococcal pharyngitis. J Pediatr 1987; 111(6): 797–806.

3. Middelton D, D'Amico F, Merenstein J. Standardized symptomatic treatment versus penicillin as initial therapy for streptococcal pharyngitis. J Pediatr 1988; 113: 1089–1094.

PROBLEM 71: A 9-MONTH-OLD INFANT WITH FEVER AND NO LOCALIZING SIGNS

A 9-month-old infant is seen in the emergency room for evaluation of fever. His mother states that he has had an intermittent fever of 39° C (rectally) for the past 24 hours. She has used acetaminophen to treat the fever, and has been able to bring it down to 38° C. The child has not been ill, and has had no symptoms of upper respiratory tract infection or other symptoms.

On examination, the child is actively playing with his toys. He does not look toxic. His temperature is 39° C rectally. The physical examination is completely normal. Your clinical judgment suggests that this child does not have a serious infection incubating.

SELECT THE ONE BEST ANSWER TO THE FOLLOWING QUESTIONS:

557. At this time, the most appropriate course would be to:
    a) order a WBC count, ESR, and blood cultures
    b) hospitalize the child for a complete evaluation, including lumbar puncture
    c) reassure the mother that there is no evidence of any serious infection, and follow-up the child's status within 24 hours
    d) change the antipyretic from acetaminophen to aspirin
    e) none of the above

558. Which of the following statements regarding the height of the fever and the incidence of bacteremia in infants is true?
    a) there is an excellent correlation between the height of the fever and the incidence of bacteremia
    b) in young infants (< 3 months), the correlation is higher than in older infants
    c) a 2-month-old infant with a fever of 38° C is almost never bacteremic
    d) caution must be exercised in using the height of fever as a screening tool for the incidence of bacteremia
    e) b and c

559. The most common organism responsible for occult bacteremia is:
    a) *Neisseria meningitidis*
    b) *Haemophilus influenzae*
    c) *Streptococcus pneumoniae*
    d) *Salmonella*
    e) *Mycoplasma pneumoniae*

ANSWER THE FOLLOWING QUESTIONS ACCORDING TO THE CODE:

A: 1, 2, and 3 are correct
B: 1 and 3 are correct
C: 2 and 4 are correct
D: Only 4 is correct
E: All of the above are correct

560. Which of the following statements regarding the presumptive use of oral antibiotics in febrile infants is(are) true?
    1) presumptive use of oral antibiotics in infants with febrile illnesses has shown to decrease morbidity from many bacteremic illnesses in all relevant studies
    2) the earlier an antibiotic is used, the greater effect it will have on reducing morbidity from bacteremic illness
    3) presumptive oral antibiotics reliably prevent meningitis as a complication of occult bacteremia
    4) none of the above statements are true

561. A 2-year-old infant developed a temperature of 39° C 2 days ago. He began complaining of a sore right ear this afternoon. His mother called you and you asked her to meet you at the hospital this evening. On the way to the hospital the child had a "convulsion."

    When the mother arrived at the hospital, the convulsion was over. The infant appeared slightly lethargic. His temperature was 39.5° C rectally. His right tympanic membrane was red and bulging. The rest of the physical examination was normal.

    Which of the following is(are) characteristic of febrile convulsions in infants and children?
    1) the onset is usually between 6 months and 5 years of age
    2) the convulsion is usually of short duration (< 15 minutes)

3) the convulsion usually presents as a generalized tonic-clonic pattern

4) there is usually no focal or lateralizing aspect to the convulsion

ANSWERS

557. C. The most appropriate course of action would be to reassure the mother that there is no evidence of any serious infection, and follow-up the child's status within 24 hours.

The three tests that have been used to predict the probability of occult bacteremia are clinical judgment, white blood cell count, and erythrocyte sedimentation rate. Although the positive predictive value of each of these tests for bacteremia is low, the negative predictive values are high (>95%). The negative predictive value for clinical judgment is just as high as the negative predictive value for the WBC or the ESR. Thus, a child who looks well clinically has at least a 95% chance of not having occult bacteremia.

Thus, in the case presented, on the basis of your clinical judgment, it is reasonable to send the child home and recheck with the parents within 24 hours. The mother should be instructed to return if there is any change in the infant's condition.[1]

558. D. In infants older than 2 or 3 months of age, there is a reasonable correlation between the height of the fever and the risk of bacteremia. In younger infants, however, the height of the fever bears no relationship to the risk of bacteremia or other serious illness.

As well, caution must be exercised in using the height of the fever since the home use of antipyretics, the effects of ambient temperature, bundling, and diurnal variation substantially decrease the sensitivity of the test.[1]

559. C. The most common cause of occult bacteremia in children is Streptococcus pneumoniae (65%). Other common causative agents include *Haemophilus influenzae* type b (25%) and *Neisseria meningitidis*. *Salmonella* and *Mycoplasma pneumoniae* are uncommon causes of occult bacteremia.[1,2]

560. D. The results of studies evaluating the presumptive use of oral antibiotics in the prevention of morbidity associated with bacteremia are controversial. While oral antibiotics may retard the emergence of some less serious focal bacterial disease (streptococcal pharyngitis, otitis media, and pneumonia), they do not reliably prevent meningitis as a complication of occult bacteremia.

There is no solid evidence that the sooner a presumptive antibiotic is used, the greater will be its effect.[1]

561. E. Febrile convulsions may accompany high fever in a child. Few children with febrile convulsions will go on to develop epilepsy in later life.

Febrile convulsions usually develop between the ages of 6 months and 5 years, occur with a rise in temperature above 39° C, last 15 minutes or less, are tonic-clonic in character, have no focal or lateralizing aspects, and do not manifest neurologic deficits postictally.[3]

Treatment of the fever and the underlying condition is usually sufficient.

SUMMARY OF THE DIAGNOSIS AND TREATMENT OF A FEBRILE INFANT WITH NO FOCUS OF INFECTION

1. Most febrile infants have nonbacteremic illnesses.

2. Young infants (<3 months) should be hospitalized as the probability of bacteremia is greater.

3. Clinical judgment is much more accurate in predicting which child does not have (rather than does have) bacteremic illness.

4. A febrile child who looks well can be discharged and followed as an outpatient.

5. White blood cell count and ESR are helpful when clinical judgment is equivocal. The ability of these tests, however, to predict the presence of bacteremia is low.

6. The use of presumptive antibiotics is not well established, nor does their use protect against subsequent severe infection.

References

1. Radetsky M. The clinical evaluation of the febrile infant. Prim Care 1984; 11 (3): 395–405.

2. Gutierrez-Nunez J, Ibanez A, Stevens M, David D. Fever without a focus. Am Fam Physician 1985; 32(1): 36, 138–144.

3. Huttenlocher P. Conditions having seizures as major manifestations. In: Behrman R, Vaughan V, eds.

Nelson's textbook of pediatrics. 13th Ed. Philadelphia: WB Saunders, 1987: 1287–1288.

PROBLEM 72: AN ANXIOUS MOTHER WITH A 3-WEEK-OLD INFANT AND MANY QUESTIONS CONCERNING FEEDING

A mother presents to the office with her 3-week-old infant. She has many questions concerning infant feeding. She is currently breast-feeding. The infant is eating every 3 hours. Her mother-in-law has suggested that she switch to cow's milk because she is getting too tired.

On examination the infant is thriving. The infant's physical examination is entirely normal.

SELECT THE ONE BEST ANSWER TO THE FOLLOWING QUESTIONS:

562. Which of the following statements comparing breast milk and cow's milk is false?
    a) cow's milk may be responsible for diarrhea, intestinal bleeding, and occult melena
    b) "spitting up," colic and atopic eczema are more common in formula fed babies
    c) human milk contains many bacterial and viral antibodies, mainly of the IgA class
    d) breast-fed infants do not require iron supplementation until 1 year of age
    e) breast milk is an adequate source of vitamin C

563. The mother has been told that she should be giving the baby "vitamins." Which of the following vitamins may need to be supplemented in a breast fed baby?
    a) vitamin A
    b) vitamin C
    c) vitamin D
    d) b and c
    e) all of the above

564. The mother has also been told by her mother-in-law that the infant should be receiving extra fluoride. Fluoride supplementation for both breast-fed and formula-fed infants is usually not required if the fluoride concentration of the water in the community exceeds:
    a) 1.0 ppm
    b) 2.0 ppm
    c) 5.0 ppm
    d) 10.0 ppm
    e) 100.0 ppm

565. Breast milk in comparison to cow's milk has:
    a) a higher fat content
    b) a lower carbohydrate content
    c) a lower protein content
    d) a greater concentration of casein
    e) a greater number of calories/gram

566. The mother is concerned that "she is doing something wrong because the baby is feeding every three hours." Her mother-in-law has told her that babies should feed no more than every 4 hours, and that they should be sleeping through the night by the age of 3 weeks.
    Which of the following statements regarding infant feeding is false?
    a) babies establish their own feeding pattern; there is a considerable variation from one baby to the other
    b) for the first 1 or 2 months of life, feedings are regularly taken throughout the 24 hour period
    c) breast-fed babies should be fed on a schedule
    d) during the first month of life, feedings average 6–8/24-hour period
    e) by 8 months of age, the average number of feedings per day is 3–4

567. The mother-in-law has also suggested the introduction of solid food at 3 weeks of age. You suggest that pablum and other solid foods do not have to be introduced into the infant's diet until:
    a) 1 month of age
    b) 2–3 months of age
    c) 4–6 months of age
    d) 9 months of age
    e) 12 months of age

568. A mother brings her 6-month-old infant to the office. She states that he has been constipated since she switched him from breast milk to formula 2 weeks ago. On careful questioning, you determine that the infant is having 1 hard bowel movement every 4 days.

The physical examination of the infant is normal.

You should advise the mother to:
a) go home and relax, the child will grow out of it
b) to supplement with extra fluids, extra foods, and prune juice
c) to use milk of magnesia at bedtime
d) to add 2 teaspoons of bran to the paplum and feed it to him every 3 hours
e) to give him a glycerine suppository at bedtime

569. A mother brings her 6-week-old infant into the office. She states that he has been spitting up all of his formula for the last 3 weeks, and is obviously malnourished. On physical examination the infant looks well. You find that he weighs 11 lbs 3 oz. His birth weight was 7 lbs 6 oz. You should advise the mother to:
a) go home and relax, the child will grow out of it
b) increase the time spent burping the infant and put him on his abdomen for a nap immediately after feeding
c) investigate the child for pyloric stenosis
d) suggest the use of a GI tract motility modifier such as metoclopramide
e) refer the child to a pediatrician

ANSWER THE FOLLOWING QUESTIONS ACCORDING TO THE CODE:

A: 1, 2, and 3 are correct
B: 1 and 3 are correct
C: 2 and 4 are correct
D: Only 4 is correct
E: All of the above are correct

570. A mother presents to your office with her 8-week-old infant. She is tearful and depressed. She has been trying to breast-feed but she states that she is not producing enough milk and the baby is "fussy all the time."

On examination, the infant looks thin. Since her last check-up 3 weeks ago, she has only gained 90 grams. The rest of the physical examination is normal.

Which of the following interventions may be appropriate in this case?
1) careful questioning about feeding technique
2) referral to the La Leche League
3) inclusion of the husband or significant other in feeding expressed breast milk by bottle

4) supplementation with an infant formula

571. Which of the following statements regarding breast feeding is (are) correct?
1) most breast-fed babies lose weight in the first week of life
2) infants should be encouraged to empty both breasts at each feeding during the first weeks of life
3) maternal fatigue may impair breast-feeding
4) 80–90% of the milk is obtained in the first four minutes of breast-feeding

572. A mother who is currently breast-feeding her 4-month-old son presents to your office with a sore right breast. On examination she has an erythematous, swollen, tender area at the 11 o'clock position in the right breast. The swelling measures 4 cm in diameter. Your initial impression is mastitis. You should advise her to:
1) apply warm compresses to the area
2) discontinue breast-feeding
3) begin antibiotic therapy with cloxacillin
4) start the baby on prophylactic penicillin

ANSWERS

562. D. Breast milk has many advantages over cow's milk for the feeding of infants. These advantages include: (1) it is easier to digest, (2) it has many bacterial and viral antibodies (especially of the IgA class) present in it, (3) it does not produce allergic manifestations such as diarrhea, GI tract bleeding, and atopic dermatitis, (4) it has a lower incidence of feeding problems including regurgitation and constipation, and (5) it is the most important method of establishing maternal-infant bonding.[1] Breast milk usually contains adequate supplies of all vitamins, with the possible exception of vitamin D (see question 563). Vitamin C is not required for supplementation.

Although breast milk contains some iron, and the iron that is present is well absorbed, the child probably should begin iron-fortified foods at 6 months of age to prevent an iron-deficiency anemia.[1]

563. C. Vitamin D is the only vitamin that may be required for supplementation in a breast-fed baby. If a baby is not exposed to adequate sunlight or has dark skin, the quantity of vitamin D may not be sufficient. It is recommended that the daily intake of vitamin D be 400 IU/day.[1]

564. A. Fluoride supplementation for infants (both breast-fed and bottle-fed) is not required if the fluoride concentration of the water supply exceeds 1.0 ppm. Additional fluoride given to formula-fed babies in a community with a fluoridated water supply could result in fluorosis.

565. C. In comparison to cow's milk, breast milk has a higher carbohydrate content; a lower protein content; lactalbumin and lactoglobulin as compared to casein as the major proteins; a qualitative (not quantitative) difference in fat (higher percentage of polyunsaturated fat); and the same caloric content (20 kcal/oz).[1]

566. C. Infants should be breast-fed on demand. An infant fed on demand will usually eat regularly throughout a 24-hour day for the first month or two.

Infants vary considerably in their feeding patterns; most infants, however, in the first month or two of life, feed 6–8 times in a 24-hour period. By the age of 8 months, this has decreased to 3–4 feedings/day.[1]

567. C. Solid foods do not have to be introduced into an infant's diet until 4–6 months of age. Pablum is the first food to be introduced. It should be followed by vegetables, fruits, and finally meats. New foods should not be introduced any more often than one every 1–2 weeks. The order of food introduction appears unimportant.[1]

568. B. Constipation is a common problem in formula-fed babies. It is extremely rare in a breast-fed baby. Constipation in a formula-fed baby may be due to an insufficient amount of food or fluid, a diet too high in fat or protein, or a diet deficient in bulk. Constipation may be alleviated by increasing the amount of fluid or sugar in the formula, or by adding or increasing the amounts of cereal, vegetables, or fruit. Prune juice (1/2-1 oz) may also be helpful.

The use of milk of magnesia and glycerine suppositories as anything but a very temporary measure is inappropriate. The addition of 2 teaspoons of bran to the pablum, although theoretically sound as a measure of increasing the bulk in the infant's diet, would be somewhat unpalatable.

Telling the mother to go home and relax is not appropriate.

569. B. Regurgitation or spitting up is a common problem in infants. The mechanism appears to be an incompetent gastroesophageal sphincter. Regurgitation can be reduced by adequate eructation of swallowed air during and after eating, by gentle handling, by avoidance of emotional conflicts, and by placing the infant on the right side or abdomen for a nap immediately after eating. The head should not be lower than the rest of the body during rest periods.Unless the child (especially a male) demonstrates projectile vomiting and has a palpable mass in the pylorus, pyloric stenosis is not likely.

Metoclopramide and other GI tract motility modifiers have no place to play in the management of regurgitation in infants. The condition should be gently explained to the mother in a calm, reassuring manner. She should be asked to try the simple measures outlined above. Inadequate explanation, along with advice to relax is inappropriate. Unless the mother is not happy with your advice, referrral to a pediatrician is not indicated.

570. E. This is a common scenario in pediatric family practice.

The mother should be carefully questioned regarding feeding technique. Before assuming that the mother has insufficient milk, three possibilities should be excluded: (1) errors in feeding technique responsible for the infant's inadequate progress; (2) remediable maternal factors related to diet, rest, or emotional distress; or (3) physical disturbances in the infant that intefere with eating or with gain in weight.[1]

Occasionally, infants who seem to be nursing well may not thrive because of milk insufficiency; in this case increased frequency of feedings may be indicated.

Referral to the La Leche League is an alternative that can be recommended to the mother. The La Leche League is a volunteer organization composed of successfully nursing mothers willing to assist other mothers desiring to nurse.

If the mother is able to successfully express sufficient milk, the husband or significant other may be able to assist the mother in feeding. This alternative is attractive because it gives the mother time to rest and recover her strength.

Supplementation with an infant formula is an alternative that should be considered in some cases. In this case, the mother is encouraged to breast-feed and supplement her baby with formula following each feeding. As long as the nipple does not have too big a hole in it (making it too easy for the infant to obtain the formula), the infant will probably continue to suck vigorously at the breast. This will allow the mother to continue breast-feeding while at the same time ensuring adequate infant nutrition.

Infant formulas provide excellent nutrition for the infant. They all combine milk, sugar, and water, and modification of a digestible curd protein. As with breast milk, infant formulas provide 20 kcal/oz.

Although "breast is best," a dogmatic approach to breast-feeding should be avoided.

571. E. Most breast-fed infants lose weight in the first week of life. This weight loss is usually reversed by 5–7 days. During the first week of life, the colostrum is gradually replaced by the much richer breast milk.

Initially, the infant should be encouraged to breast feed from both breasts. This will ensure maximal milk production. After breast-feeding has been well established, the breasts may be alternated at successive feedings.

Maternal fatigue may impair breast-feeding. In this situation, expression of milk with feeding by the husband or significant other, or supplementation with commercial formula can be recommended.

Some infants will empty a breast in 5 minutes; others nurse at a more leisurely pace for 20 minutes or more. Most of the milk is obtained early in the feeding; 50% in the first 2 minutes and 80–90% in the first 4 minutes.[1]

572. B. Mastitis is a common complaint in breast-feeding mothers. Treatment should begin with analgesics, warm compresses, and an anti-staphylococcal antibiotic such as cloxacillin. Breast-feeding should be continued. It is very unlikely that the baby will develop an infection because of the infection in the mother, and thus prophylactic antibiotics in the infant are not recommended.

SUMMARY OF INFANT FEEDING

1. **Breast-feeding is preferable**: Advantages include convenience, digestibility, transfer of antiviral and antibacterial antibodies, no allergic phenomenon, maternal-infant bonding, low incidence of regurgitation, and no constipation

2. Vitamins are unnecessary in all formula-fed infants and probably in most breast-fed babies. If the mother is not exposed to sufficient sunlight or is darkly pigmented, supplemental vitamin D is recommended.

3. Fluoride supplementation is unnecessary if community water supply is fluoridated; this applies to breast-fed and formula-fed infants.

4. Breast feeding should be encouraged: before assuming milk production is insufficient for the infant consider errors in feeding technique, remediable maternal factors, and physical disturbances in the infant.

5. Supplementation with formula and formula feeding provide excellent nutrition; a dogmatic approach to breast-feeding should be avoided.

6. Solid foods need not be introduced until 4–6 months of age; after that time introduce 1 new food every 1–2 weeks. The order of introduction appears unimportant.

Reference

1. Barness L. Feeding of infants. In: Behrman R, Vaughan V, eds. Nelson's textbook of pediatrics, 13th Ed. Philadelphia: WB Saunders, 1987: 123–138.

PROBLEM 73 : A FULL-TERM INFANT WHO DEVELOPS JAUNDICE ON THE SECOND DAY OF LIFE

A full-term infant weighing 3800 grams develops jaundice on the 2nd day of life. The infant appears healthy and is breast-feeding well. Vital signs are normal. The mother and infant are group A Rh positive. The infant's hemoglobin is 180 g/L. The direct and indirect Coombs' tests are negative. The infant's total bilirubin is 171 µmol/L (10 mg/dl) and the indirect bilirubin is 154 µmol/L (9 mg/dl).

SELECT THE ONE BEST ANSWER TO THE FOLLOWING QUESTIONS:

573. The most likely diagnosis in this infant is:
    a) undiagnosed neonatal sepsis
    b) breast milk jaundice
    c) physiologic jaundice
    d) jaundice due to a minor antigen blood group incompatibility
    e) ABO blood group incompatibility

574. The treatment of choice for the infant described in question 573 at this time is:
    a) phototherapy
    b) exchange tranfusions
    c) withdrawal of breast-feeding
    d) supplementation with water
    e) none of the above

575. A full-term infant weighing 3700 grams develops jaundice on the 4th day of life. He is being breast-fed and is feeding well. Vital signs are normal. The mother and infant are group A Rh positive. The infant's hemoglobin is 175 g/L. The direct and indirect Coombs' tests are negative. The total serum bilirubin is 256 µmol/L (15 mg/dl). The indirect bilirubin is 242 µmol/L (14.15 mg/dl).

    The most likely diagnosis in this infant is:
    a) undiagnosed neonatal sepsis
    b) breast milk jaundice
    c) physiologic jaundice
    d) jaundice due to minor antigen blood group incompatibility
    e) ABO incompatiblity

576. The treatment of choice for the infant described in question 575 at this time is:
    a) phototherapy
    b) exchange transfusions
    c) withdrawal of breast-feeding
    d) supplementation with water
    e) none of the above

577. A 2900-gram infant born at term develops jaundice during the first 24 hours of life. The infant's bilirubin at 24 hours of age is 220 µmol/L (12.9 mg/dl). The indirect bilirubin is 205 µmol/L (12 mg/dl). The infant is group A Rh positive and his mother is group O Rh positive. The direct Coombs' test is positive. The infant's hemoglobin is 180 g/dl. The reticulocyte count is 10%.

    The most likely diagnosis in this infant at this time is:

    a) undiagnosed neonatal sepsis
    b) breast milk jaundice
    c) physiologic jaundice
    d) jaundice due to minor antigen blood group incompatibility
    e) ABO incompatibility

578. The treatment of choice for the infant described in question 577 at this time is:
    a) phototherapy
    b) exchange transfusions
    c) withdrawal of breast-feeding
    d) supplementation with water
    e) none of the above

579. Jaundice in the newborn period develops in what percentage of full-term infants?
    a) 20%
    b) 40%
    c) 60%
    d) 80%
    e) 95%

ANSWER THE FOLLOWING QUESTION ACCORDING TO THE CODE:

A: 1, 2, and 3 are correct
B: 1 and 3 are correct
C: 2 and 4 are correct
D: Only 4 is correct
E: All of the above are correct

580. Which of the following is/are complications of phototherapy in the treatment of newborn infants with jaundice?
    1) frequent loose stools
    2) a transient rash
    3) lethargy and abdominal distention
    4) hyperthermia and flushing

ANSWERS

573. C. The most likely diagnosis in this infant is physiologic jaundice. Physiologic jaundice usually begins on the 2nd or 3rd day of life. It is due to the accumulation of unconjugated bilirubin in the skin.

    Jaundice in a newborn is not physiologic if (1) it appears in the first 24 hours of life, (2) there is an increase in total bilirubin concentration of more than 86 µmol/L (5 mg/dl) per day, (3) the total serum bilirubin concentration is greater than 256 μmol/L (15 mg/dl) in a full-term infant or 220 μmol/L (12.9 mg/dl) in a preterm infant, (4) the direct bilirubin concentration exceeds 34 μmol/L (2 mg/dl), or (5) jaundice persists for more than 1 week in a full-term infant or more than 2 weeks in a premature infant.[1]

Physiologic jaundice or exaggerated jaundice usually disappears by the 5th day of life.

The other causes of neonatal jaundice will be discussed in subseqeunt questions.

574. E. None of the above.

No treatment should be instituted at this time.

The levels at which phototherapy should be instituted for physiologic jaundice are controversial.[1,2] Kernicterus does not develop in children with physiologic jaundice, and thus the level at which treatment is initiated should probably be high. It is reasonable to suggest that phototherapy should be withheld in an otherwise healthy infant with physiologic jaundice unless the serum bilirubin exceeds 290 μmol/L– 320 μmol/L (17 mg/dl–18.8 mg/dl).

575. B. The most likely diagnosis is this infant is breast milk jaundice.

Breast milk jaundice usually begins between the fourth and seventh day of life. Bilirubin levels range from 171 μmol/L (10 mg/dl) – 520 μmol/L (30.4 mg/dl).

Breast milk jaundice can be due to either caloric deprivation (early breast milk jaundice) or enzyme inhibition (late breast milk jaundice).[1]

576. E. None of the above.

The infant has a total bilirubin level of 256 μmol/L (15 mg/dl). As stated earlier, bilirubin levels secondary to breast milk jaundice may reach 520 μmol/L. Although interruption of breast-feeding during the first week of life may improve the jaundice, it may also result in earlier termination of breast-feeding. Water supplementation alone does not appear to be helpful in reducing breast milk jaundice.[1]

Although phototherapy would be initiated by some clinicians at this level, it is not necessary.

Exchange tranfusion is inappropriate.

577. E. This infant most likely has ABO incompatibility. Maternal antibody may be formed against B cells if the mother is type A or against A cells if the mother is type B. Usually, however, the mother is Type O and the infant is type A or type

B. Although ABO incompatibility occurs in 20–25% of pregnancies, hemolytic disease (as in this case) develops in only about 10% of those infants with possible blood group incompatibility.[1,3]

578. A. The treatment of choice in this infant is phototherapy. It is generally accepted that if an infant with an ABO incompatibility develops a significant hemolytic he/she should be treated with phototherapy. If phototherapy is unsuccessful in keeping the serum bilirubin below 342 μmol/L (20 mg/dl), exchange transfusions should be considered. Kernicterus can result from untreated hemolytic anemia secondary to blood group incompability.[1,3]

579. C. Jaundice is extremely common in newborn infants. Under usual nursery conditions jaundice is observed during the lst week of life in approximately 60% of term infants and 80% of breast-fed infants.

580. E. The potential complications of phototherapy include: (1) frequent and loose stools, (2) transient rash, (3) lethargy and abdominal distension, (4) bronze baby syndrome— a gray brown discoloration of the skin in those infants with some degree of cholestasis, (5) hyperthermia, (6) flushing, and (7) potential dehydration.[1-3]

The risk/benefit ratio of phototherapy must always be considered. It is a reasonable conclusion to suggest that physiologic jaundice should only be treated with phototherapy if the serum bilirubin exceeds 320 μmol/L (18.7 mg/dl), and that breast milk jaundice should rarely be treated with phototherapy.

SUMMARY OF THE DIAGNOSIS AND TREATMENT OF NEONATAL JAUNDICE

1. **Physiologic jaundice (exaggerated jaundice):** Commonly begins on the 2nd or 3rd day of life and is usually resolving by the 5th day. Treatment: Phototherapy is probably not indicated unless the total bilirubin level exceeds 320 μmol/L (18.7 mg/dl).

2. **Breast milk jaundice:** Usually begins on the 4th–7th day of life. Breast milk jaundice can be "early" or "late." It may not clear for up to 8 weeks. Treatment: no therapy is usually needed. Supplementation with water is not useful by itself in reducing the degree of breast milk jaundice. Sup-

plementation with formula may be used but the risks of decreased effectiveness of breast-feeding and decreased maternal-infant bonding probably outweigh the benefits.

3. **Hemolytic disease of the newborn**: Most commonly due to ABO incompatibility where the mother is type O and the infant is Type A or Type B. Jaundice usually develops within the first 24 hours. Treatment with phototherapy is indicated in many cases.

4. The other causes of neonatal jaundice (e.g., neonatal sepsis) must always be kept in mind but are uncommon.

References

1. Greenwald J. Hyperbilirubinemia in otherwise healthy infants. Am Fam Physician 1988; 38(6): 151–158.

2. Dixon A. Babies and bilirubin—a jaundiced view. Can Fam Physician 1984; 30: 1979–1982.

3. Behrman R, Kliegman R. Jaundice and hyperbilirubinemia in the newborn. In: Behrman R, Vaughan V, eds. Nelson's textbook of pediatrics. 13th Ed. Philadelphia: WB Saunders, 1987: 405–407, 413.

PROBLEM 74: A 1-YEAR-OLD MALE WITH A RASH AND A HIGH FEVER

A 1-year-old male is brought to your office by his mother. The child was well until 3 days ago when he developed a fever of 40° C. The child's mother has been trying to keep the fever down with acetaminophen. Today, his temperature suddenly dropped and he developed a skin rash over his entire body.

On physical examination the child does not look ill. His temperature is 38° C. He has a fine maculopapular eruption over his entire body. The rest of the physical examination is normal.

SELECT THE ONE BEST ANSWER TO THE FOLLOWING QUESTIONS:

581. The most likely diagnosis in this child is:
    a) exanthem subitum
    b) erythema infectiosum
    c) adenoviral exanthem
    d) rubella
    e) rubeola

582. A 5-year-old male presents to your office with his mother. He has been running a low-grade fever for the past 24 hours. This afternoon, he suddenly developed a bright red rash on both cheeks.

    On examination, the child has a livid erythema of the cheeks, and has the beginnings of a maculopapular rash on the trunk and the extremities. No other abnormalities are noted on physical examination.

    The most likely diagnosis in this child is:
    a) exanthem subitum
    b) erythema infectiosum
    c) adenoviral exanthem
    d) rubella
    e) rubeola

583. A 4-year-old unimmunized female presents with her mother for assessment of fever and a skin rash. The child had mild upper respiratory symptoms for 1 week prior to developing a sensation of "being sore behind my ears." This morning, a maculopapular rash began on the face and began spreading to the trunk. The child's temperature at that time was 38.3° C.

    On examination, the child does not appear to be sick. The child has very tender posterior auricular lymph nodes bilaterally. There is a discrete maculopapular eruption present over the entire body. There are also large areas of flushing. The pharyngeal mucosa and conjunctiva are slightly injected. There are no other abnormalities on physical examination.

    The most likely diagnosis in this child is:
    a) exanthem subitum
    b) erythema infectiosum
    c) adenoviral exanthem
    d) rubella
    e) rubeola

584. A 4-year-old male, who has not been immunized, presents with a 5-day history of fever, a dry hack-

ing cough, coryza, and conjunctivitis. This morning the child's temperature rose to 40° C. and a fine maculopapular rash appeared on the face, upper arms, and upper part of the chest. The child has significant photophobia.

On examination, there is signficant posterior cervical lymphadenopathy. There is marked conjunctival injection bilaterally. There is a diffuse maculopapular eruption over the face, arms, and chest that appears to be spreading on the back and the thighs.

The most likely diagnosis in this patient is:
a) exanthem subitum
b) erythema infectiosum
c) adenoviral exanthem
d) rubella
e) rubeola

585. An 8-year-old male presents to your office with his mother. The child has been ill for 3 days. The illness began as a fever of 39° C, with chills, vomiting, and headache.

On examination, the child has hyperemic tonsils, that are edematous and covered with exudate. The dorsum of the tongue has a white coat and also appears edematous. There is a generalized, finely papular skin rash that has the texture of coarse sandpaper. The child's forehead and cheeks are flushed, and the area around the mouth is pale.

The most likely diagnosis in this child is:
a) erythema infectiosum
b) adenoviral exanthem
c) rubella
d) rubeola
e) none of the above

ANSWER THE FOLLOWING QUESTION ACCORDING TO THE CODE:

A: 1, 2, and 3 are correct
B: 1 and 3 are correct
C: 2 and 4 are correct
D: Only 4 is correct
E: All of the above are correct

586. Which of the following viruses is/are associated with viral exanthems?
1) coxsackie A
2) coxsackie B
3) adenovirus
4) echovirus

ANSWERS

581. A. The most likely diagnosis in this child is exanthem subitum (roseola infantum).

Exanthem subitum is a viral infection of infants and young children that initially presents with a high fever that typically lasts 3–4 days. Usually, there are no physical findings to explain the fever, and the child looks well. As the fever falls, a maculopapular rash appears that eventually covers the entire body. The rash fades within 24 hours.

The treatment of exanthem subitum is symptomatic. Acetaminophen should be administered if the fever reaches 40° C.[1]

582. B. Erythema infectiosum is a human parvovirus infection of childhood that begins with a low-grade fever and produces a livid erythema on the cheeks, giving the child a "slapped-cheek" appearance. An erythematous maculopapular eruption then appears on the trunk and the extremities. The rash fades with central clearing producing a reticular or lacy pattern. The rash may last from a few days to several weeks. It is frequently pruritic. Recurrences after exercise, or the application of heat or emotional upset are not uncommon.

There are no diagnostic laboratory tests.

The differential diagnosis includes rubella, other viral exanthems, atypical measles, and drug rashes.

Complications are rare.

Treatment is symptomatic.[1]

583. D. This child has rubella. Rubella immunization, usually offered at 12–15 months, affords full protection against the disease. This child, however, missed her immunizations.

Rubella usually begins with symptoms of mild upper respiratory tract infection. Tender retroauricular, posterior cervical, and postoccipital lymphadenopathy is prominent and characteristic of the disease. In some cases, an enanthem covering the soft palate and fauces may appear prior to the onset of the skin rash.

The exanthem usually begins on the face, and spreads to the trunk. The rash is maculopapular, with areas of confluence and flushing. Mild pruritis is common. The rash usually clears by the third day.

Photophobia is absent, and fever is mild.

Complications are rare.

Treatment is symptomatic.[1]

584. E. This child has rubeola.

The prodromal phase of rubeola (red measles) is characterized by low-grade to moderate fever, a dry hacking cough, coryza, and conjunctivitis. Photophobia is prominent. These symptoms precede the enanthem that begins as a red mottling on the hard and soft palates. Koplik spots on the buccal mucosa (i.e., small grayish white dots with reddish areolae that may be hemorrhagic) are pathognomonic for rubeola.

The temperature rises as the rash appears. The maculopapular rash usually begins on the face and neck and spreads over the entire body from the neck down. By the time the rash reaches the feet the child has begun to clinically improve.

Cervical lymphadenopathy may be prominent.

The major complications of rubeola are otitis media, bronchopneumonia, and gastrointestinal symptoms including diarrhea and vomiting.

Treatment of rubeola is symptomatic.

Prevention with active immunization at 12-15 months is much preferrable to passive immunization (with gamma globulin) for disease attentuation.[1]

585. E. This child has scarlet fever.

Scarlet fever usually begins with the abrupt onset of fever, vomiting, headaches, pharyngitis, and chills. The temperature usually peaks on the 2nd day and gradually returns to normal within 5 to 7 days. The tonsils are hyperemic and edematous and may be covered with an exudate. The throat is inflamed and may be covered with a membrane. The dorsum of the tongue often initially has a white coat, with projecting edematous papillae.

The exanthem is usually finely papular or punctate. It is sometimes described as having the consistency of coarse sandpaper. The rash generally begins in the axillae, groin, and neck and within 24 hours becomes generalized. The forehead and cheeks may appear to be flushed, and the area around the mouth is pale.

Desquamation usually begins on the face and proceeds to the hands and feet, and may continue for up to 6 weeks.

The treatment of choice for all streptococcal infections is penicillin. Amoxicillin is a better tasting and acceptable alternative. For children allergic to penicillin, erythromycin is the drug of choice.[2]

586. E. All of the viruses listed in the question may be associated with viral exanthems. The enteroviruses that may produce viral exanthems include coxsackie A, coxsackie B, and echoviruses. The respiratory tract viruses that are commonly associated with viral exanthems include adenoviruses and reoviruses.[1]

SUMMARY OF COMMON VIRAL EXANTHEMS IN CHILDREN:

1. **Exanthem subitum (roseola infantum)**: High fever followed by defervescence, and appearance of rash and clinical improvement

2. **Erythema infectiosum**: Low-grade fever followed by appearance of rash— "slapped-cheek appearance" followed by appearance of lacy or reticular rash

3. **Rubella**: Mild fever; significant tender retroauricular, posterior, and postoccipital lymphadenopathy

4. **Rubeola**: Prodromal symptoms: the three C's— cough, coryza, conjunctivitis. Koplik spots are pathognomonic. Photophobia is common. The temperature rises abruptly as the rash appears. The severity of the disease is directly related to the extent and confluence of the rash

5. **Scarlet fever**: Fever, chills, headache, vomiting, and pharyngitis. Exanthem has texture of coarse sandpaper. Circumoral pallor is common. Penicillin is drug of choice.

References

1. Phillips C. Viral infections and those presumed to be caused by viruses. In: Behrman R, Vaughan V, eds. Nelson's textbook of pediatrics. 13th Ed. Philadelphia: WB Saunders, 1987: 655–668.

2. Feigin R. Streptococcal infections. In: Behrman R, Vaughan V, eds. Nelson's textbook of pediatrics. 13th Ed. Philadelphia: WB Saunders, 1987: 576–583.

PROBLEM 75 : AN 18-MONTH-OLD INFANT WHO APPEARS MALNOURISHED

An 18-month-old infant is brought to the emergency department by his mother for an assessment of an upper respiratory tract infection. He has been coughing for the past 3 days and has had a runny nose.

On examination, his temperature is 37.5 ° C. He looks malnourished, has thin extremities, a narrow face, prominent ribs, and wasted buttocks. He has a prominent diaper rash, unwashed skin, a skin rash that resembles impetigo on his face, uncut fingernails, and dirty clothing. His weight is below the 3rd percentile for age.

SELECT THE ONE BEST ANSWER TO THE FOLLOWING QUESTIONS:

587. The most likely diagnosis in the infant described above is:
    a) nonorganic failure to thrive
    b) organic failure to thrive
    c) child neglect
    d) a and c
    e) b and c

588. The treatment of choice in this infant at this time is:
    a) to provide the mother with a high-calorie formula and reassess the infant in 1 week
    b) to initiate outpatient investigations to exclude serious organic disease
    c) to treat the respiratory tract infection and instruct the mother in correct feeding practices
    d) all of the above
    e) none of the above

589. A 5-year-old girl is brought to your office for assessment of short stature. On examination, she has a weight below the 5th percentile, a webbed neck, lack of breast bud development, a high-arched palate, and a low-set hairline.
    The most likely diagnosis in this child is:
    a) Noonan's syndrome
    b) Trisomy 21
    c) Turner's syndrome
    d) Fragile X syndrome
    e) constitutional delay of growth

590. The most common cause of short stature in children is:
    a) familial short stature
    b) chromosomal abnormality
    c) constitutional delay of growth
    d) hypothyroidism
    e) psychosocial dwarfism

591. Bone age can sometimes be used to differentiate certain causes of short stature in children. With respect to bone age, which of the following statements is true:
    a) bone age is normal in both familial short stature and constitutional delay of growth
    b) bone age is normal in familial short stature and delayed in constitutional delay of growth
    c) bone age is normal in constitutional delay of growth and delayed in familial short stature
    d) bone age is delayed in both familial short stature and constitutional delay of growth
    e) bone age is variable in these two situations and cannot be used to differentiate them

592. Psychosocial dwarfism is a situation in which poor physical growth may be associated with an unfavorable psychosocial situation. With respect to psychosocial dwarfism, which of the following statements is FALSE?
    a) sleep and eating aberations occur in these children
    b) growth usually returns to normal when the stress is removed
    c) growth hormone levels are always normal in these children
    d) behavioral problems are common

ANSWER THE FOLLOWING QUESTION ACCORDING TO THE CODE:

A: 1, 2, and 3 are correct
B: 1 and 3 are correct
C: 2 and 4 are correct
D: Only 4 is correct
E: All of the above are correct

593. Which of the following investigations should be performed in a child with failure to thrive or a child in which short stature is unlikely to be familial in nature?
    1) complete blood count
    2) urinalysis
    3) creatinine
    4) stool for ova and parasites

ANSWERS

587. D. This infant most likely has nonorganic failure to thrive secondary to child neglect.

Failure to thrive (FTT) may be due to organic causes, nonorganic causes, or both. Nonorganic causes predominate. [1] Nonorganic FTT includes psychologic FTT (maternal deprivation), child neglect, and lack of education or errors in feeding.

Nonorganic failure to thrive is most often attributable to maternal deprivation or lack of a nuturing environment at home.

588. E. None of the above.

The treatment of choice is to hospitalize the child and give the child unlimited feedings for a minimum of 1 week. At the same time, a careful physical examination and certain routine investigations including complete blood count, urinalysis, and renal function testing can be completed. If the child lives in a poor inner-city neighborhood a serum lead level should also be done.

The family physician can begin to involve social services and initiate a detailed assessment of the home environment.

Before the child is discharged home, the home environment must be assessed and the parents must be given explicit instructions in feeding practices. The child should then be followed very closely on an outpatient basis. [1,2]

589. C. The most likely cause of this child's short stature is Turner's syndrome. [3] Noonan's syndrome (an autosomal dominant trait with widely variable expressivity), also has short stature as its most common presentation, but it can be easily distinguished from Turner's syndrome because of the normal chromosomal analysis. Turner's syndrome will have a 45 XO chromosome complement or else will present as a mosaic.

Trisomy 21 will usually be recognized long before the age of 13 years. The fragile X syndrome is a syndrome associated with mental retardation and macro-orchidism in males.

590. A. The most common cause of a short child is short parents. When a short child who is growing at a normal rate and has a normal bone age is found to have a strong family history of short stature, familial short stature is the most likely cause. Other causes of short stature include constitutional delay of growth, chromosomal abnormalities, intrauterine growth retardation, chronic diseases such as renal disease or inflammatory bowel disease, hypothyroidism, adrenal hyperplasia, growth hormone deficiency, bioinactive growth hormone, and psychosocial dwarfism. [4]

591. B. Bone age determination can distinguish between the two most common causes of short stature: familial short stature and constitutional delay of growth. Children with familial short stature have normal bone ages. Constitutional delay of growth, which is really a delay in reaching ultimate height and sexual maturation, presents with delayed bone age and delayed sexual maturation. [4]

592. C. Inadequate growth in children may be associated with an unfavorable psychologic environment. In this situation, the child may show transiently low human growth hormone levels during periods of stress. They may also have behavioral, sleep, and eating disturbances. Both growth and growth hormone levels return to normal when the psychologic stressors are removed. [4]

593. E. Recommended investigations in a child with failure to thrive or a child in which short stature is unlikely to be familial in nature should include a complete blood count, a urinalysis, serum creatinine, an ESR, serum thyroxine, serum lead level, stool for ova and parasites, and x-rays of the hands and wrists. [4]

SUMMARY OF THE DIAGNOSIS AND TREATMENT OF FAILURE TO THRIVE AND SHORT STATURE

1. **Failure to thrive:**
    a) may be nonorganic (psychologic FTT (maternal deprivation), child neglect, or lack of education or errors in feeding; or organic
    b) treatment: hospitalization, investigation for other causes and unlimited feedings. When the child goes home the parents must be instructed in proper feeding practices and the child must be observed closely

2. **Short stature:**
    a) most common cause: familial short stature
    b) familial short stature can be differented from constitutional delay of growth (the second most common cause) by bone age
    c) other causes of short stature include chromosomal abnormalities, intrauterine growth retardation, hypothyroidism, psychosocial

dwarfism, bioinactive growth hormone, and true growth hormone deficiency

d) investigation of a child with short stature should include complete blood count, urinalysis, serum creatinine, an ESR, serum thyroxine, serum lead level, stool for ova and parasites, and x-rays of the hands and wrists

References

1. Schmitt B, Krugman R. Nonorganic failure to thrive. In: Behrman R, Vaughan V, eds. Nelson's textbook of pediatrics. 13th Ed. Philadelphia: WB Saunders, 1987: 83–84.

2. Frank D, Ziesel S. Failure to thrive. Pediatr Clin North Am 1988; 35(6): 1187–1206.

3. Digeorge A. Turner syndrome. In: Behrman R, Vaughan V, eds. Nelson's textbook of pediatrics. 13th Ed. Philadelphia: WB Saunders, 1987: 1236–1237.

4. Kritzler R, Plotnick L. The short child: a matter of time or cause for concern? Postgrad Med 1985; 78(4): 51–59.

PROBLEM 76 : AN ADOLESCENT GIRL WITH BILATERAL KNEE PAIN AFTER PERIODS OF STRENUOUS ACTIVITY

A 15-year-old girl presents to your office with a 6-month history of bilateral knee pain, which she localizes to the region of the patella. The pain comes on after periods of strenuous activity, especially running, jumping, or squatting, and usually clears with rest. She states that she often develops a sharp pain in her knees after she has been sitting down and gets ups to move, but the pain subsides after a short distance.

On examination, there is bilateral patellar tenderness. On examination, crepitus is felt on flexion and extension when the hand is over the anterior aspect of the patella.

SELECT THE ONE BEST ANSWER TO THE FOLLOWING QUESTIONS:

594. The most likely diagnosis in this patient is:
    a) chondromalacia patellae
    b) patellofemoral arthralgia
    c) Osgood-Schlatter disease
    d) medial meniscal tear
    e) partial collateral ligament disruption

595. Which of the following statements regarding the diagnosis of the condition described in question 594 is/are true?
    a) the knee x-ray is likely to be abnormal
    b) arthrography is the diagnostic tool of choice
    c) arthroscopy provides the most comprehensive evaluation of the condition
    d) a and b
    c) a and c

596. The treatment of choice for the patient described in question 595 is:
    a) serial casting
    b) bilateral osteotomies
    c) rest
    d) quadriceps strengthening
    e) c and d

597. A 14-year-old male presents for assessment of a 6-month history of a painful left knee that is aggrevated by activity and relieved by rest.
    On examination, there is tenderness and pain at the insertion of the patellar tendon and at the adjacent tibial tubercle.
    The most likely diagnosis in this boy is:
    a) osteogenic sarcoma
    b) chrondomalacia patellae
    c) Osgood-Schlatter disease
    d) stress fracture
    e) fracture of the intercondylar eminence of the tibia

598. The treatment of choice for the patient described in question 597 is:
    a) quadriceps strengthening exercises
    b) rest
    c) active physiotherapy
    d) above knee cast
    e) none of the above

ANSWER THE FOLLOWING QUESTIONS ACCORDING TO THE CODE:

A: 1, 2, and 3 are correct
B: 1 and 3 are correct

C: 2 and 4 are correct

D: Only 4 is correct

E: All of the above are correct

599. A mother presents with her 6-year-old boy who has "flat feet." You are the sixth doctor that she has consulted about the case. She has had three different types of custom-molded inserts, three pairs of corrective shoes, and numerous other orthopedic devices.

On physical examination, the child appears to have flat longitudinal arches when viewed from the lateral angle. When viewed from behind, the heels are in mild valgus. When the child stands on tiptoe, the heels roll into varus and an arch is formed.

Which of the following statements regarding this child is/are true?

1) this child has flexible flat feet

2) this child should have a special orthopedic device made to try and strengthen the longitudinal arch

3) no orthopedic devices are needed in the treatment of this child

4) because the heel rolls into varus, some surgical strengthening of the loose ligaments may be required

600. A mother presents to your office with her 6-year-old daughter who has "had growing pains for the past 3 years." These pains appear to be centered in the front of the thighs, in the calves, and behind the knees. The pains are deep and localized in areas distant from the major joints.

The child has, in the past, had numerous x-rays (at least 10), and complete blood evaluations. All have been negative.

On physical examination the child appears healthy. There is no evidence of musculoskeletal disease.

Which of the following statements regarding this child is/are true?

1) this child should go through another "complete work-up"

2) growing pains usually disappear by the age of 6 years

3) a CT scan or an MRI scan should be performed to "rule out" any other pathology

4) reassurance and symptomatic treatment are the only interventions that are indicated in this case

ANSWERS

594. A. This young girl has chondromalacia patella. Chondromalacia, or "softening of the cartilage" results from repetitive trauma from physical activity that induces a strain on the patellofemoral mechanism.[1]

The most common symptom of chondromalacia is pain. The pain typically comes on after periods of strenuous activity and is relieved by rest. Occasionally, the patient will describe knee locking or buckling.[1]

On physical examination, the most specific sign is tenderness on palpating the articular surface of the patella. A grating sensation (crepitus) on knee flexion may be felt. There may be secondary atrophy and weakness of the quadriceps muscle. Limitation of knee movement is unusual.[1]

Osgood-Schlatter's disease will be discussed in a subsequent question.

Meniscal tears and ligament disruptions will be discussed in another chapter in this book.

Patellofemoral arthralgia, although sometimes used synonymously with chondromalacia patella, is a nonspecific term.

595. C. The routine knee x-ray is likely to be normal in a patient with chondromalacia patella. Although arthrography will often demonstrate softened and split articular cartilage, the diagnostic procedure of choice is arthroscopy. Arthroscopy will provide a comprehensive evaluation of the status of the knee joint, by allowing inspection of the articular cartilage of the patella and the associated patellofemoral relationships.[1]

596. E. The treatments of choice for this patient are rest and quadriceps strengthening exercises. The patient should refrain from running, jumping, climbing, and other activities that produce high patellofemoral compressive force. Walking and swimming should be encouraged.

Quadriceps strengthening exercises, in the form of straight-leg raising against increasing amounts of resistance are recommended.

If the condition is severe, a cylinder cast or splint may be indicated. Serial casts, however, are not indicated.[1]

597. C. Osgood-Schlatter disease is a painful enlargement of the tibial tubercle and the insertion of the patellar tendon. It is most likely due to repetitive

stress imposed by the pull of the quadriceps muscle, and is most common in adolescent boys.[1]

The most common symptom is pain in the area of the tibial tubercle that is aggrevated by activity and relieved by rest. On examination, there may be tenderness and swelling of the tibial tubercle and adjacent patellar tendon. [1]

In this case, an x-ray of the knee would rule out osteogenic sarcoma or any fracture.

598. B. Osgood-Schlatter's disease is treated by restriction of physical activity for 2–3 weeks. When activity is resumed, it should be done so gradually.

Above knee casting or surgical excision of an associated tendon ossicle is rarely necessary.[1] Osgood-Schlatter's disease will disappear when growth is completed.

599. B. This child has flexible flat feet. Flexible flat feet are associated with ligamentous laxity, and hyperextendible knees, elbows, and fingers.

If, when standing on tiptoe, an arch forms and the heel rolls into varus, good muscle power in the ankle and foot is confirmed, and no serious problem exists.

Although the treatment of flat feet is controversial, there is no evidence that custom-molded inserts, corrective shoes, or other orthopedic devices are helpful. Ordinary shoes should be worn in the absence of signficant symptoms or severe shoe wear problems. Special shoes should only be recommended when there is associated foot pain, or deformities that cause rapid wearout of the shoe.[2]

600. D. Growing pains in children are intermittent pains or aches that are localized to the muscles of the legs and thighs.[3] Restlessness often accompanies the pain. The most common sites are the front of the thighs, the calves, and behind the knees.[3] The pain is usually described as localized, deep, and bilateral. The pains usually occur at night and awaken the child from sleep. They may be accentuated by increased running during the day.

Growing pains are very common in children and young adolescents. They usually commence before the age of 5 years, are most prominent between the ages of 8 and 12, and disappear when the child reaches maturity.

The pain is not associated with tenderness, erythema, or swelling. Results of physical examination, laboratory studies, and x-rays are normal.

The etiology is unknown.

If after a thorough examination in this child no abnormalities are found, no further investigations should be performed. The parents and the child should be reassured that the pains will eventually disappear. Supportive treatments such as heat, massage, and mild analgesics are the only appropriate treatments.[3]

SUMMARY OF COMMON PEDIATRIC MUSCULOSKELETAL COMPLAINTS

1. **Chondromalacia patella:**
    a) etiology: repetitive trauma: usually from strenuous repetitive activity
    b) chief symptom: pain in region of patella
    c) treatment: rest, quadriceps strengthening exercises

2. **Osgood-Schlatter disease:**
    a) etiology: painful enlargement of tibial tubercle
    b) chief symptoms: pain in region of tibial tubercle and insertion of patellar tendon
    c) treatment: rest

3. **Flexible Flat feet:**
    a) etiology: ligamentous laxity
    b) test for flexibility: conversion from valgus to varus on tiptoe
    c) treatment: reassurance, no "special" orthopedic shoes or inserts necessary

4. **Growing pains:**
    a) definition: intermittent pain or ache, localized to the muscles of legs and thighs and not due to any other cause
    b) treatment: rest, massage, mild analgesics

References

1. Smith J. Knee problems in children. Pediatr Clin North Am 1988; 33(6): 1439–1456.

2. Wenger D, Leach J. Foot deformities in infants and children. Pediatr Clin North Am 1988; 33(6): 1411–1427.

3. Peterson H. Growing pains. Pediatr Clin North Am 1988; 33(6): 1365–1371.

PROBLEM 77: AN ANXIOUS MOTHER WITH A 3-MONTH-OLD INFANT WHO HAS CROOKED FEET

A 3-month-old infant is brought to the office by his mother. She states that he has "crooked feet." She has been told by her friend that he will need a number of casts to correct this.

On examination, the infant's feet deviate laterally. The heel position as viewed from behind with his feet dorsiflexed is valgus.

SELECT THE ONE BEST ANSWER TO THE FOLLOWING QUESTIONS:

601. The most likely diagnosis is this infant is:
    a) calcaneovalgus
    b) metatarsus valgus
    c) metatarsus varus
    d) talipes equinovarus
    e) clubfoot

602. The treatment of choice in this child is:
    a) serial casts
    b) bilateral osteotomies
    c) Dennis-Browne splints
    d) immediate referral to an orthopedic surgeon
    e) reassurance and foot exercises

603. A mother brings her 3-month-old infant into the office concerned about the child's "toeing in." She states that another physician has told her that this will probably require serial casts to correct.

    On physical examination, both feet deviate medially. The feet dorsiflex easily and the heel position is dorsiflexion in valgus.

    The most likely diagnosis in this child is:
    a) calcaneovalgus
    b) metatarsus varus
    c) metatarsus valgus
    d) talipes equinovarus
    e) clubfoot

604. The treatment of choice in this patient is:
    a) serial casts
    b) bilateral osteotomies
    c) Dennis-Browne splints
    d) immediate referral to an orthopedic surgeon
    e) reassurance and foot exercises

605. A mother brings her 15-month-old toddler into your office for an assessment of "his bowlegs." She states that he has been "bowlegged" since he began to walk 3 months ago.

    On examination, the feet point inward while the knees point straight ahead.

    The most likely diagnosis is this child is:
    a) internal tibial torsion
    b) internal femoral torsion
    c) metatarsus varus
    d) fixed tibia varum
    e) calcaneovalgus

606. The treatment of choice in this child is:
    a) serial casts
    b) bilateral osteotomies
    c) Dennis-Browne splints
    d) immediate referral to an orthopedic surgeon
    e) reassurance and leg exercises

ANSWERS

601. A. This child has calcaneovalgus.[1] This is the most common newborn foot deformity. In this deformity the foot folds against the anterolateral surface of the tibia. The deformity will correct spontaneously.

602. E. Although treatment of calcaneovalgus is not necessary, the parents can be encouraged to exercise the foot each time they change the diaper. Reassurance about the benign nature of the condition is most important.[1]

603. B. This child has metatarsus varus. In a child with metatarsus varus, the foot can easily be dorsiflexed (the heel cord is not tight) and when viewed from behind with the forefoot dorsiflexed, the heel is in valgus. A mild clubfoot (talipes equinovarus), on the other hand, cannot be dorsiflexed and the heel remains fixed in varus.[1]

    Metatarsus varsus, which may be unilateral or bilateral, is probably the result of intrauterine position.

604. E. As with calcaneovarus, the treatment of choice for metatarsus varus is reassurance and foot exercises. Foot exercises involve firmly grasping and stabilizing the heel to avoid producing even more heel valgus. The forefoot is stretched laterally.

This exercise should be repeated five times with each diaper change.[1]

If there is any fixation, difficulty in dorsiflexion, or failure to produce heel valgus on dorsiflexion, the child should be referred to an orthopedic surgeon for serial casting.[1]

605. A. This child has internal tibial torsion. Internal tibial torsion is a physiologic bowing of the lower extremities that is produced by the external rotation of the femur and internal rotation of the tibia.[2]

606. E. The treatment of choice for internal tibial torsion is also reassurance and leg exercises. The parents should be assured that this is a transient deformity that will correct itself.[2]

If, after six months, there is still an obvious deformity, the parents can be shown how to externally rotate the tibia in relationship to the long axis of the femur with the knee flexed at 90 degrees. This simple exercise can be performed at each diaper change.

Only if this exercise cannot be effectively performed by the parents should a Dennis-Browne splint be considered.[2]

SUMMARY OF EVALUATION OF FOOT AND LEG DEFORMITIES IN YOUNG CHILDREN

1. **Foot deformities:** Calcaneovalgus (most common), metatarsus varus and talipes equinovarus (clubfoot)

2. **Intoeing in young children:** Three common reasons for in-toeing are: (1) the forepart of the foot is turned medially (metatarsus varus or adductus); (2) the entire foot points inwards while the knee points straight ahead (medial tibial torsion); and (3) the entire leg turns in so that both the knee and the foot are facing medially (medial femoral torsion or increased anteversion of the hips).

3. Treatment of foot and leg deformities in children (except clubfoot): reassurance and passive exercises

References

1. Wenger D, Leach J. Foot deformities in infants and children. Pediatr Clin North Am 1988; 33(6): 1411–1427.

2. Wilkins K. Bowlegs. Pediatr Clin North Am 1988; 33(6): 1429–1438.

PROBLEM 78: A 6-YEAR-OLD BOY WITH A NOSE THAT IS CONSTANTLY RUNNING

A mother presents to your office with her 6-year-old son. She states that for the past 1 year, his nose has been "constantly" running. As you are taking the history, you note that the child is rubbing his nose and eyes.

On examination, after instillation of a vasoconstrictor, the mucosa appears edematous and congested. There is a mucoid material noted in the nasal cavity and on the posterior pharyngeal wall.

SELECT THE ONE BEST ANSWER TO THE FOLLOWING QUESTIONS:

607. The most likely diagnosis in this child is:
a) vasomotor rhinitis
b) allergic rhinitis
c) chronic infectious rhinitis
d) primary atrophic rhinitis
e) eosinophilic nonallergic rhinitis

608. Which of the following immunoglobulins are associated with the condition described in question 607?
a) IgA
b) IgG
c) IgE
d) IgM
e) none of the above

609. The patient lives in a cold climate (Canada). Which of the following would be most likely to be an etiologic factor in this patient's condition?
a) tree pollen
b) grass pollen
c) ragweed
d) nonflowering, wind-pollinated plants
e) house dust/house dust mite

610. The single most important aspect of the treatment of the patient described above is:

a) topical corticosteroids
b) topical disodium cromoglycate
c) systemic antihistamines
d) systemic adrenergic drugs
e) none of the above

ANSWER THE FOLLOWING QUESTIONS ACCORDING TO THE CODE:

A: 1, 2, and 3 are correct
B: 1 and 3 are correct
C: 2 and 4 are correct
D: Only 4 is correct
E: All of the above are correct

611. Which of the following may be useful in the diagnostic evaluation of the patient discussed in question 609?
    1) examination of nasal secretions
    2) epicutaneous prick tests
    3) radioallergosorbent (RAST) tests
    4) CT scan of the nasal and sinus cavities

612. Which of the following topical medications is/are associated with rhinitis medicamentosa?
    1) oxymetazoline
    2) disodium cromoglycate
    3) phenylephrine
    4) beclomethasone

613. Which of the following is/are true regarding the treatment of the condition described above?
    1) H1-receptor antagonists generally do not give satisfactory relief of nasal congestion
    2) a combination of H1 and H2 receptor provides greater relief of nasal congestion than either drug alone
    3) disodium cromoglycate may provide significant relief of nasal congestion
    4) inhaled corticosteroids should not be used for longer than 12 months

614. Which of the following statements regarding immunotherapy is/are correct?
    1) immunotherapy should only be considered for patients who are poorly controlled by optimal modification of the environment
    2) immunotherapy should only be considered for patients who are poorly controlled by optimal pharmacologic management
    3) immunotherapy is based on the development of IgG blocking antibodies

4) immunotherapy is virtually devoid of side effects

ANSWERS

607. B. This child most likely has allergic rhinitis.

Allergic rhinitis is an inflammatory disorder of the nasal mucosa initiated by an IgE- mediated hypersensitivity.[1] It is the most common chronic disease of the respiratory tract.

The symptoms of allergic rhinitis include nasal congestion (stuffy nose), sneezing, itching, and rhinorrhea, nasal discharge, mouth breathing, and snoring.[1] Exposure to cigarette smoke, paint fumes, strong odors, and allergens may precipitate the symptoms.

Physical examination may show an "allergic salute" (rubbing and dorsal manipulation of the nose resulting in a transverse wrinkle externally), edematous and congested nasal mucosa, or "allergic shiners" (obstruction of venous drainage in the periorbital region). Hypertrophied tonsils and adenoids may be seen. Serous otitis media is common. Allergic rhinitis often is associated with atopic dermatitis or asthma.

Eosinophilic nonallergic rhinitis may manifest the same symptoms as allergic rhinitis, but is much less common and may be distinguished by the absence of positive skin tests or radioallergosorbent tests (RAST).

Vasomotor rhinitis is a nonallergic, noninfectious rhinitis characterized by increased parasympathetic activity and pathologic hyperreactivity of the nasal mucosa. It is uncommon in children.

Chronic infectious rhinitis results in mucopurulent rhinorrhea, often associated with low-grade fever, cough, sore throat, and malaise. Sinusitis and recurrent purulent otitis media may be present.

Primary atrophic rhinitis, with autosomal-dominant inheritance, rarely occurs in children.[1]

608. C. IgE is produced as an antibody response to patients with allergic rhinitis.[1]

609. E. This child has had a "constantly running nose" for the last year. Therefore, in a cold climate, the allergen(s) associated with the condition would have to be present all year round. Perennial allergic rhinitis is usually caused by house dust, house dust mite, animal danders, and molds.[1]

Seasonal allergic rhinitis in temperate climates is most often produced by tree pollens, grass pollens, ragweed, and nonflowering, wind-pollinated plants.[1]

Food allergens are unlikely to be associated with chronic allergic rhinitis.

610. E. The single most important factor is the elimination from the environment (as much as possible) of the provoking factor(s) for the allergic rhinitis.[1]

611. A. Examination of nasal secretions for eosinophils is a valuable test for the confirmation of allergic rhinitis.In patients with allergic rhinitis the eosinophil count and the IgE level may also be elevated; however, a normal count does not rule out the diagnosis.[1]

Epicutaneous prick tests, and the measurement of allergen-specific IgE in the patient's serum by the radioallergosorbent test (RAST) may also be helpful in the diagnosis of allergic rhinitis.[1]

A CT scan of the nasal cavity and sinuses is not a reasonable test for the evaluation of allergic rhinitis.

612. B. Rhinitis medicamentosa results from prolonged overuse of drugs that have a pronounced vasoconstrictive effect on the nasal mucosa, such as the topical imidazoline derivatives naphazoline, oxymetazoline, or xylometazoline; or the phenylamines, phenylephrine or ephedrine, or cocaine.[1] As well, the prolonged use of vasoconstrictors will eventually result in "rebound congestion" in which the nasal mucosa rebounds to a more congested state after the effect of the vasoconstrictor has worn off.

Disodium cromoglycate and beclomethasone are not associated with rhinitis medicamentosa or rebound congestion.[1]

613. B. H1-receptor antagonists (such as chlorotripolon, terfenadine, astemizole) generally do not provide satisfactory relief of nasal congestion in children. A combination of an H-1 receptor antagonist and an H-2 receptor antagonist does not produce greater relief from nasal congestion than either agent alone; the combination is not recommended in children.[1]

Sodium cromoglycate suppresses antigen-induced mediator release and may provide significant relief of nasal congestion.[1]

The inhaled synthetic glucocorticosteroids like beclomethasone are very effective in the treatment of both seasonal and perennial allergic rhinitis. They are the most potent drugs available for relief of seasonal and perennial allergic rhinitis symptoms.[1]

614. A. Immunotherapy should only be considered for patients who are poorly controlled by other methods such as environmental manipulation and pharmacologic therapy.[1]

Immunotherapy consists of a series of injections of increasing doses of specific antigens identified on the basis of the patient's history, and the results of skin and RAST tests.

Immunotherapy has multiple immunologic effects, but the main effect is through the production of an antigen-specific IgG blocking antibody.[1]

The duration of treatment required is not well defined. A 1–2 year trial of therapy seems reasonable. If signficant improvement occurs, the patient may continue for 3–5 years before reevaluation.

Adverse effects from immunotherapy including anaphylaxis and serum sickness do occur. Patients should wait for at least 20 min in the physician's office after receiving an allergy shot.

SUMMARY OF THE DIAGNOSIS AND TREATMENT OF ALLERGIC RHINITIS

1. Allergic rhinitis is the most common chronic disease of the respiratory tract.

2. **Symptoms:** Nasal congestion (stuffy nose), sneezing, itching, and rhinorrhea or nasal discharge.

3. **Diagnosis:** History is most important. Confirmation by physical examination, examination of nasal smear for eosinophils, and epicutaneous and RAST tests.

4. **Treatment:** Most important treatment is the avoidance, whenever possible, of sensitizing allergens.
Pharmacologic treatment:
a) intranasal disodium cromoglycate
b) intranasal synthetic glucocorticosteroids
c) systemic antihistamines (do not substantially relieve nasal stuffiness)
d) adrenergic agents: (1) topical agents may cause rhinitisa medicamentosa and rebound congestion
e) oral agents have significant side effects and should only be used on a short term basis
f) immunotherapy: should be considered only when symptoms are poorly controlled by op-

timal modification of the environment and optimal pharmacologic management

Reference

1. Simons F. Allergic rhinitis: recent advances. Pediatr Clin North Am 1988; 35(5): 1053–1071.

PROBLEM 79: A 6-MONTH-OLD INFANT WHO FELL OFF A SOFA AND FRACTURED HIS HUMERUS

A 6-month-old infant presents to the hospital emergency room with his mother. She says that he fell off the sofa this evening and injured his right arm.

On examination, the infant has a swollen, bruised right arm. An x-ray reveals a spiral fracture of the right humerus. The remainder of the physical examination is normal. The mother says that the child has been well since birth, and has had no significant medical illnesses.

SELECT THE ONE BEST ANSWER TO THE FOLLOWING QUESTIONS:

615. Given the history, physical examination, and x-ray report you should now:
    a) obtain an orthopedic consultation
    b) prescribe a sling for the child's arm
    c) investigate the child for possible osteogenesis imperfecta
    d) suggest that the mother purchase a walker instead of laying her child on a sofa
    e) discuss the details of the incident more fully with the mother and contact the hospital social worker

616. After your initial intervention or recommendation, you should then:
    a) ask the mother to return with the child for follow-up in 3 weeks
    b) ask the mother to return with the child for follow-up in 1 week
    c) arrange for the family physician to see the child at home the next day
    d) hospitalize the child
    e) none of the above

617. A 1-year-old child is admitted to the hospital for investigation of failure to thrive. The child's weight is below the 5th percentile for age. The child appears scared and clings to anyone who is present in his room. His mother says that "there is something wrong with him," and she can't understand why she "had to get a kid like this."

    Apart from being below the 5th percentile for weight, no other abnormalities are found on physical examination. A complete blood count, urinalysis and electrolytes are within normal limits.

The most likely diagnosis for this child's behavior is:
    a) the "white-coat syndrome"
    b) psychotic depression
    c) child abuse or neglect
    d) childhood schizophrenia
    e) acute paranoia of childhood

618. If your diagnosis is correct for the child described in question 615, you would except that the child:
    a) will not gain significant weight during the initial hospitalization period
    b) will gain weight slowly during the initial hospitalization period
    c) will gain weight during the initial hospitalization period only if put on a signficant antipsychotic agent
    d) will gain weight quickly during the initial hospitalization period
    e) will lose weight during the initial hospitalization period

619. Which one of the following statements most accurately reflects the situation in a family in which there has been documented child abuse?
    a) in most cases the child has to be permanently removed from the family
    b) rehabilitation of parents that have been involved in child abuse is usually unsuccessful
    c) with comprehensive, intensive treatment of the entire family, 80–90% of families involved in child abuse or neglect can be rehabilitated
    d) in most cases, child abuse will have a lasting, permanent effect on the child's personality
    e) in a situation in which one child in a family has been abused, there is usually no increased risk to other children in the family

ANSWER THE FOLLOWING QUESTIONS ACCORDING TO THE CODE:

A: 1, 2, and 3 are correct
B: 1 and 3 are correct
C: 2 and 4 are correct
D: Only 4 is correct
E: All of the above are correct

620. Which of the following statements regarding child abuse and spousal abuse is true?
    a) women who are abused are unlikely to abuse their children
    b) men who abuse there wives are unlikely to abuse their children
    c) men who abuse their wives are much more likely to abuse their children than men who do not
    d) there is no correlation between the various forms of family violence
    e) parents who abuse their children are unlikely to have come from families in which abuse occurred.

621. Which of the following is/are clues to the diagnosis of child abuse or neglect?
    1) discrepant history
    2) delay in seeking care
    3) family crisis
    4) higher socioeconomic class

622. An 8-month-old child presents to the hospital emergency room with a large burn in the shape of an iron on his buttocks. The child's father states that the child dropped the iron on himself as he was reaching for his toys. As the casualty officer in charge, your next step(s) would be to:
    1) treat the burn and contact the hospital social worker
    2) call the police and have the father arrested
    3) try to obtain a more detailed history of the child's present injury and his previous health
    4) use a confrontation approach and accuse the father of concealing information and abusing the child

623. Child abuse or neglect includes which of the following:
    1) physical abuse
    2) physical neglect
    3) sexual abuse
    4) emotional neglect

ANSWERS

615. E. This child is a victim of child abuse. Child abuse is defined as any maltreatment of children or adolescents by their parents, guardians, or other caretakers.[1] The definition includes physical abuse, sexual abuse, physical neglect, medical neglect, emotional abuse, and emotional neglect.[1]

    The physician must be able to distinguish accidental from nonaccidental injury. Clues to nonaccidental injury include:[1]
    1) A discrepant history: The explanation given by the parents or significant other does not fit the pattern and severity of the medical findings. Thus, the "baby rolling off the sofa" is a totally inadequate explanation for a fractured humerus.
    2) A delay in seeking care
    3) A concurrent family crisis
    4) A triggering behavior such as excessive crying
    5) Unrealistic expectations of the child
    6) Increasing severity of injuries
    7) A history of the parent(s) being abused as children
    8) Families that are socially isolated
    The treatment of the fracture itself, although important, is not the highest priority. An orthopedic consultation may be appropriate, depending on the severity of the fracture.

    It would be inappropriate to suggest the purchase of a walker at the best of times as this is associated with an increased incidence of falls and injuries.

    There are no associated findings to suggest the diagnosis of osteogenesis imperfecta.

616. D. If you suspect that a child has been abused or neglected, the child should be hospitalized. This removes the child to a safe environment and permits time for a complete evaluation.[1] A complete evaluation should include a skeletal survey.

617. C. The most likely diagnosis in this child is child abuse or neglect. Child abuse or neglect is one of the most common causes of failure to thrive.[1,2]

618. D. A child with failure to thrive, which is suspected to be due to neglect, should be hospitalized for 1 week and given unlimited feedings. The child should gain significant weight during the initial hospitalization period.

619. C. With comprehensive, intensive treatment of the entire family, 80–90% of families involved in child abuse or neglect (excluding incest) can be rehabilitated to provide adequate care for their children. Approximately 10–15% of such families can only be stabilized, and will require an indefinite continuation of support services until the child is independent. In only 2–3% of cases is termination of parental rights or continued foster care necessary.[1]

620. C. Men who abuse their wives are more likely to abuse their children than men who do not.

Women who are abused are also more likely to abuse their children than women who do not.

Parents who abuse their children are more likely than not to have come from nuclear families in which abuse occurred. In many cases, they were abused themselves. In other cases, they witnessed abuse of their mother by their father.[3]

621. A. Child abuse or neglect is increased in lower socioeconomic groups. See the critique of question 615 for a more detailed explanation of the clues to diagnosis.

622. B. The most appropriate step in the situation would be to determine as accurately as possible the circumstances surrounding the accident. If possible, the other parent should be interviewed as well. It is also appropriate to contact the hospital social worker who will go about reporting the case to the authorities.

It is unwise to use a confrontational approach in dealing with the father. Accusations almost guarantee a poor outcome.[1]

623. E. The definition of child abuse includes physical abuse, physical neglect, sexual abuse, and emotional neglect.[1]

SUMMARY OF THE DIAGNOSIS AND TREATMENT OF CHILD ABUSE

1. Suspect child abuse if there is a discrepant history, a delay in seeking care, a crisis, a trigger factor, unrealistic expectations of the child, increasing severity of injuries, a parent who was abused as a child, and families that are isolated.

2. In cases of physical abuse and neglect hospitalize the child for safety and for complete assessment of her injuries.

3. In most cases of physical abuse and neglect rehabilitation is possible; it is unlikely that the child will have to be placed in a foster home.

References

1. Krugman R. Child abuse and neglect. Prim Care 1984; 11(3): 527–534.

2. Schmitt B, Krugman R. Child abuse and neglect. In: Behrman R, Vaughan V, eds. Nelson's textbook of pediatrics. 13th Ed. Philadelphia: WB Saunders, 1987: 79–84.

3. Swanson R. Battered wife syndrome. Can Med Assoc J 1984; 130: 709–713.

PROBLEM 80: A 3-YEAR-OLD CHILD WITH A HEART MURMUR

A 3-year-old child is brought to your office for a complete physical examination. The child has been well and has no history of significant medical illness. He has reached all of his developmental milestones.

On physical examination he is found to have a Grade I/VI systolic heart murmur heard maximally along the left sternal edge. There is no radiation of the murmur. The child's pulse is 84/minute and regular. The femoral artery pulses are normal. The blood pressure is 90/70 mm Hg. You suspect an "innocent systolic murmur."

SELECT THE ONE BEST ANSWER TO THE FOLLOWING QUESTIONS:

624. Which of the following signs or symptoms IS NOT associated with an innocent cardiac murmur?

a) low frequency
b) an associated thrill
c) short ejection systolic
d) grade I or II
e) increases with increasing heart rate

625. At this time, which of the following investigations should be done on the child discussed in question 624?
   a) CXR
   b) ECG
   c) echocardiogram
   d) a and b
   e) all of the above

626. The results of the investigations performed are normal. At this time, you should tell the mother that:
   a) the child has a heart murmur, but you think everything is all right
   b) the child has a heart murmur, but you will watch it carefully
   c) the heart sound that you hear is innocent and is a very common occurrence in over half of all the healthy children that you see
   d) the child has a heart murmur that will require extensive further testing
   e) you should tell the mother nothing

627. An 18-month-old infant is brought in for a complete assessement. You have not seen the child before, as the family has just moved into the area. The mother states that the child has been well, and has had no medical problems.

   On examination, the child has a Grade III/VI systolic murmur heard along the left sternal edge. There is no radiation of the murmur. The heart rate is 72/min and regular. There is no thrill palpable. The blood pressure is 80/60 mm Hg.

   At this time, which of the following investigations should be performed on this infant?
   a) CXR
   b) ECG
   c) echocardiogram
   d) a and b
   e) all of the above

628. The frequency of cardiac murmurs in childhood is:
   a) 5%
   b) 10%
   c) 20%
   d) 50%
   e) 90%

629. The most common congenital heart lesion in childhood is:
   a) atrial septal defect
   b) tetralogy of Fallot
   c) ventricular septal defect

   d) transposition of the great arteries
   e) aortic stenosis

ANSWER THE FOLLOWING QUESTION ACCORDING TO THE CODE:

A: 1, 2, and 3 are correct
B: 1 and 3 are correct
C: 2 and 4 are correct
D: Only 4 is correct
E: All of the above are correct

630. Which of the following is/are common innocent cardiac murmurs in infancy and childhood?
   1) neonatal pulmonary artery branch murmur
   2) venous hum of late infancy
   3) Still's aortic vibratory murmur
   4) pulmonary valve area "flow" murmur

ANSWERS

624. B. The characteristics of an innocent cardiac murmur are: (1) low frequency, (2) short systolic ejection murmur, (3) localized murmur, and (4) accentuation with heart rate. An innocent cardiac murmur is never associated with a thrill.[1]

625. D. A child between the ages of 1 and 5 who is found to have a heart murmur of intensity ≤2, and who you suspect has an innocent murmur, should have a CXR and ECG performed. An echocardiogram is not necessary. Clinical examination, along with a CXR and an ECG is a sufficiently sensitive screening examination to rule out cardiac disease.[1]

626. C. The parents should be told that a heart murmur has been heard and that your investigations confirm your impression that this is simply a common heart sound heard in at least one-half of normal children.[1–3]

   The way the information is delivered is critical. You want to tell the parents that their child has a clinical finding that on investigation is not significant; this will ensure that the parents do not worry unnecessarily.

   It is not appropriate to tell the parents nothing; if you do not mention the heart murmur, some other physician very likely will and the parents will question you as to why you did not tell them.

627. E. In an infant with a heart murmur that is greater than Grade II/VI, an echocardiogram probably

should be added to the routine investigations of CXR and ECG. This is a sensitive investigation that will allow differentiation of an innocent from a pathologic murmur.[1]

628. D. The frequency of cardiac murmurs in children is at least 50%. To the sensitive ear, the prevalence may be substantially higher.[1]

629. C. The most common organic cardiac murmur in childhood is a ventricular septal defect.[1] Ventricular septal defects are usually silent at birth, and are first heard on the discharge examination or at the first well-baby examination.[1]

630. E. The common functional or innocent cardiac murmurs of infancy and childhood are (1) neonatal pulmonary artery branch murmur, (2) venous hum of late infancy and early childhood, (3) Still's aortic vibratory systolic murmur, and (4) pulmonary valve area "flow" murmur of late childhood and adolescence.[2]

SUMMARY OF THE DIAGNOSIS AND INVESTIGATION OF CHILDHOOD CARDIAC MURMURS

1. **Prevalence of childhood cardiac murmurs**: At least 50%

2. Clinical assessment is a sensitive test for distinguishing innocent from pathologic murmurs.

3. **Investigation:**
   a) newborn–1 year:
      intensity ≤ II/VI: Review in 3 months
      intensity > II/VI:
      i) without a thrill: CXR/ECG—if normal review in 3 months
      ii) with a thrill: refer to pediatric cardiologist
   b) age 1–age 5:
      intensity ≤ II/VI: pulses, BP, CXR, ECG. If normal see annually
      intensity > II/VI: as above plus echocardiogram
      If any abnormalities refer to pediatric cardiologist
   c) age greater than 5:
      check pulses, BP, CXR, ECG, echocardiogram
      If any abnormalities refer to pediatric cardiologist

References

1. Duncan W. Childhood cardiac murmurs. Innocent of not? Can Fam Physician 1985; 31: 1047–1049.

2. McNamara D. The pediatrician and the innocent heart murmur. Am J Dis Child 1987; 141: 1161.

3. Hersher L. Avoiding anxiety about 'innocent' heart murmur. Am J Dis Child 1988; 142: 586–587.

PROBLEM 81:   A 6-WEEK-OLD INFANT WHO CRIES AT LEAST 5 HOURS A DAY

An anxious mother presents with her 6-week-old baby. She states that he is is "constantly crying." When questioned carefully concerning the child's history, she states that her infant cries at least 5 hours a day, mostly between the hours of 3 PM and 12 midnight. The crying began at age 2 weeks. This crying does not seem to be associated with any particular activities, including feeding. She says that there is nothing she can do to improve it.

The infant smiles at you when being examined. There are no abnormalities found on physical examination.

SELECT THE ONE BEST ANSWER TO THE FOLLOWING QUESTIONS:

631. The most likely cause of this child's excessive crying is:
   a) infantile psychiatric disturbance
   b) infantile colic
   c) early otitis media
   d) occult intestinal obstruction
   e) parental tension

632. The problem discussed above is common in infants until the age of:
   a) 6 weeks
   b) 3–4 months
   c) 6 months
   d) 9 months
   e) 1 year

ANSWER THE FOLLOWING QUESTIONS
ACCORDING TO THE CODE:

A: 1, 2, and 3 are correct
B: 1 and 3 are correct
C: 2 and 4 are correct
D: Only 4 is correct
E: All of the above are correct

633. Which of the following have been suggested as
etiologies of the condition described above?
1) protein allergy
2) parental tension
3) interaction between parents and child
4) functional causes

634. Which of the following conditions must be considered in the differential diagnosis of the condition discussed above?
1) urinary tract infection
2) intussusception
3) constipation
4) milk allergy

635. Which of the following have been shown to be
effective in the treatment of the disorder discussed
above?
1) dietary modifications
2) reassurance
3) antihistamines
4) application of heat to the abdomen

ANSWERS

631. B. This child has infantile colic.

Colic typically begins in the first 3 weeks of life
and may be seen as early as 3 days. Patients are
usually substantially better by 3 or 4 months of age.

Infantile colic can be defined as a syndrome of
unexplained paroxsyms of irritability, fussing, or
crying that may develop into agonizing screaming
in a child under the age of 6 months, which is not
due to other organic causes.[1] These episodes must
be excessive (probably greater than 3 or 4 hours in
a 24-hour period) before the diagnosis of colic can
be made.[2] In this child, there were no abnormalities
on physical examination to suggest otitis media or
intestinal obstruction.

Parental tension has been discussed as a potential cause for colic, but has not been shown to be
significant.

Infantile psychiatric disturbance is not a diagnosis.

632. B. Infantile colic is usually substantially improved
by 3 to 4 months of age.[1]

633. E. All of the above.

Protein allergy, parental tension, infant-parent
interaction, and functional causes have all been
suggested as potential causes of infantile colic.[1]
The evidence for all of these theories is tenuous.
Also, there appears to be difference between
breast- and bottle-fed infants in the incidence of
infantile colic. When parents ask, the best response
is: "we really don't know what causes colic."

634. E. The differential diagnosis of infantile colic infectious causes, especially urinary tract infections;
infantile seizures; abdominal obstruction including intussusception and volvulus; acute appendicitis; gastroesophageal reflux; milk allergy;
lactose intolerance; and constipation.[1] Before a
diagnosis of colic is made, these conditions should
be ruled out by a careful history and physical
examination.

635. C. Reassurance about the benign, self-limited nature of infantile colic is the cornerstone of therapy.
Specific suggestions for managing severe episodes
of infantile colic include introducing a well-
greased rectal thermometer to break rectal spasm
and allow the passage of gas; applying heat to the
abdomen (warm bath or warm water bottle
wrapped in a towel); only bottle feeding in the
upright position to avoid swallowing air; limiting
breast-feeding to 10 min on each side with frequent
burping; and walking the child or taking the child
for a car ride.[1]

Dietary alterations have little beneficial effect
in the treatment of infantile colic.[1]

Pharmacologic agents such as anticholinergics,
antispasmodics, barbiturates, antiflatuents, and
sedatives should not be used in the treatment of
infantile colic. There is no evidence that they work,
and they all have the potential for serious side
effects in a young infant.[1] Acetaminophen may
provide sympomatic relief.

SUMMARY OF THE DIAGNOSIS AND
TREATMENT OF INFANTILE COLIC

1. **Diagnosis:** Unexplained paroxysms of irritability,
fussing, or crying that may develop into agonizing
screaming in a child under the age of 6 months,
which is not due to any organic cause. The duration

of these episodes must be clearly excessive (greater than 3 or 4 hours/day).

2. **Treatment:**
   a) reassurance: usually significantly improves by 3–4 months
   b) specific suggestions: relief of intestinal gas with a rectal thermometer, application of heat to the abdomen, bottle feed in the upright position, avoiding breastfeeding longer than 10 minutes on each side, walking the child, or taking the child for a car ride.

c) avoid medications other than acetaminophen.

References

1. Adams L, Davidson M. Present concepts of infant colic. Pediatr Ann 1987; 16(10): 817–820.

2. Hunziker U, Barr R. Increased carrying reduces infant crying. A randomized controlled trial. Pediatrics 1986;77: 641–647.

PROBLEM 82: A 2-MONTH-OLD INFANT WITH A RASH ON HIS CHEEKS

A 2-month-old infant presents to your office with his mother. He developed a erythematous, dry, skin rash on both cheeks 1 week ago. Apparently, the rash becomes worse after feeding. The child was breast-fed for 4 weeks but the mother decided to switch him to whole milk at that time.

On examination, the child appears healthy. He has an erythematous eruption that covers both cheeks. He appears to be developing erythematous, dry, patches on his neck, both wrists, and both hands. The rest of the physical examination is normal.

SELECT THE ONE BEST ANSWER TO THE FOLLOWING QUESTIONS:

636. The most likely diagnosis in this infant is:
   a) atopic dermatitis
   b) allergic contact dermatitis
   c) seborrheic dermatitis
   d) infectious eczematoid dermatitis
   e) none of the above

637. Recommended treatment of the infant discussed in question 636 may include:
   a) wet dressings
   b) local corticosteroid therapy
   c) systemic antihistamines
   d) antibiotics
   e) all of the above

638. A 1-month-old infant is brought into your office by his mother. She says the infant has had a "diaper rash" for the past 2 weeks that has not cleared up with zinc oxide paste. She feels she is "doing something wrong" and is extremely upset.

On examination the infant has an erythematous, weeping, oily eruption in the diaper area. As well, he has a scaly eruption on the scalp, involving the ear and contiguous skin, the sides of the nose, and the eyebrows and eyelids. The rest of the physical examination is normal.

The most likely diagnosis in this infant is:
   a) atopic dermatitis
   b) allergic contact dermatitis
   c) seborrheic dermatitis
   d) infectious eczematoid dermatitis
   e) none of the above

639. The treatment(s) of choice for the condition described in question 638 is/are:
   a) wet compresses
   b) topical corticosteroids
   c) topical ketoconazole
   d) a and b
   e) all of the above

640. An 8-month-old infant presents to your office with a diaper rash. His mother has tried corn starch, talcum powder, vitamin E cream, zinc oxide, and three different prescribed corticosteroid creams. In frustration, she is coming to you for a second opinion.

On examination, the infant has an intensely erythematous diaper dermatitis that has a scalloped border and a sharply demarcated edge. There are numerous "satellite lesions" present on the lower abdomen and thighs.

The most likely diagnosis in this infant is:
   a) atopic dermatitis
   b) allergic contact dermatitis

c) seborrheic dermatitis
d) infectious eczematoid dermatitis
e) none of the above

641. The treatment of choice in this infant is a:
a) topical corticosteroid
b) topical antibiotic
c) systemic antibiotic
d) topical antifungal
e) none of the above

642. A 4-month-old infant is brought to your office by her mother. Her mother complains the child has a "diaper rash" that is probably related to "her lack of changing by the babysitter." Apparently, the infant would be wet for long periods of time while the babysitter sat on the couch watching television. Needless to say, the babysitter is no longer employed.

On examination, the infant has a erythematous, scaly, papulovesicular diaper dermatitis with numerous bullous lesions, fissures, and erosions.

The most likely diagnosis is this infant is:
a) atopic dermatitis
b) primary irritant contact dermatitis
c) seborrheic dermatitis
d) fungal dermatitis
e) allergic contact dermatitis

643. The treatment(s) of choice for this dermatitis is(are):
a) zinc oxide paste
b) topical hydrocortisone
c) systemic antibiotics
d) a and b
e) all of the above

ANSWERS

636. A. This child has atopic dermatitis. Atopic dermatitis is an inflammatory skin disease characterized by erythema, edema, pruritis, exudation, crusting, and scaling.[1]

Atopic dermatitis usually begins in infancy. The areas most affected include the cheeks, neck, wrists, hands, and extensor aspects of the extremities. Spread to the flexural areas usually occurs later. Pruritis may lead to intense scratching and secondary infection.

Atopic dermatitis may be precipitated by or exacerbated by the introduction of certain foods into the infant's diet, particularly cow's milk, wheat, or eggs. Environmental factors such as dust,

mold, cat dander etc. may also trigger the condition.[1]

Generally, a remission begins by 3–5 years of age. There is often a family history of asthma, hay fever, or atopic dermatitis.

Serum IgE concentrations are usually elevated.

The other common forms of infant dermatitis will be discussed in subsequent questions.

637. E. The treatment of atopic dermatitis begins with the avoidance of environmental factors that precipitate or aggrevate the condition. Allergens, including foods, that aggrevate the condition should be avoided.[1]

A warm climate of moderate humidity is optimal for the majority of patients.

Garments should be made of a smooth-textured cotton; wool should be avoided.

The use of soaps and detergents that defat the skin should be avoided whenever possible. Bathing without the addition of a bath oil should be avoided. Ideally, the child should be in the tub for at least 15 minutes before the bath oil is added to the water.[1]

Atopic dermatitis is best managed with local therapy. Flare-ups of the disease are best managed with wet dressings (e.g., aluminum acetate 1:20). As well as providing symptomatic relief, wet dressings immobilize and protect the affected parts and prevent scratching. In addition, the fingernails should be kept cut short.[1]

Topical corticosteroid creams or lotions can be applied between dressing changes. Percutaneous absorption of corticosteroid does occur, and atrophy of the skin should be watched for.

Systemic antihistamines such as diphenhydramine, promethazine, and hydroxyzine may have to be used to control pruritis. As discussed in another chapter, these agents can be toxic to young children and should be used with extreme caution.

Infected atopic dermatitis is best managed by antibiotic therapy. Systemic antibiotics have, in the past, been the mainstay of treatment. However, with the introduction of newer, nonsensitizing local antibiotic preparations such as fusidic acid, the need for systemic antibiotics has significantly decreased.

638. C. This infant has seborrheic dermatitis.

Seborrheic dermatitis is an inflammatory disorder that often begins in the first month of life. The initial manifestation of the condition is often a diffuse or focal scaling and crusting of the scalp, often known as "cradle cap." A dry, scaly, erythematous, papular dermatitis, which is usually nonpruritic, may develop to involve the face, neck, retroauricular areas, axillae, and diaper area. The dermatitis may be patchy or focal, or may spread to involve almost the entire body.[2]

639. E. Wet compresses are an effective first line of treatment for seborrheic dermatitis. A soft brush can be used to remove some of the scales associated with "cradle cap." Scalp lesions may also be controlled with an antiseborrheic shampoo, such as selenium sulfide.

Topical corticosteroids (hydrocortisone 1%), may be applied to inflammatory lesions.[2] Recently, the use of topical ketoconazole (2%) has been shown to be effective in the treatment of seborrheic dermatitis.

640. E. This infant has candidal diaper dermatitis.

Candidal diaper dermatitis presents as an erythematous confluent plaque, formed by papules and vesiculopustules, with a scalloped border and a sharply demarcated edge. Candidal diaper dermatitis can usually be distinguished from other childhood diaper dermatoses by the presence of "satellite lesions" that are produced at some distance from the primary eruption.[3]

641. D. The treatment of choice in this infant is a topical antifungal agent. Topical miconazole, clotrimazole, or ketoconazole can be used after soaking the inflamed area with wet aluminum acetate compresses.[3] In an infant with a severe inflammatory reaction, a topical corticosteroid may be mixed 50/50 with a topical antifungal agent and applied on a regular basis for a few days.

642. B. This child has a primary irritant contact dermatitis.

Irritant contact dermatitis is a reaction to friction, maceration, and prolonged contact with urine and feces. It usually presents as an erythematous, scaly, dermatitis with papulovesicular or bullous lesions, fissures, and erosions. The eruption can be either patchy or confluent. The genitocrural folds are often spared. Secondary infection with either bacteria or yeasts can occur. The infant can be in considerable discomfort because of the marked inflammatory reaction that is sometimes associated with this type of diaper rash.[1]

643. D. Diaper dermatitis should be managed by frequent changing of diapers and thorough washing of the genitalia with warm water and a mild soap. Occlusive plastic pants that promote maceration should be avoided. Disposable diapers should be used instead of cloth diapers.

An occlusive topical agent such as zinc oxide or petroleum jelly should be applied after washing. A mild hydrocortisone cream with or without zinc oxide can be applied until healing occurs. Systemic antibiotics are not indicated in the treatment of primary irritant dermatitis.

SUMMARY OF THE DIAGNOSIS AND TREATMENT OF CERTAIN INFANTILE SKIN AND DIAPER RASHES

1. **Atopic dermatitis**: Diagnostic clue: usually begins or is more prominent on the cheeks of infants. Treatment: wet dressings, moisturization, topical corticosteroids, systemic antihistamines (with caution), and topical antibiotics for secondary infection

2. **Seborrheic dermatitis**: Diagnostic clue: " cradle cap" is often associated with diaper dermatitis. Treatment: wet compresses, topical hydrocortisone, topical ketoconazole

3. **Candidal dermatitis**: Diagnostic clue: "satellite lesions." Treatment: topical miconazole, topical ketoconazole. Topical hydrocortisone can be mixed 50/50 when severe inflammation present

4. **Primary irritant dermatitis**: Diagnostic clue: maceration, often a history of the use of cloth diapers and/or plastic pants. Treatment: occlusive topical agent such as zinc oxide or petroleum jelly. With severe inflammation, zinc oxide can be applied over hydrocortisone base.

References

1. Ellis E. Atopic dermatitis. In: Behrman R, Vaughan V, eds. Nelson's textbook of pediatrics. 13th Ed. Philadelphia: WB Saunders, 1987: 501–504.

2. Esterley N. Eczema. In: Behrman R, Vaughan V, eds. Nelson's textbook of pediatrics. 13th Ed. Philadelphia: WB Saunders, 1987: 1404-1407.

3. Esterley N. Candidal infections. In: Behrman R, Vaughan V, eds. Nelson's textbook of pediatrics. 13th Ed. Philadelphia: WB Saunders, 1987: 1434-1435.

PROBLEM 83: A 6-YEAR-OLD CHILD WITH ENURESIS

A mother presents to the office with her 6-year-old boy. The child is, and always has been, enuretic at night. The child has no other significant past medical history. Specifically, the child has no history of urinary tract infections or other urinary tract disease.

The child appears healthy. There are no abnormalities found on physical examination.

SELECT THE ONE BEST ANSWER TO THE FOLLOWING QUESTIONS:

644. Which of the following statements regarding enuresis is FALSE?
    a) at age 6 years 10% of children are enuretic
    b) enuresis is more common in children of whom one or both parents were enuretic
    c) the functional bladder capacity in enuretic children is significantly less than normal
    d) enuresis usually implies significant psycho-pathology in the child
    e) urethral valves, neurogenic bladder, and ectopic ureter may be associated with enuresis

645. A child is defined as enuretic if he has not attained full bladder control by the age of:
    a) 3 years
    b) 4 years
    c) 5 years
    d) 6 years
    e) 8 years

646. Which of the following investigations is the MOST IMPORTANT investigation to be done in a child with enuresis?
    a) urinalysis
    b) urine culture
    c) complete blood count
    d) complete cystometric evaluation
    e) intravenous pyelogram

647. Which of the following statements most accurately reflects the treatment of enuresis?
    a) most therapies have been shown to be superior to placebo
    b) behavior modification has been shown to be superior to all other therapies
    c) pharmacologic therapy is superior to all other therapies

    d) because of the high spontaneous remission rate, and the high placebo improvement rate, the efficacy of therapy has been difficult to prove
    e) because of the lack of efficacy, no treatment can be recommended in the persistently enuretic child

648. Pharmacologic treatment is sometimes effective in treating enuresis that does not spontaneously regress, and for which education and supportive counseling is not sufficient. Which of the following medications is the treatment of choice in this situation?
    a) Ditropan
    b) imipramine
    c) chloropheniramine
    d) diazepam
    e) hydroxyzine

ANSWER THE FOLLOWING QUESTIONS ACCORDING TO THE CODE:

A: 1, 2, and 3 are correct
B: 1 and 3 are correct
C: 2 and 4 are correct
D: Only 4 is correct
E: All of the above are correct

649. Which of the following is/are correct regarding behavior modification approaches to the treatment of enuresis?
    1) behavior modification programs can increase bladder capacity
    2) behavior modification programs are enhanced by responsibility reinforcement programs
    3) a urinary alarm system may be part of a behavior modification program
    4) with behavior modification programs the child is rewarded for having a dry night

650. In supportive counseling of parents of children with enuresis, which of the following approaches is/are suggested?
    1) provide information about the high prevalence rate
    2) provide information about the high spontaneous cure rate
    3) provide information about the unconscious nature of enuresis
    4) encourage the child to keep a journal or chart

ANSWERS

644. D. Enuresis is defined as the involuntary discharge of urine after the age of which bladder control should usually have been established.[1] Enuresis is defined as nocturnal if it only occurs at night and diurnal if it occurs both during the day and night. It is defined as 'primary' if the child has never been dry and 'secondary' if the child has had at least one 3-month period of dryness. The prevalence of enuresis is 12–25% at 4 years, 10–13% at 6 years, 7–10% at 8 years, 3–5% at 10 years, 2–3% at 12 years, and 1–3% at 14 years.

    Enuresis is more common in children of which one or both parents were enuretic.

    There appears to be a developmental immaturity leading to decreased functional bladder capacity in enuretic children.[2]

    Uropathies may be associated with enuresis. Urethral valves, neurogenic bladder, and ectopic ureter may occasionally be the cause of primary enuresis.

    Urinary tract infections are a more common organic cause of enuresis, especially of secondary enuresis in girls. Although psychologic factors have been implicated as a cause of enuresis in some children, there does not appear to be a cause and effect relationship between enuresis and various forms of serious psychopathology in children.[2]

645. C. A child is defined as enuretic if he has not attained full bladder control by the age of 5 years.[1] After the age of 5 years, 15% of the nocturnal enuretics convert per year to dryness.

646. A. The only laboratory evaluation that is mandatory in every enuretic child is a urinalysis.[2] White blood cells in urinary tract infection, low specific gravity in diabetes insipidus, proteinuria or hematuria in kidney disease, and glycosuria in diabetes mellitus, are important abnormalities that may be associated with enuresis. Urine culture, complete blood count, intravenous pyelogram and cystometric evaluation should be performed if there are specific indications from the history or physical examination.

647. D. Because of the high spontaneous remission rate and the high rate of improvement on placebo medication, the efficacy of therapy has been difficult to prove. No treatment has been consistently shown to be superior to placebo. However, numerous therapies do exist; these include pharmacologic therapy, behavior modification therapy, and alarm systems.[2]

648. B. At this time, a tricyclic antidepressant is the pharmacologic treatment of choice for enuresis. The most commonly used agents are imipramine and amitriptyline. The alpha- and beta-adrenergic stimulation that occurs with these agents may increase the functional bladder capacity of the enuretic child. Tricylics, however, remain one of the leading causes of drug-related deaths (from accidental overdose) in children. They should be used with caution.[2]

    Ditropan and other anticholinergics have not consistently been shown to be any more effective than placebo.[2]

    Chlorpheniramine, hydroxyzine, and diazepam are not recommended for the treatment of enuresis.

    Desmopressin, an analogue of vasopressin, is being used with considerable success as a treatment for enuresis in some countries.[2]

649. E. Behavior modification programs are aimed at slowly increasing time intervals between voiding so that bladder capacity is effectively enlarged.[2] Positive reinforcement is provided for longer intervals between voidings and for larger measured voiding volumes.

    This program can be enhanced by the addition of a treatment modality known as a responsibility reinforcement program.[2] With this program, the child keeps a progress record, and is rewarded for dry nights. He or she is also responsible for changing his bed and washing his sheets following enuretic nights.

    Urinary alarm systems are sometimes used in conjunction with behavior modification programs. A wet bed will automatically trigger the alarm. This awakens the child and inhibits the voiding reflex. The child completes voiding in the washroom. The success rate of the alarm method in primary enuretics in whom there is no element of daytime instability is 70% with a 30% relapse rate.[2]

650. E. Supportive counseling of parents with enuretic children is often the only form of therapy needed. Supportive counseling should: (1) provide information about enuresis, its high prevalence and cure rate; (2) advise parents to avoid shaming or punishing the child; (3) encourage responsibility reinforcement; (4) advise simple maneuvers such as reducing fluids prior to bed, having the child void before going to bed, and awakening the child to void during the night.[1,2]

SUMMARY OF THE DIAGNOSIS AND TREATMENT OF ENURESIS

1. **Definition:** Involuntary voiding of urine after the age of 5 years.

2. **Investigation:** Urinalysis should be performed on all children.

3. **Treatment:**
   a) supportive: education about the condition and the high spontaneous cure rate should be given to parents

b) pharmacologic: tricyclic antidepressants are still drugs of choice

c) behavior modification: should utilize responsibility reinforcement program with or without an alarm system

NOTE: A recent report in the *Medical Letter* [3] reports the sudden death of three children treated with the tricyclic antidepressant desipramine, which is a metabolite of imipramine. It would seem prudent to use caution in the prescription of this class of drugs in children until further information is available.

References

1. Vaughan V. Disorders related to vegetative functions. In: Behrman R, Vaughan V, eds. Nelson's textbook of pediatrics. 13th Ed. Philadelphia: WB Saunders, 1987: 56.

2. McLorie G, Husmann D. Incontinence and enuresis. Pediatr Clin North Am 1987; 34(5): 1159–1172.

3. Sudden death in children treated with a tricyclic antidepressant. The Medical Letter 1990; 32(819):53.

PROBLEM 84:   AN 18-MONTH-OLD INFANT WITH DIARRHEA

A mother presents to the office with her 18-month-old infant son, who has had "diarrhea" for the past 5 days. When asked about the diarrhea, the mother states that the infant has had six to eight loose bowel movements per day. There has been no blood in the stools. The infant has had a mild fever (38° C) and appears to have some abdominal discomfort. The child vomited several times in the first 3 days of the illness but this has subsided. On examination, the child is active, and does not appear to be significantly dehydrated. There are no other abnormalities on physical examination.

SELECT THE ONE BEST ANSWER TO THE FOLLOWING QUESTIONS:

651. The most likely cause of this infant's diarrhea is:
    a) Norwalk agent
    b) rotavirus
    c) coxsackievirus
    d) echovirus
    e) *Shigella*

652. The treatment of choice in the patient described in the question would be:
    a) admission to hospital for intravenous fluid therapy

    b) admission to hospital for observation and oral rehydration therapy
    c) treatment at home with fluids including fruit juices and uncarbonated beverages
    d) treatment at home with an oral rehydrating solution
    e) none of the above

653. Which of the following represents the composition of an ideal rehydrating solution for moderate dehydration? (All numbers are represented in mEq/L except CHO that is given in %)
    a) Na-23, K- 3, Cl-15, CHO- 3.0%
    b) Na-40, K- 10, Cl-20, CHO- 3.0%

c) Na-75, K-20, Cl-65, CHO-2.0%
d) Na-140, K-50, Cl-80, CHO-5.0%
e) Na-100, K-40, Cl-100, CHO- 7.5%

654. The most common bacterial cause of diarrhea in the pediatric age group is:
a) *Salmonella*
b) *Shigella*
c) *Campylobacter*
d) *E.coli*
e) enterococcus

655. The most common cause of antibiotic-associated diarrhea in the pediatric age group is:
a) ampicillin
b) clindamycin
c) erythromycin
d) penicillin
e) none of the above

ANSWER THE FOLLOWING QUESTIONS ACCORDING TO THE CODE:

A: 1, 2, and 3 are correct
B: 1 and 3 are correct
C: 2 and 4 are correct
D: Only 4 is correct
E: All of the above are correct

656. The investigations that should be done on all children who present with diarrhea include:
1) urine specific gravity
2) stool culture
3) stool evaluation for blood and leukocytes
4) serum osmolarity

657. Which of the following pediatric infections often present with diarrhea?
1) acute appendicitis
2) otitis media
3) urinary tract infections
4) pneumonia

ANSWERS

651. B. The most common cause of pediatric gastro-enteritis is rotavirus.[1] Symptoms of rotavirus infection include low grade fever, anorexia, nausea, vomiting, diarrhea, and abdominal cramps. Dehydration may occur.[1] The disease typically runs a 4–10 day course. Other causes of viral diarrhea in children include small round viruses (SRV) such as Norwalk virus and calicivirus.

Shigella will usually produce a much more toxic presentation, with blood in the stool often being a prominent feature.

652. D. Since this child does not appear to be significantly dehydrated, hospitalization is not required. The treatment of choice is home treatment with an oral rehydrating solution. Fruit juices (undiluted) and commercial beverages are not recommended because of the high osmolarity, and the danger of hypernatremia.

Oral rehydrating solutions are discussed in question 653.

653. C. Oral rehydration therapy will effectively treat most cases of pediatric gastroenteritis.

The World Health Organization standard for oral rehydration therapy recommends 90 mEq/L sodium, 20 mEq/L potassium, 80 mEq/L chloride, 30 mEq/L of other anions, and 2 % carbohydrate. Among the common oral rehydration solutions used, Gastrolyte has the identical composition to the WHO formula. Pedialyte, on the other hand, contains 45 mEq/L instead of 90 mEq/L and 2.5% CHO.

"Clear liquid" solutions should not be used in infants with diarrhea because they contain low sodium, low potassium and high carbohydrate content.[2]

Oral rehydration therapy by itself should not exceed 24 hours.[2]

654. C. The most common cause of bacterial gastro-enteritis in both the pediatric and adult populations is *Campylobacter jejuni*.[3]

Campylobacter typically begins with fever and malaise, followed by nausea, diarrhea, and abdominal pain. The diarrhea is often profuse, and may be bloody. The illness is self-limited, lasting less than 1 week in 60% of cases. Recurrences and chronic symptoms can occur, especially in infants. Infection with *Campylobacter jejuni* usually occurs due to the production of an endotoxin. Invasive strains also occur and produce disease. Most cases of *Campylobacter* do not require antibiotic treatment; severe cases are effectively treated with erythromycin.[3]

Salmonella gastroenteritis begins with watery diarrhea, accompanied by fever and nausea. As with *Campylobacter,* the diarrhea may be bloody. *Salmonella* produces disease both by mucosal invasion and enterotoxin production. Most cases do not require antibiotic therapy.[3]

Shigella gastroenteritis begins with watery diarrhea, high fever and malaise; this is usually followed in 24 hours by tenesmus and frank dysentery. Mucosal invasion with frank ulceration and hemorrhage often occurs. Dehydration is common. *Shigella* gastroenteritis should be treated with trimethoprim-sulfamethoxazole.[3]

E. coli gastroenteritis may occur as an enteropathic infection, an enterohemorrhagic infection, an enterotoxigenic infection, or an enteroinvasive infection. Enteropathogenic *E. coli* usually produces a mild self-limited illness. Enterohemorrhagic *E. coli* produces a diarrhea that is initially watery, which later becomes bloody. Enterotoxigenic *E. coli* is the most common cause of traveler's diarrhea. Enteroinvasive *E. coli* invades the mucosa and produces a dysentery like illness.[3]

In children, *Yersinia enterocolitica* may produce acute and chronic gastroenteritis and mesenteric lymphadenitis. Mesenteric lymphadenitis is often difficult to distinguish from acute appendicitis. Diarrhea, fever, and crampy abdominal pain are the most common presenting symptoms. Treatment is symptomatic only; antibiotic therapy is unnecessary.[3]

Enterococcus is not a cause of bacterial gastroenteritis in children.

655. A. The most common cause of antibiotic-associated diarrhea in children is ampicillin. Ampicillin induced diarrhea is probably due to the presence of *Clostridium difficile* toxin. Most cases are mild and resolve on discontinuation of the drug. Treatment of severe cases consists of vancomycin hydrochloride or metronidazole.

656. B. The investigations that should be performed on all children with diarrhea include a complete urinalysis including urine specific gravity, and stool analysis for blood and fecal leukocytes. A urine specific gravity below 1.015 suggests adequate hydration.[3]

If a patient presents with bloody diarrhea, high fever, persistent symptoms, tenesmus, or a history of foreign travel, then a stool culture and an examination for ova and parasites should be performed. Routine stool culture is not cost-effective.[3]

Other investigations that should be considered in a toxic child include a complete blood count, serum electrolytes, and serum osmolarity. However, in most milder cases, they are unlikely to change your management.[3]

657. E. Some nonenteric infections may produce diarrhea. These include otitis media, urinary tract infections, acute appendicitis, and lower lobe pneumonia.[4]

SUMMARY OF THE DIAGNOSIS AND TREATMENT OF GASTROENTERITIS IN CHILDREN

1. Rotavirus is the most common cause.

2. **Bacterial gastroenteritis:** *Campylobacter jejuni* is the most common cause. Other common bacterial agents include *Salmonella*, *Shigella*, *Yersinia*, and *E. coli*. Diarrhea in children may also be caused by the parasite *Giardia lamblia*.

3. **Diagnosis:** All children should be evaluated by complete urinalysis including specific gravity, and a stool examination for blood and fecal leukocytes. Specific gravity less than 1.015 suggests adequate hydration. If there is bloody diarrhea, persistent symptoms, fever, tenesmus, or recent foreign travel a stool culture should be done. Otherwise, stool culture is not cost-effective.

4. **Treatment:** Most children can be managed with 24 hours of oral rehydration therapy with a solution containing 75–90 mEq/L Na, 20 mEq/L K, 65–80 mEq/L Cl, 30 mEq/L citrate, and 2 % CHO. Antibiotic therapy should be initiated for *Shigella* (TMP-SMX) and possibly for *Campylobacter jejuni* (erthyromycin).

References

1. Hamilton J. Viral enteritis. Pediatr Clin North Am 1988; 35(1): 89–99.

2. Ghishan F. Electrolyte transport and rehydration solutions. Pediatr Clin North Am 1988; 35(1): 44–48.

3. Bishop W, Ulshen M. Bacterial gastroenteritis. Pediatr Clin North Am 1988; 35(1): 69–81.

4. Paisley J. Acute gastroenteritis syndromes in children. Prim Care 1984; 11(3): 513–526.

PROBLEM 85: A 6-YEAR-OLD CHILD WHO IS " ALWAYS ON THE GO," "INTO EVERYTHING," AND "EASILY DISTRACTIBLE"

A mother brings her 6-year-old boy into the office for a complete assessment. She states "there is something very wrong with him." He just sprinkled baby powder all over the house, and last night opened a bottle of ink and threw it on the floor. He is unable to sit still at school, is easily distracted, has difficulty waiting his turn in games, has difficulty in sustaining attention in play situations, talks all the time, always interrupts others, does not listen when talked to, and is constantly shifting from one activity to another.

As you enter the examining room the child is in the process of destroying it.

SELECT THE ONE BEST ANSWER TO THE FOLLOWING QUESTIONS:

658. The most likely diagnosis in this patient is:
    a) mental retardation
    b) childhood depression
    c) attention deficit-hyperactivity disorder
    d) maternal deprivation
    e) childhood schizophrenia

659. The estimated prevalence of this condition in the pediatric population is:
    a) 3–6%
    b) <1%
    c) 8–10%
    d) 12–15%
    e) 18–20%

ANSWER THE FOLLOWING QUESTIONS ACCORDING TO THE CODE:

A: 1, 2, and 3 are correct
B: 1 and 3 are correct
C: 2 and 4 are correct
D: Only 4 is correct
E: All of the above are correct

660. Which of the following statements regarding the above condition is/are TRUE?
    1) it may be associated with epilepsy
    2) it may be associated with cerebral palsy
    3) it may be associated with infantile autism
    4) it may be associated with conduct disorder

661. Which of the following is/are particularly important in making the diagnosis of this condition?
    1) developmental history of the child
    2) family history of psychiatric illness
    3) history of family dysfunction
    4) corroborating evidence from school personnel

662. Which of the following is/are recommended in the management of this condition?

1) behavior modification using a reward system
2) environmental manipulation
3) self-monitoring skills
4) placement in special schools with other individuals with the same problem

663. The drug(s) of choice for children with this condition include:
    1) methylphenidate
    2) tricyclic antidepressants
    3) dextroamphetamine
    4) monoamine oxidase inhibitors

664. Which of the following is(are) TRUE regarding dietary therapy for this condition?
    1) synthetic flavorings have been shown to be causally related to the condition
    2) high dietary sugar content has been shown to be causally related to the condition
    3) synthetic colorings have been shown to be causally related to the condition
    4) none of the above statements are true

ANSWERS

658. C. This child has attention deficit-hyperactivity disorder. Attention deficit-hyperactivity disorder should be considered if a child has a 6-month history of the following symptoms: fidgeting and squirming, easy distractibility, difficulty following instructions, difficulty sustaining attention, difficulty playing quietly, shifting from one task to another before completion, excessive talking, interrupting or intruding on others, difficulty remaining seated, and a tendency to engage in physically dangerous activities without consideration of possible consequences.[1]

Attention deficit-hyperactivity disorder may be associated with conduct disorder.[1] Symptoms of conduct disorder include stealing, running away from home, school truancy, breaking and entering, destroying others' personal property, rape, robbery, and physical violence.[1]

659. A. The prevalence of attention deficit-hyperactivity disorder is 3–6%. Thus, an average of 1 child in a classroom of 20-25 students will have the disorder.[1]

660. E. A minority of patients with attention deficit-hyperactivity disorder have associated epilepsy, cerebral palsy, or infantile autism.[2] As previously discussed, attention deficit-hyperactivity is associated with conduct disorder.[1]

661. E. The diagnosis of attention deficit-hyperactivity disorder should only be made after a careful history has been elicited. Of particular importance in the history are: (1) a developmental history of the child, (2) a family history of pyschiatric illness, and (3) a history of family dysfunction. The school teacher should also be interviewed.[2]

The parents should be carefully questioned regarding all of the child's behaviors. After that, the child's behavior in the office should be documented.[2] Only after considering all of the evidence should a diagnosis of attention deficit-hyperactivity disorder be made.

662. A. The management of attention deficit-hyperactivity disorder includes: (1) a behavior modification program to reward good behavior, (2) environmental manipulation to eliminate extraneous noise and activity, and (3) the teaching of self-monitoring skills to older children.

The placement of children with this condition in special schools is not recommended.

Drug therapy of attention deficit-hyperactivity disorder is discussed in a subsequent question.[2]

663. B. Not all children with attention deficit-hyperactivity disorder need pharmacologic therapy. Non-pharmacologic management should be tried first. If pharmacotherapy is needed, the drugs of choice are methylphenidate and dextroamphetamine.[2] Toxicity with these agents is minimal. Pharmacologic therapy is most successful in helping a child with this disorder pay attention in class.

To maximize efficacy, the drug selected should be administered in the morning. Adverse effects such as sleep disturbance, decreased appetite, irratibility, and mild abdominal pain usually do not necessitate discontinuation of the drug. The physician should consider stopping the medication during the summer holidays, and reevaluating the child before school starts in the fall again.

Tricyclic antidepressants and MAO inhibitors have been shown to be effective in attention deficit-hyperactivity disorder, but because of their side effects they should be regarded as second line agents.[2]

664. D. None of the above statements are true.

There is no evidence to support a relationship between attention deficit-hyperactivity disorder and synthetic flavorings, synthetic colorings, or high dietary sugar content.[2] A recommendation to decrease the refined sugar content in a child's diet may, however, be made on other grounds such as dental hygiene.

SUMMARY OF THE DIAGNOSIS AND TREATMENT OF ATTENTION DEFICIT-HYPERACTIVITY DISORDER

1. Attention deficit-hyperactivity disorder will likely affect at least one child in every class.

2. Attention deficit-hyperactivity disorder may be associated with conduct disorder.

3. **Therapy:**
   a) first line- educational and behavioral therapy
   b) second line- pharmacotherapy: methylphenidate and dextroamphetamine.
   c) dietary therapy is unproved

References

1. American Psychiatric Association. Diagnostic and statistical manual of mental disorders. 3rd Ed. Revised (DSM-III-R). Washington: APA Press, 1987.

2. Meller W, Lyle K. Attention deficit disorder in childhood. Primary Care 1987; 14(4): 745–759

PROBLEM 86: A 2-MONTH-OLD INFANT WITH A HIGH FEVER 1 DAY AFTER IMMUNIZATION

A mother presents with her 2-month-old infant 1 day after the child received his first immunization. The infant started running a fever 8 hours after the immunization. It is now 40.6° C. The child is screaming and irritable.

On physical examination, there are no localizing signs of infection.

You assume that the fever and the irritability is due to the immunization.

SELECT THE ONE BEST ANSWER TO THE FOLLOWING QUESTIONS:

665. The most likely cause of the fever and the irritability is the immunizing agent against:
    a) poliomyelitis
    b) pertussis
    c) diptheria
    d) tetanus
    e) none of the above

666. Considering the condition of this infant, at this time you should:
    a) hospitalize the child
    b) advise the mother to use aspirin to bring down the temperature
    c) advice the mother to use acetaminophen to bring down the temperature
    d) obtain stat blood cultures and a lumbar puncture
    e) none of the above

667. Considering the cause of this child's condition, which of the following statements regarding future immunizations is true?
    a) all future DTP-polio immunizations should be canceled
    b) future immunizations should omit diptheria toxoid
    c) future immunizations should omit tetanus toxoid
    d) future immunizations should not be affected; DTP-polio should be given as before
    e) none of the above

668. Measles, mumps, and rubella vaccine is usually given at:
    a) 6 months
    b) 12 months
    c) 2 years
    d) 4 years
    e) 6 years

ANSWER THE FOLLOWING QUESTION ACCORDING TO THE CODE:

A: 1, 2, and 3 are correct
B: 1 and 3 are correct
C: 2 and 4 are correct
D: Only 4 is correcy
E: All of the above are correct

669. Which of the following is/are part of the recommended schedule for active immunization of normal infants and children?
    1) DTP, oral polio at age 2 months
    2) DTP, oral polio at age 4 months
    3) DTP, oral polio at age 6 months
    4) *Haemophilus influenzae* type b at age 4 years

ANSWERS

665. B. Pertussis vaccine is the most likely cause of the adverse reaction.[1] Pertussis vaccine may produce minor reactions such as local discomfort, induration, and fever in up to 75% of vaccine recipients. Drowsiness, anorexia, persistent crying, screaming, and febrile convulsions may also occur.[1]

    Adverse reactions from the poliomyelitis vaccine, the diptheria vaccine, and the tetanus vaccine are much less common.[1]

666. C. With a normal physical examination, it is reasonable to assume that there is a cause and effect relationship between the administration of the pertussis vaccine and the onset of fever.

    Hospitalization is not necessary, nor is an intensive septic work-up.

    Acetaminophen is the analgesic of choice for the treatment of fever in children. Aspirin should not be given because of its possible link with Reye's syndrome. The child should be reassessed within 24 hours if the symptoms do not improve, or before if any other symptoms or signs develop.

667. E. Future immunizations should not include the pertussis component. Pertussis vaccine should not be given to children who (a) have had high fever

(more than 40.5° C), convulsions, screaming episodes, shock, symptoms of encephalopathy, or thrombocytopenia following a previous dose of pertussis vaccine; or (b) are suffering from an evolving neurologic disorder.[1]

668. **B.** Measles, mumps, and rubella immunization should be given to all infants at 12 months of age.[1] A second immunization for measles at 4–6 years of age has recently been recommended.[2]

669. **A.** Diptheria, tetanus, pertussis and oral polio (DTP, OPV) is recommended at 2 months, 4 months, 6 months, 18 months, and at 4–6 years. Diptheria, tetanus, and polio should again be given at 14–16 years.[1]

   Measles, mumps, and rubella (MMR) should be given at 12 months of age.

   Haemophilus influenzae b should be given at 18 months of age.[1]

SUMMARY OF CHILDHOOD IMMUNIZATIONS

1. Follow immunization schedule discussed above.

2. Eliminate pertussis vaccine from DTP if significant fever, screaming episodes, or convulsions.

3. Most adverse effects to childhood immunizations are mild; treat high fever in infants and children with acetaminophen.

References

1. Canadian Immunization Guide. 3rd Ed. Health and Welfare Canada, 1989.

2. Centers for Disease Control. Measles prevention: recommendations of the Immunization Practices Advisory Committee. MMWR 1989; 38(no. S–9).

PROBLEM 87: A 6-MONTH-OLD CHILD WITH AN UPPER RESPIRATORY TRACT INFECTION

A 6-month-old infant presents with his mother to your office for assessment of an upper respiratory tract infection. The child has had a runny nose and an occasional cough for the last 5 days. He has had no fever. On examination, the tympanic membranes and throat are normal. There are no adventitious breath sounds. There is signficant rhinorrhea and an occasional cough. You decide to prescribe an antihistamine to relieve the rhinorrhea.

ANSWER THE FOLLOWING QUESTIONS ACCORDING TO THE CODE:

A: 1, 2, and 3 are correct
B: 1 and 3 are correct
C: 2 and 4 are correct
D: Only 4 is correct
E: All of the above are correct

670. Which of the following statements regarding the prescription of an antihistamine to this child is/are TRUE?
   1) antihistamines shorten the duration of respiratory tract illness in children
   2) antihistamines reduce the incidence of otitis media following upper respiratory tract infections
   3) the prescription of an antihistamine to this child is a reasonable treatment
   4) antihistamines may produce seizures in children of this age

671. The mother returns for follow-up 3 days later. She states that despite your treatment the child has not improved. He now has significantly greater nasal congestion and is having a difficult time breathing at night.

   On examination the ears and throat remain clear. The lungs are clear. There is now signficant nasal congestion.

   Which of the following statements regarding the treatment of this child is/are true?
   1) a decongestant to relieve the nasal congestion is a reasonable therapeutic maneuver
   2) decongestants have been shown to reduce the duration of respiratory tract illness
   3) topical sympathomimetics are unlikely to be systemically absorbed
   4) overstimulation is a common side effect when decongestant preparations are given to children

672. A mother presents to your office with her 6-month-old infant for assessment of a persistent cough. The cough has been present for the past 10 days. It is nonproductive, and the mother feels it is interfering significantly with the child's sleep. You are considering prescribing an antitussive and or an expectorant.

Which of the following statements regarding the use of antitussives and expectorants in children is/are true?
1) dextromethorphan suppresses cough and is unlikely to produce any significant adverse reactions
2) the combination of a cough suppressant and an expectorant is a logical combination to try in a child with persistent cough
3) dextromethorphan has been shown to significantly decrease the duration of respiratory tract infection in children
4) respiratory depression in children has been reported with dextromethorphan

673. A mother brings her 13-month-old infant to the office for assessment of nausea and vomiting. She stopped in at the local emergency department 24 hours previously and was told to purchase childrens dimenhydrinate suppositories for the nausea. Apparently, the emergency physician did a complete work-up and found no other significant findings.

The nausea and vomiting continue. The child appears to be approximately 5% dehydrated. On physical examination there are no other abnormalities found. The child appears somewhat sedated and lethargic.

You decide to admit the child for observation, reevaluation, and rehydration.

Which of the following statements regarding the use of antiemetics in children is/are true?
1) dimenhydrinate is generally effective for the treatment of the nausea and vomiting associated with gastroenteritis
2) the sedation that is seen in this infant may be secondary to the dimenhydrinate
3) the dimenhydrinate suppository is unlikely to produce significant side effects
4) dimenhydrinate toxicity may be difficult to distinguish from worsening of the illness

674. A mother brings her 8-month-old infant into the office for assessment of fever, diarrhea, and "red cheeks" that she attributes to "teething." She was advised by her neighbor to purchase a preparation of topical benzocaine. This hasn't helped.

On examination, the infant has a temperature of 39° C. There are no abnormalities on physical examination.

Which of the following statements regarding this infant is/are true?
1) the symptoms described probably are due to teething
2) acetaminophen is a reasonable treatment for a child that is teething
3) topical benzocaine preparations are virtually devoid of side effects
4) teething often begins at 4–6 months and carries on intermittently up to the age of 2 years

ANSWERS

670. D. Most cough and cold remedies contain antihistamines. Antihistamines, however, have never been shown to be of value in the treatment of the common cold.[1] Antihistamines do not shorten the duration of respiratory tract illness in children, and do not reduce the incidence of otitis media following upper respiratory infection. They may, however, produce seizures in children if given in toxic amounts. This is a particular concern in young infants.[1]

Treatment of a viral upper respiratory tract infection in a child should consist of reassurance, and the suggestion of the use of cool steam if significant nasal congestion is present.

671. D. Decongestants have not been shown to shorten the duration of respiratory tract illness. Topical sympathomimetic agents are systemically absorbed, and may result in hypertension, tachycardia, and overstimulation of the central nervous system leading to irratibility, insomnia, and sometimes even frank psychosis.[1] Overstimulation is a particularly common side effect in children. Thus, as with antihistamines, the risks of using decongestants in children outweigh any potential benefits.

672. D. Dextromethorphan is the most common ingredient of over the counter cough medicines. As well as producing drowsiness, it has been reported to produce respiratory depression in children.[1] As with antihistamines and decongestants, dextromethorphan has not been shown to shorten the duration of respiratory tract illness in children or adults.[1]

Many cough preparations also contain an expectorant. The combination of a cough suppressant and an expectorant does not make sense.

Time remains the best cure for the common cold. The use of a nasal aspirator (bulb syringe) will help to clear a young infant's nasal secretions and make feeding easier. Saline nasal drops may also be used. In infants who are irritable and feverish from symptoms of the common cold, the use of acetaminophen is probably the safest over the counter medication to use.[1]

673. C. Dimenhydrinate should not be used for the treatment of nausea and vomiting secondary to gastroenteritis in children. Even in adults the use of this agent is questionable; it has only been shown to be of value in the treatment of motion sickness.[1] Dimenhydrinate may produce significant sedation (and even a semicomatose state) in children. The pediatric suppository contains 50 mg of dimenhydrinate (the same as the adult oral dose).

It may be difficult for the physician to differentiate dimenhydrinate toxicity from a worsening of the illness itself. This makes the use of this agent in children dangerous.[1]

674. C. Teething usually begins at 4–6 months and continues until the age of 2 years. Although often blamed on teething, there is no good evidence that rash, fever, diarrhea, vomiting, nasal congestion, irratibility or sleeplessness are related to teething.[1]

Although topical benzocaine usually does not produce any side effects, cases of methemoglobinemia have been reported in children who ingested too much of this agent.[1]

Teething is best treated with reassurance and appropriate doses of acetaminophen.[1]

SUMMARY OF THE ABUSE OF OVER-THE-COUNTER DRUGS IN INFANTS AND YOUNG CHILDREN

1. **Upper respiratory tract infections**: No evidence to suggest that antihistamines, decongestants, and cough suppressants are of any value in the treatment of upper respiratory tract infections in children. Potential toxicity is present with all of these medications.

2. **Nausea and vomiting**: Dimenhydrinate is not useful and is potentially toxic

3. **Diarrhea**: Kaolin/pectin may change the appearance of the stool slightly, but has no effect on water loss— the major hazard of protracted diarrhea

4. **Teething**: No evidence to suggest that rash, diarrhea, vomiting, nasal congestion, irratability and sleeplessness are associated with teething. Benzocaine preparations should be avoided. Reassurance and judicious use of acetaminophen is indicated.

Reference

1. Goldbloom A. Hazards of over-the-counter medications in children. Med North Amer 1986; 2: 392–405.

PROBLEM 88:   A 2-YEAR-OLD MALE WITH A FEVER, COUGH, AND DYSPNEA

A 2-year-old boy is brought to you office by his mother. He developed rhinitis, cough, fretfulness and diminshed appetite 3 days ago. Last night, he developed dyspnea (respiratory rate 40/min), a productive cough, and a temperature of 40° C. The cough is productive of purulent sputum.

On examination, the left lower lobe is dull to percussion and bronchial breath sounds are heard in that lobe. A chest x-ray demonstrates consolidation in the left lower lobe.

SELECT THE ONE BEST ANSWER TO THE FOLLOWING QUESTIONS:

675. The most likely diagnosis in this child is:
   a) pneumococcal pneumonia
   b) *H. influenzae* pneumonia

   c) viral pneumonia
   d) *Mycoplasma* pneumonia
   e) *Klebsiella* pneumonia

676. The treatment of choice in this child is:
   a) penicillin

b) erythromycin
c) symtomatic treatment
d) gentamicin
e) clindamycin

677. A 3-year-old female presents to your office with her mother. She developed rhinitis and a non-productive cough 4 days ago, which has become worse in the last 24 hours. She started to run a fever 12 hours ago. Two other siblings at home are ill with upper respiratory tract symptoms.

The child's temperature is 38.5° C. There is slight dyspnea and nasal flaring. On auscultation, wheezing is heard in all lobes.

The chest x-ray reveals a diffuse infiltrate, especially in the perihilar areas. The white blood cell count is 14,000 mm³

The most likely diagnosis is this child is:
a) pneumococcal pneumonia
b) *H. influenzae pneumonia*
c) viral pneumonia
d) *Mycoplasma* pneumonia
e) *Klebsiella* pneumonia

678. The most common etiologic agent causing the clinical picture discussed in question 677 is:
a) *Mycoplasma pneumoniae*
b) *Streptococcus pneumoniae*
c) respiratory syncytial virus
d) parainfluenza virus
e) none of the above

679. A 7-year-old girl presents with her mother to your office. She has had a headache, a mild fever, a sore throat, and a nonproductive, harsh cough for the last 10 days. She has coughed to the point of vomiting on three occasions.

On examination she has a temperature of 38° C. She has a few fine rales in all lobes. As well, she has a bullous myringitis on the right side. The chest x-ray reveals bilateral bronchopneumonia.

The most likely diagnosis in this child is:
a) pneumococcal pneumonia
b) *Klebsiella* pneumonia
c) viral pneumonia
d) *Mycoplasma* pneumonia
e) *H. influenzae* pneumonia

680. The most appropriate treatment for the child discussed in question 679 is:
a) tetracycline
b) erthyromycin
c) penicillin

d) amoxicillin
e) cefaclor

ANSWERS

675. A. Pneumococcus is the most common bacterial pathogen between the ages of 1 month and 4 years.[1,2] The history and physical examination suggesting lobar consolidation favor pneumoccal pneumonia.

The classic history of a shaking chill followed by a high fever, cough, and chest pain that is described in adults with pneumococcal pneumonia is rarely seen in infants and young children.[2]

In infants and young children early symptoms include stuffy nose, fretfulness, and diminished appetite. These mild symptoms usually end with the abrupt onset of high fever, restlessness, apprehension, and respiratory distress.[2]

The physical examination reveals signs of consolidation including dullness, increased fremitus, and tubular breath sounds.

The white blood cell count is usually elevated to 15,000–40,000 cells/mm², with neutrophil predominance.

Consolidation may be demonstrated by chest x-ray before it is detectable by physical examination, and resolution of the infiltrate may not be complete until several weeks after the child is clinically well.[2]

H. influenzae pneumonia (type b) is the second most common cause of bacterial pneumonia in children.

Klebsiella pneumonia is uncommon in children with normal immune systems.

Mycoplasma pneumonia usually occurs after the age of 4 and will be discussed in a subsequent question.

Viral pneumonia is, overall, the most commmon cause of pneumonia in children and will be considered in a subsequent question.

676. A. The drug of choice in pneumococcal pneumonia is penicillin. In children that are allergic to penicillin, alternative drugs include erythromycin or a cephalosporin.[2] Treatment should be given for 7–10 days in uncomplicated cases.

677. C. This child has a viral pneumonia. Viral pneumonia in childhood usually begins with upper respiratory tract symptoms including rhinitis and cough. Fever is usually lower than in bacterial pneumonia. Often, other family members are ill.[3]

On physical examination nasal flaring (especially in younger children and infants) and tachypnea are found. Rales may be present.

The chest x-ray usually reveals a diffuse infiltrate, especially in the perihilar areas. Lobar infiltrates may occur with viral pneumonia. Hyperinflation is common.

The white blood cell count is usually under 20,000/mm³.[3]

678. C. Between 1 month and 4 years of age, most pneumonias are viral in origin. Respiratory syncytial virus is the most common agent, followed by parainfluenza viruses, adenovirus, enteroviruses, rhinovirus, influenza virus, and herpes simplex virus.[1]

Treatment of viral pneumonia is symptomatic. Humidified oxygen and intravenous fluids may be necessary in more severe cases. There may be some benefit from continuous treatment with aerosolized ribavirin if RSV infection is documented.[1,2]

679. D. Above the age of 4, pneumococcus and *Mycoplasma* pneumoniae are the most frequent causes of pneumonia and viruses of lesser importance.[1]

The patient described in this case has a typical *Mycoplasma* pneumonia. *Mycoplasma pneumoniae* is a major cause of respiratory infections in school-age children and young adults. Clinically significant disease is unusual before the age of 4–5 years, the peak incidence occurs from 10–15 years.[3]

Mycoplasma pneumonia is characterized by the gradual onset of headache, malaise, and fever; cough is prominent, and sore throat is frequent.

On physical examination, fine, crackling rales are sometimes heard, although it is not uncommon for auscultation to be completely normal. Extrapulmonary findings, including bullous myringitis (as in this patient) may occur.

Bilateral bronchopneumonia is the most common chest x-ray finding. A bilateral bronchopneumonia may be seen on x-ray in the absence of physical signs.

Most *M. pneumoniae* illnesses are mild and hospitalization is infrequent.

Cold hemagglutinins in a titer of 1:64 or greater support the diagnosis.[3]

680. B. The treatment of choice for *Mycoplasma pneumoniae* is either erythromycin or tetracycline. Erythromycin is the drug of choice in children under the age of 10 years. Treatment should be given for 7–10 days. As well as antibiotic treatment, symptomatic treatment including rest, acetaminophen, fluids, and increased humidity are indicated.[3]

SUMMARY OF THE ETIOLOGY AND TREATMENT OF CHILDHOOD PNEUMONIA

1. **Age 3 weeks– 3 months:** *Chlamydia trachomatis* most common agent: Treatment—Erythromycin

2. **Age 3 months– 4 years:** Viral pneumonia is most common: Treatment—symptomatic. Pneumococcal pneumonia is most common bacterial pneumonia: Treatment—penicillin

3. **Age greater than 4 years:** *Mycoplasma pneumoniae* is the most common etiologic agent: Treatment—erythromycin below the age of 10, erythromycin or tetracycline are equally effective agents.

References

1. Editorial. Pneumonia in childhood. Lancet 1988; l: 741–743.

2. Boat T. Bacterial and viral pneumonia. In: Behrman R, Vaughan V, eds. Nelson's textbook of pediatrics. 13th Ed. Philadelphia: WB Saunders, 1987: 898–904.

3. Denny F. *Mycoplasma* infections. In: Behrman R, Vaughan V, eds. Nelson's textbook of pediatrics. 13th Ed. Philadelphia: WB Saunders, 1987: 654–655.

PROBLEM 89:   A 6-MONTH-OLD INFANT WITH A 2-DAY HISTORY OF WHEEZING

A 6-month-old infant is brought into your office by his mother. He presents with a 2-day history of wheezing, a mild fever (38.5° C), and rhinorrhea.

The child has no known allergies but there is a history of allergies in the family.

On examination, the child's respiratory rate is 60/minute. There is rhonchi and moist rales heard throughout the chest. The chest x-ray shows evidence of hyperaeration.

SELECT THE ONE BEST ANSWER TO THE FOLLOWING QUESTIONS:

681. The most likely diagnosis in this child is:
    a) *Mycoplasma pneumoniae* infection
    b) allergic bronchitis
    c) viral tracheitis
    d) bacterial tracheitis
    e) bronchiolitis

682. The etiologic agent that is most likely responsible for this infection is:
    a) respiratory syncytial virus
    b) parainfluenza virus
    c) adenovirus
    d) *Mycoplasma pneumoniae*
    e) rhinovirus

683. The treatment of choice for the patient described in question 681 is:
    a) erythromycin
    b) ampicillin
    c) cold, humidified, oxygen
    d) systemic corticosteroids
    e) an inhaled beta-agonist

684. Which of the following statement(s) regarding wheezing in infancy is(are) true?
    a) it is sometimes difficult to differentiate bronchial asthma from bronchiolitis by clinical assessment
    b) children with bronchiolitis who do not develop asthma may be inappropriately labeled with the stigma of asthma
    c) the relationship between bronchiolitis and ongoing hyperreactivity is unclear; ongoing bronchial hyperreactivity or "asthma" may be precipitated by an acute episode of bronchiolitis
    d) all of the above statements are true

685. A 6-year-old male presents to the emergency room with an acute asthmatic attack. He developed a respiratory tract infection 3 days ago and began wheezing 24 hours ago. He had his first asthmatic attack 2 years ago and usually has 1 attack per month. He is on no prophylactic medications.

    On examination, the child is in marked respiratory distress. His respiratory rate is 48/minute. He has marked indrawing of the accessory muscles of respiration. Generalized wheezes are heard throughout the lung fields.

    The treatment of first choice in this patient at this time is:
    a) intravenous theophylline
    b) inhaled corticosteroid
    c) nebulized beta-agonist with or without ipratropium bromide
    d) humidified oxygen and intravenous corticosteroid
    e) humidified oxygen only

686. Pulmonary function tests are performed on the patient described in question 685. Which of the following parameters of pulmonary function would be expected to increase after administration of a bronchodilator?
    a) FVC (forced vital capacity)
    b) FEV_1 (forced expiratory volume in 1 second)
    c) MEF_{25-75} (maximum expiratory flow between 25 and 75% of the vital capacity)
    d) TLC (total lung capacity)
    e) b and c

687. The patient described in question 685 is stabilized and you decide to begin prophylactic therapy. Which of the following is the prophylactic agent of choice?
    a) inhaled beta-agonist
    b) oral theophylline
    c) inhaled corticosteroid
    d) sodium cromoglycate
    e) oral corticosteroid

688. A 12-year-old boy presents for assessment of exercise-induced asthma. The child is fine when at rest, and develops shortness of breath and wheezing at the end of any vigorous exercise session.

    The treatment of first choice in this child is:
    a) sodium cromoglycate

b) inhaled beta-agonist
c) oral theophylline
d) inhaled corticosteroid
e) oral corticosteroid

ANSWERS

681. E. This infant has bronchiolitis. Acute bronchiolitis is a lower respiratory tract infection of infants resulting from inflammatory obstruction of the small airways. It is most common in the first 2 years of life.

    Acute bronchiolitis usually begins with nasal discharge and fever. This is followed by the gradual development of respiratory distress characterized by paroxysmal wheezy cough, dyspnea, and irratibility.[1]

    Examination reveals tachypnea, and sometimes severe air hunger and cyanosis. Nasal flaring and use of the accessory muscles of respiration is common.[1] End inspiratory rales and expiratory rales and rhonchi are heard.

    Allergic bronchitis is not really a diagnosis.

    Mycoplasma pneumoniae and rhinoviruses may be associated with wheezing in school-age children.

    The clinical picture presented in not one of tracheitis.

682. A. Respiratory syncytial virus is the most common cause of bronchiolitis. Other causes include para-influenza virus, *Mycoplasma,* some adenoviruses and some rhinoviruses.[1]

683. C. The treatment of choice for the patient described in question 681 is cold, humidified, oxygen. Oral intake must often be supplemented to offset the dehydrating effect of tachypnea.[1]

    Ribavirin (Virazole), an antiviral agent, is effective in reducing the severity of bronchiolitis due to RSV infection when administered early in the course of the illness. It is used in children under the age of 2 years who have severe infection.[1]

    Antibiotics have no therapeutic value unless there is secondary bacterial pneumonia.

    Most controled studies with corticosteroids have failed to demonstrate any therapeutic efficacy in bronchiolitis.

    Bronchodilators may have a role in establishing whether or not the child has bronchial hyperreactivity. At this time, however, they are not considered as an established treatment for bronchiolitis.[1]

684. D. All of the above statements are true. It is sometimes difficult to diffierentiate bronchial asthma from bronchiolitis by clinical assessment. Thus, an inappropriate diagnosis of "asthma" may be made, and the child may be labeled as having this disease. The relationship, however, between bronchiolitis and asthma is unclear; young infants with bronchiolitis may be at increased risk of developing asthma. Bronchial asthma may be precipitated by an acute episode of bronchiolitis.[1]

685. C. The treatment of choice in this patient at this time is nebulized beta-agonist (albuterol or salbutamol) with or without nebulized ipratropium bromide.[2]

    If the initial treatment does not suffice, another treatment is given in 20 minutes. If this does not produce a response, epinephrine by subcutaneous injection can be tried. If there is no response, intravenous theophylline and intravenous corticosteroids should be administered.

    Inhaled corticosteroids and humified oxygen by itself would not be appropriate for treatment of an acute asthmatic attack.[2]

686. D. Pulmonary function testing before and after administration of an aerosol bronchodilator will assess the degree of reversibility of airway obstruction Normally, the administration of a bronchodilator will result in an increase in FEV_1 and MEF_{25-75}. FVC and TLC, which may already be increased in patients with bronchial asthma, will not increase further after administration of a bronchodilator.[2]

687. A. The prophylactic agent of choice in bronchial asthma is an inhaled beta-agonist.[2] Two inhalations of albuterol, metaproterenol, or terbutaline three or four times a day from a metered dose inhaler will control a significant number of asthmatic patients.

    As asthma has become recognized as an inflammatory disorder, the administration of an anti-inflammatory agent in aerosol form has become accepted second line therapy. The two most commonly used agents are inhaled sodium cromoglycate and inhaled corticosteroids.[2,3]

688. A. Exercise induced asthma may be manifested by both an early (in terms of time following exercise) and late bronchoconstriction. Early bronchoconstriction begins 3–8 minutes following exercise and late bronchoconstriction occurs 4–6 hours

after exercise. Inhaled sodium cromoglycate will block both early and late bronchoconstriction. An inhaled beta-agonist will only block early bronchoconstriction. Corticosteroids will only block late bronchoconstriction.[3]

SUMMARY OF THE DIAGNOSIS AND TREATMENT OF THE WHEEZING CHILD

1. Wheezing in infancy is usually due to either bronchiolitis or bronchial asthma. The distinction between the two is often difficult to make clinically. Bronchiolitis may predispose to the later development of asthma

2. Bronchiolitis is mainly caused by respiratory syncytial virus. Treatment is humidified oxygen, and sometimes ribavirin.

3. Bronchial asthma can be more easily diagnosed in older children and adults. FEV_1 and MEF_{25-75} will increase after bronchodilator therapy in patients with asthma.

Management of Bronchial Asthma:
a) remove any precipitating allergens
b) first choice: inhaled beta-agonists with or without ipratropium bromide
c) second choice: inhaled sodium cromoglycate or inhaled corticosteroid
d) third choice: theophylline preparations
e) acute asthma is best managed by nebulized beta-agonist with or without ipratropium bromide. If not successful, intravenous corticosteroids and theophylline should be given.
f) a short course of oral corticosteroids may prevent the progression of an acute asthma attack to a life-threatening conditon.

References

1. Skoner D, Caliguiri L. The wheezing infant. Pediatr Clin North Am, 35(5): 1011–1030.

2. Ellis E. Asthma: current therapeutic approach. Pediatr Clin North Am 1988; 35(5): 1041–1050.

3. Pierson W. Exercise-induced broncospasm in children and adolescents. Pediatr Clin North Am 1988; 35(5): 1031–1039.

General Surgery and Surgical Specialties

PROBLEM 90: A 27-YEAR-OLD MALE WITH NAUSEA, VOMITING, AND RIGHT LOWER QUADRANT ABDOMINAL PAIN

A 27-year-old male presents to your office with a 24-hour history of abdominal pain, initially periumbilical, but with movement to the right lower quadrant within the past 3 hours. The patient also describes anorexia for the past 2 days, and nausea that began 8 hours ago. The patient has vomited once.

On examination the patient has a temperature of 38.5° C. There is mild cough tenderness and in the right lower quadrant. There is no rebound tenderness. The rectal examination is normal.

SELECT THE ONE BEST ANSWER TO THE FOLLOWING QUESTIONS:

689. At this time you should:
    a) advise the patient to go home and return for follow-up in 24 hours
    b) hospitalize the patient and order a CT scan
    c) order a WBC count
    d) order a plain film of the abdomen
    e) c and d

690. The laboratory investigation(s) that you performed heighten your suspicions of the diagnosis in this patient. You should now:
    a) advise the patient to go home and return for follow-up in 24 hours
    b) hospitalize the patient for observation
    c) consult a surgeon for the performance of a definitive surgical procedure
    d) order further laboratory investigations
    e) begin therapy with a broad spectrum antibiotic

ANSWER THE FOLLOWING QUESTIONS ACCORDING TO THE CODE:

A: 1, 2, and 3 are correct
B: 1 and 3 are correct
C: 2 and 4 are correct
D: Only 4 is correct
E: All of the above are correct

691. Which of the following may be associated with the condition described above?
    1) diarrhea
    2) urinary frequency
    3) hematuria
    4) poorly localized epigastric pain

692. In which of the following groups are the signs and symptoms of the condition described above likely to be classical and not confused with other illnesses?
    1) infants and young children
    2) young adult females
    3) elderly patients
    4) young adult males

693. Which of the following is/are complications of the condition described above?
    1) perforation
    2) peritonitis
    3) appendiceal abscess
    4) pylephlebitis

ANSWERS

689. E. To further evaluate this patient's condition you should order a WBC count and a plain film of the abdomen. The diagnosis until proven otherwise is acute appendicitis. In acute appendicitis, the average leukocyte count is 15,000/mm^3, and 90%

of patients have a leukocyte count of greater than 10,000/mm^3. In 75% of patients, the differential count shows more than 75% neutrophils.[1] However, 10% of patients with acute appendicitis have both a normal white blood cell count and a normal differential[1].

Abdominal x-rays are of value in detecting other causes of abdominal pain. They may also show localized air-fluid levels, localized ileus, increased soft tissue density in the right lower quadrant, a fecalith, an altered right psoas shadow, or an abnormal right flank stipe; all radiologic signs that may be associated with acute appendicitis.[1]

690. C. In the patient discussed, both an elevated white blood cell count and a localized air-fluid level in the right lower quadrant heighten your suspicions of acute appendicitis. At this time, a surgeon should be consulted and an appendectomy should be performed. Advising the patient to go home and return in 24 hours is unwise because of the risk of perforation and peritonitis. Further investigations are unlikely to be of any help. Broad spectrum antibiotics may be indicated prior to and after appendectomy to decrease the risk of septic complications, but they are unlikely to eliminate the need for appendectomy. Further observation in hospital will just increase the probability of a septic complication.

691. E. The typical history of appendicitis is vague abdominal discomfort followed by anorexia, nausea, vomiting and indigestion. The pain, which is continuous but usually not severe, begins as a vague discomfort, often central in location, and then moves into the right lower quadrant. The pain is usually aggrevated by moving, walking, or coughing. There may be tenesmus.[1]

On examination, there is usually cough tenderness localized in the right lower quadrant. There may be well-localized one-finger tenderness, and sometimes muscular rigidity. Rebound tenderness is often referred to the same area. Peristalsis may be normal or slightly reduced. Rectal and pelvic examinations are likely to be normal. Unless perforation has occurred, there is likely to only be a mild elevation of temperature.[1]

Retrocecal or retroileal appendicitis usually begins with poorly localized epigastric pain, which does not shift to the right lower quadrant. Nausea and vomiting are mild. There may be mild diarrhea, and urinary frequency and hematuria may occur from a retrocecal appendix that is lying adjacent to the ureter. Tenderness may not be present in the right lower quadrant, and one-finger palpation is negative unless the flank is examined.[1]

692. D. Only in young adult males is the diagnosis not likely to be mistaken for other illnesses.

Infants and young children may present with lethargy, irratibility, and anorexia in the early stages. Vomiting, fever, and pain usually become apparent as the disease progresses.

In the elderly, classical symptoms may not be elicited and the diagnosis is often not considered. The course of appendicitis is more virulent in the elderly, and suppurative complications are more frequent.

Women in the age group 20–40 provide the greatest diagnostic challenge. The highest incidence of false-positive diagnosis occurs in this age group because of the prevalence of pelvic inflammatory disease and other gynecologic conditions. If a careful history and physical examination is performed, the false-positive rate can be substantially reduced. Compared with appendicitis, pelvic inflammatory disease is usually bilateral, has associated left adnexal tenderness, begins within 5 days of the last menstrual period, and is not associated with nausea and vomiting. Cervical motion tenderness is common in both diseases.[1]

693. E. All of the above are complications of acute appendicitis.

Perforation, peritonitis, appendiceal abscess, and pylephlebitis (suppurative thrombophlebitis of the portal venous system) may all occur as complications of acute appendicitis.[1]

SUMMARY OF THE DIAGNOSIS AND TREATMENT OF ACUTE APPENDICITIS

1. **Classical symptoms:** Abdominal pain, initially vague but later localized to the right lower quadrant; anorexia, nausea, and vomiting; localized abdominal tenderness; low-grade fever; and leukocytosis.

Retrocecal or retroileal appendicitis: poorly localized abdominal pain, mild nausea and vomiting, mild diarrhea, urinary frequency, and hematuria.

2. **Diagnosis:** High index of suspicion (especially in infants, children, and the elderly), presenting symptoms and signs, elevated white blood cell

count, and sometimes changes on the plain abdominal x-ray.

3. **Complications:** Perforation, peritonitis, appendiceal abscess, and pylephlebitis

Reference

1. Way L. Appendix. In: Way L, ed. Current surgical diagnosis and treatment. 8th Ed. Norwalk: Appleton & Lange, 1988: 556–559.

PROBLEM 91: A 32-YEAR-OLD FEMALE WITH RIGHT UPPER QUADRANT ABDOMINAL PAIN

A 32-year-old female presents with a 24-hour history of right upper quadrant abdominal pain. This is accompanied by nausea, vomiting, and a low-grade fever. She has had two similar attacks within the last 6 months.

On examination, the patient's temperature is 38.5°C. Her blood pressure is 150/100 mm Hg and her pulse is 72 and regular. Examination of the abdomen reveals tenderness in the right upper quadrant with associated voluntary guarding. There is radiation of the pain to the right scapula. Murphy's sign is positive.

SELECT THE ONE BEST ANSWER TO THE FOLLOWING QUESTIONS:

694. The most likely diagnosis in this patient is:
    a) biliary colic
    b) acute cholecystitis
    c) ascending cholangitis
    d) perforated peptic ulcer
    e) acute pancreatitis

695. The treatment of choice for the patient described in question 694 is:
    a) nasogastric suction, parenteral fluids, analgesics, IV antibiotics, and elective cholecystectomy in 3–6 months
    b) nasogastric suction, parenteral fluids, analgesics, IV antibiotics and urgent cholecystectomy
    c) nasogastric suction, parenteral fluids, analgesics, IV antibiotics and cholecystectomy as soon as the inflammation has been controlled
    d) nasogastric suction, parenteral fluids, analgesics, IV antibiotics, and repair of perforated ulcer
    e) none of the above

696. You have decided to place the patient described above on an IV antibiotic. Which of the following would be the antibiotic of first choice in the situation described?
    a) cefazolin
    b) penicillin
    c) erthyromycin
    d) metronidazole
    e) gentamicin

697. Which of the following statements regarding the condition described above is false?
    a) the condition usually results from obstruction of the cystic duct by a gallstone impacted in Hartmann's pouch
    b) most patients will have experienced previous attacks of biliary colic
    c) the leukocyte count is usually elevated
    d) a plain film of the abdomen will usually reveal the diagnosis
    e) ultrasonic evaluation is the diagnostic procedure of choice.

698. Which of the following statements about biliary colic is FALSE?
    a) oral cholecystography is the diagnostic procedure of choice
    b) biliary colic has cholelithiasis as its cause
    c) biliary colic may be produced by ingestion of the oral contraceptive pill
    d) biliary colic implies supersaturation of bile with cholesterol
    e) cholesterol gallstones are responsible for most cases of biliary colic

699. Which of the following is/are complications of acute cholecystitis?
    a) empyema
    b) perforation
    c) gangrene
    d) a and b
    e) all of the above

700. Which of the following statements regarding choledocholithiasis and cholangitis is false?
    a) choledocholithiasis occurs in approximately 15% of patients who harbor calculi in their gallbladders
    b) choledocholithiasis should be suspected if intermittent chills, fever, or jaundice accompany biliary colic
    c) Charcot's triad (the common symptoms of cholangitis) consists of biliary colic, chills, and high fever
    d) the most common bacterial organism involved in cholangitis is *E. coli*
    e) the primary treatment of acute cholangitis is medical management with IV antibiotics; definitive surgical management follows later in most cases

ANSWERS

694. B. The patient described in the question has a typical history of acute cholecystitis.

Symptoms of acute cholecystitis include right upper quadrant pain, nausea, vomiting, and fever. Examination usually reveals a tender right upper quadrant with voluntary guarding. Pain may be referred to the scapula, and the gallbladder may be palpable. Mild icterus may occur.

Acute cholecystitis is really an extension of biliary colic, with the latter term applied to recurrent right upper quadrant pain associated with blockage of the cystic duct or the ampullary end of the gallbladder by a stone, but not associated with actual gallbladder inflammation (manifested by systemic signs).

Murphy's sign is frequently positive in acute cholecystitis. In this test, the patient is instructed to breathe deeply during palpation in the right subcostal region; with acute cholecystitis, the patient experiences accentuated tenderness and sudden inspiratory arrest.

Ascending cholangitis usually presents a much more toxic picture, with right upper quadrant pain accompanied by high fever, chills, jaundice, and other systemic symptoms.

Perforated peptic ulcer, acute pancreatitis, strangulating small bowel obstruction, pneumonia, myocardial infarction, congestive cardiac failure, and pulmonary embolism are also causes of right upper quadrant pain but are distinctly less common than acute cholecystitis.[1]

695. C. Acute cholecystitis should be treated with nasogastric suction, parenteral fluids, analgesics, and IV antibiotics. Cholecystectomy should be performed as soon as the infection and inflammation associated with the acute cholecystitis has been controlled.[1]

696. A. The antibiotic of choice for acute cholecystitis of average severity is a third generation cephalosporin such as cefotaxime.[1,2] In severe infections, a combination of an extended spectrum penicillin such as piperacillin and an aminoglycoside (such as gentamicin) should be given.

697. D. Acute cholecystitis most often results from obstruction of the cystic duct by a gallstone impacted in Hartmann's pouch.

Most patients will have experienced previous attacks of either acute cholecystitis or biliary colic.

The WBC is usually elevated to 12,000 to 15,000/µl, with a predominance of neutrophils. A mild elevation in serum bilirubin and alkaline phosphatase levels may occur. The serum amylase level may also have been significantly elevated.

Plain x-rays of the abdomen are of limited value. An enlarged gallbladder may occasionally be seen on the plain film. In 15% of patients, the gallstones contain enough calcium to be seen on the plain film.

The gallbladder ultrasound is the diagnostic procedure of choice. A gallbladder ultrasound in a patient with acute cholecystitis may show gallstones, sludge, and thickening of the gallbladder wall. If a patient suspected of having acute cholecystitis has a negative gallbladder ultrasound, a radionuclide excretion scan (e.g., HIDA scan) should be performed. Although this investigation cannot demonstrate gallstones, it can and does exclude acute cholecystitis if the gallbladder is visualized.[1]

698. A. Biliary colic implies preexisting cholelithiasis. Repeated minor episodes of obstruction of the cystic duct cause intermittent biliary colic and contribute to inflammation and subsequent scar formation.

Biliary colic, the most characteristic symptom, is caused by transient gallstone obstruction of the cystic duct. The pain of biliary colic usually begins abruptly and subsides gradually, lasting from a few minutes to several hours. The pain of biliary colic is usually steady—not intermittent, like that of intestinal colic. The relationship of biliary colic to food is quite variable. Biliary colic is usually described as a pain in the right upper quadrant; but epigastric, left abdominal, and even precordial pain may occur. Dyspepsia (epigastric discomfort following meals) is common.

Cholelithiasis results from a supersaturation of bile with the excess cholesterol being deposited in the gallbladder and leading to the formation of cholesterol gallstones, the most common type. Young women taking the oral contraceptive pill are at increased risk for biliary colic, as estrogen increases the saturation of bile with cholesterol and subsequent gallstone formation.

The diagnostic procedure of choice for biliary colic is abdominal ultrasound. If an abdominal ultrasound is negative, oral cholecystography is indicated as a second test.[1]

699. E. The major complications of acute cholecystitis are empyema, gangrene, and perforation. Gangrene is usually associated with perforation.[1]

700. C. Approximately 15% of patients with stones in the gallbladder are found to have common bile duct stones as well (choledocholithiasis). Approximately 50% of patients with choledocholithiasis remain asymptomatic. The other 50% usually present with biliary colic, often accompanied by chills, fever, and/or jaundice. Pancreatitis may also be diagnosed.

Cholangitis (bacterial infection of the biliary ducts) always implies biliary obstruction. The principal causes are choledocholithiasis, biliary stricture, and neoplasm. By far the most common cause is choledocholithiasis. The symptoms of cholangitis (sometimes referred to as Charcot's triad) consist of biliary colic, jaundice, and chills and fever. Laboratory findings include leukocytosis, and elevated serum bilirubin and alkaline phosphatase levels.

The predominant organisms in bile in decreasing order of frequency are *E. coli, Klebsiella pneumonia, Pseudomonas, enterococci,* and *Proteus, Bacteroides fragilis,* and other anaerobes. Multiorganism infection is common.[1,2]

SUMMARY OF ACUTE CHOLECYSTITIS AND BILIARY COLIC

1. **Acute cholecystitis:** Symptoms and signs:
   a) acute right upper quadrant pain and tenderness
   b) mild fever and leukocytosis
   c) nausea and vomiting
   d) palpable gallbladder in one-third of cases
   e) gallstones on ultrasound scan
   Treatment: Nasogastric suction, parenteral fluids, analgesics, IV antibiotics, and cholecystectomy as soon as the inflammation has subsided.

2. **Biliary Colic:** (Gallstones/chronic cholecystitis) Symptoms and signs:
   a) recurrent abdominal pain (usually RUQ)
   b) dyspepsia
   c) gallstones on ultrasound
   Treatment: Cholecystectomy.

3. **Choledocholithiasis/Cholangitis:** Choledocholithiasis occurs in 15% of patients with gallstones. Choledocholithiasis is the major cause of cholangitis.
   Symptoms of cholangitis (Charcot's triad): biliary colic, jaundice, fever, and chills.
   Treatment of cholangitis: IV antibiotics followed by elective cholecystectomy and exploration of the common bile duct.

References

1. Way L. Biliary tract. In: Way L, ed. Current surgical diagnosis and treatment. 8th Ed. Norwalk: Appleton & Lange, 1988: 495–507.

2. Dunagan W, Powderly W. Antimicrobials and infectious diseases. In: Dunagan W, Ridner M, eds. Manual of medical therapeutics. 26th Ed. Boston: Little, Brown, 1989: 239–245.

PROBLEM 92: A 35-YEAR-OLD FEMALE WITH A BREAST LUMP

A 35-year-old female presents to your office for a routine physical examination. She states that she has felt a fullness in both breasts for the last 6 months. The fullness appears to be confined to the last week of the menstrual cycle. There is significant tenderness associated with the fullness. On self-examination, the patient says that her breasts feel "lumpy."

On physical examination, there is a 2 cm mass present in the upper outer quadrant of the right breast, and numerous smaller lumps felt throughout both breasts. There is no axillary lymphadenopathy.

SELECT THE ONE BEST ANSWER TO THE FOLLOWING QUESTIONS:

701. The most likely diagnosis in this patient is:
    a) carcinoma of the breast
    b) fibroadenoma
    c) multiple intraductal papillomas
    d) fibrocystic breast changes
    e) premenstrual tension syndrome

702. The most appropriate diagnostic procedure at this time is:
    a) excisional biopsy
    b) bilateral breast ultrasound
    c) mammography
    d) breast cyst aspiration
    e) none of the above

703. Which of the following may be indicated in the treatment of the condition described above:
    a) oral progesterone
    b) vitamin E
    c) low dose oral contraceptives
    d) a and c
    e) all of the above

704. A 25-year-old female presents to your office for assessment of a breast lump that has been present for the past 6 months. It is painless, and does not vary throughout the menstrual cycle.
    On examination, there is a 2 cm mass present in the upper outer quadrant of the left breast. It is rubbery in consistency, freely mobile, and round in shape. There is no axillary lymphadenopathy.
    The most likely diagnosis is this patient is:
    a) carcinoma of the breast
    b) fibroadenoma
    c) intraductal papilloma
    d) fibrocystic breast disease
    e) none of the above

705. The treatment of choice for the patient described in question 704 is:
    a) do nothing; reassess the mass in 6 months

    b) perform a mammogram; if it confirms your suspicions, reassess in 1 year
    c) perform a breast cyst aspiration
    d) perform a fine needle biopsy or schedule an excisional biopsy
    e) schedule ultrasound examination every 3 months to document the growth of the mass.

706. A 33-year-old female presents with a 2-month history of a bloody unilateral left nipple discharge. She has also noted a very small soft lump just beneath the areola.
    On examination, there is a 3 mm soft mass located just inferior to the left areola. No other abnormalities are found in either breast.
    The most likely diagnosis in this patient is:
    a) carcinoma of the breast
    b) fibroadenoma
    c) intraductal papilloma
    d) fibrocystic breast disease
    e) none of the above

707. A 54-year-old female presents to your office for assessment of a breast lump that she noted 2 weeks previously. The lump is located in the upper outer quadrant of the left breast.
    On examination, the patient has a 4 cm, hard, irregular mass that is nonmobile. It is present at the 2 oclock position in the left breast. It is not fixed to any underlying structures. Two lymph nodes are palpable, 1 cm each in diameter, in the left axilla.
    The most likely diagnosis in this patient is:
    a) carcinoma of the breast
    b) fibroadenoma
    c) intraductal papilloma
    d) fibrocystic breast disease
    e) sarcoma of the breast

ANSWER THE FOLLOWING QUESTIONS ACCORDING TO THE CODE:

A: 1, 2, and 3 are correct
B: 1 and 3 are correct

C: 2 and 4 are correct
D: Only 4 is correct
E: All of the above are correct

708. Which of the following is(are) risk factors for the development of carcinoma of the breast?
      1) older age
      2) present or previous use of oral contraceptives
      3) family history of breast cancer
      4) fibrocystic disease of the breast

709. Which of the following is(are) reasonable therapeutic options for the patient discussed in question 707?
      1) modified radical mastectomy
      2) breast irradiation alone
      3) lumpectomy with postoperative radiation
      4) reassessment of the mass in 3 months to demonstrate any change in size

710. Which of the following groups of patients should receive postoperative adjunctive chemotherapy or hormonal therapy for the management of breast cancer?
      1) premenopausal patients with positive axillary nodes
      2) premenopausal patients with negative estrogen and progesterone receptors
      3) postmenopausal patients with positive nodes and positive hormone receptors
      4) premenopausal patients with negative nodes and positive estrogen receptors

711. Which of the following statements regarding screening for breast cancer by the family physician is(are) true?
      1) several studies have demonstrated a decreased mortality from breast cancer in women who were screened by mammography
      2) breast self-examination has been shown to reduce breast cancer mortality in all studies that have been performed to date
      3) the usefullness of mammography greatly depends upon the definition of an abnormal mammogram and who reads it
      4) the American Cancer Society recommends a baseline mammogram at age 30

ANSWERS

701. D. This patient has fibrocystic breast changes. All breasts contain cysts, and thus "fibrocystic breast

disease," as the condition was previously called, is inappropriate.[1]

Fibrocystic breast changes are probably hormonal in origin, perhaps related to an estrogen-progesterone imbalance or a prolactin excess.[1]

The most common presenting symptom of fibrocystic breast disease is pain. The pain usually begins 1 week prior to menstruation, and is relieved following menstruation. The pain is usually bilateral, and is most common in the upper outer quadrants.[1] It may be associated with breast swelling, and yellow to green breast discharge.

The other diagnoses offered in this question will be discussed in subsequent questions.

702. D. The most appropriate diagnostic procedure at this time is breast cyst aspiration. The fluid that is withdrawn is usually amber to green in color. If blood is withdrawn, a biopsy is indicated.[1] Breast ultrasound and mammography are also useful in the assessment of suspected fibrocystic disease. However, a discrete lump that disappears after withdrawal of yellow to greenish fluid is diagnostic of fibrocystic disease.

703. D. Fibrocystic breast changes can be effectively treated by (a) wearing a well-padded brassiere, (b) a low-dose oral contraceptives that contains a potent progesterone (e.g., Loestrin 1/20), or c) medroxyprogesterone from days 15–25 of the calendar month.

Danazol is occasionally used for severe fibrocystic breast changes. It is expensive, however, and has numerous side effects.

Vitamin E has not been shown to be of value in the treatment of fibrocystic breast changes.[1]

704. B. This patient has a fibroadenoma or "breast mouse." Fibroadenomas are the most frequent solid benign tumors of the breast. They are most prevalent in women under the age of 25. They are usually painless, well-circumscribed, completely round, and freely mobile. They are usually described as being rubbery in consistency.[1]

705. D. The treatment of choice is to perform either a fine needle biopsy or an excisional biopsy. Although rare, malignancies have occasionally been found in fibroadenomas.[1]

706. C. This patient has an intraductal papilloma. Intraductal papillomas are small, soft tumors that occur below the areola. If a patient presents with a

bloody nipple discharge associated with a soft mass, there is a 95 % chance that this is an intraductal papilloma.[1] If physical examination reveals no mass, Paget's disease of the nipple, adenoma of the nipple, and a breast carcinoma with ductal invasion must be considered in the differential diagnosis.

The treatment of choice is surgical removal. This is often facilitated by mammography or a ductogram.

707. A. This patient most likely has a carcinoma of the breast. The most common presenting symptom of breast cancer is a painless breast lump. Most breast lumps are discovered by patients themselves. Other symptoms include breast pain; nipple discharge; erosions; retraction; enlargement or itching of the nipple; and redness, generalized hardness, enlargement or shrinking of the breast.[2]

708. B. Factors associated with increased risk of breast cancer include white race, older age, family history of breast cancer, previous history of endometrial cancer or cancer in the other breast, early menarche (under age 12), late menopause (after age 50), nulliparous status, and a late first pregnancy (after age 35).[1,2]

Fibrocystic breast disease and a present or previous use of oral contraceptives have not definitively been shown to be associated with an increased risk of carcinoma of the breast.

709. B. The National Surgical Adjunctive Breast Project (NSABP) has concluded that segmental mastectomy (lumpectomy) followed by breast irradiation in all patients and adjunctive chemotherapy in women with positive nodes is appropriate therapy for stage I and stage II breast tumors less than 4 cm in diameter, provided that the margins are free of resected specimens of tumor. Stages I and II tumors include those that are less than 5 cm in diameter, and nodes, that if palpable, are not fixed to each other or to any other structure, and with no evidence of distant metastases.[3] This is the alternative to modified radical mastectomy.

710. A. Patients who should receive adjunctive therapy include: (1) premenopausal patients with positive axillary lymph nodes—combination chemotherapy; (2) premenopausal patients without positive lymph nodes if they have negative estrogen and progesterone receptors—combination chemotherapy; and (3) postmenopausal patients with positive axillary lymph nodes and positive estrogen and progesterone receptors—tamoxifen therapy.

711. B. There is considerable controversy over the use of mammography and breast self-examination in the prevention of breast cancer death in women.

One large American study, the Health Insurance Plan (HIP) Study, and several other studies have demonstrated decreased mortality from breast cancer in women who were screened by routine mammography.[1] There are, however, several concerns about mammography. These concerns include the cost, and the fact that physicians may be lulled into a false sense of security. Mammography may miss breast cancer, and it is only as good as the definition of what constitutes normal and abnormal, who reads the mammogram, and how good the equipment used to perform the mammogram is. Mammography will also lead to unnecessary surgery with wider biopsy use.[1]

Breast self-examination (BSE) has been assessed by retrospective studies; some have shown a benefit from BSE, others have not.[1]

The American Cancer Society recommends a baseline mammogram at age 35–40, mammograms every 1 or 2 years from ages 40–49, and annual mammograms from age 50 onward. As well, they recommend monthly breast self-examination starting at age 20, physical examination of the breast at 3 year intervals between the ages of 20 and 40, and annually thereafter.[2]

SUMMARY OF THE DIAGNOSIS AND MANAGEMENT OF BREAST LUMPS AND BREAST CANCER SCREENING

1. **Fibrocystic breast changes:**
   Etiology: hormonal factors
   Symptoms: breast pain and fullness premenstrually, with or without discharge
   Diagnosis: breast cyst aspiration; supplemented by mammography and ultrasound
   Treatment: supportive measures, oral contraceptives with low estrogenic activity and potent progestin, medroxyprogesterone acetate

2. **Fibroadenoma:** Most frequent solid benign tumor of breast. Painless, well-circumscribed, round, rubbery, freely mobile lesion. Common in young women.
   Treatment: excisional biopsy

3. **Intraductal papilloma**: Bloody, unilateral nipple discharge with a soft mass.

Treatment: surgical removal

4. **Carcinoma of the breast:**

Symptoms: most common symptom is painless lump diagnosed by patient herself.

Treatment: lumpectomy with radiation for Stage I or Stage II, or modified radical mastectomy. Adjuvant chemotherapy for premenopausal patients with positive nodes, those with negative nodes and negative estrogen and progesterone receptor, and hormonal therapy (tamoxifen) therapy for postmenopausal patients with positive nodes and positive receptors.

5. Breast self-examination and mammography are still being assessed in terms of cost/benefit ratio.

Routine mammography, however, appears to decrease mortality from breast cancer in women over the age of 50 years.

References

1. Bachman J. Breast problems. Prim Care 1988: 15(3):643–644.

2. Giuliano A. Breast. In: Way L, ed. Current surgical diagnosis and treatment. 8th Ed. Norwalk: Appleton & Lange: 1988:258–275.

3. Fisher B, Bauer M, Margolese R. Five-year results of a randomized clinical trial comparing total mastectomy and segmental mastectomy with or without radiation in the treatment of breast cancer. N Engl J Med 1985, 312:665.

PROBLEM 93: A 42-YEAR-OLD MALE WITH RECTAL BLEEDING

A 42-year-old male presents to your office with a 3-week history of rectal bleeding. He states this is his first episode of rectal bleeding. He attributes the bleeding to hemorrhoids and asks you for a cream or an ointment to alleviate the problem. On further questioning, he says the bleeding is bright red, not mixed in with the stool, and is not sufficient in amount to color the toilet water.

On anoscopic examination, the patient has significant internal hemorrhoids in the right anterior, right posterior, and left lateral positions. No other abnormalities are seen.

SELECT THE ONE BEST ANSWER TO THE FOLLOWING QUESTIONS:

712. Considering the history and physical examination of the patient described in the question above you should now:
    a) order a therapeutic hemorrhoidal ointment
    b) tell the patient to take a hot bath and the hemorrhoids will go away
    c) book the patient for a complete work-up: complete blood profile, air-contrast barium enema, and colonscopy
    d) tell the patient to relax, get more rest, and eat a high fiber diet
    e) perform a flexible sigmoidoscopy

713. With regard to hemorrhoids, which of the following statements is false?
    a) internal hemorrhoids are a plexus of superior hemorrhoidal veins
    b) internal hemorrhoids usually occur in the right anterior, right posterior, and left lateral positions

    c) the most common reason for hemorrhoids becoming symptomatic is straining in the squatting position at the time of a bowel movement
    d) suppositories and rectal ointments have been shown to be of significant therapeutic value in the treatment of hemorrhoids
    e) bleeding from internal hemorrhoids may produce a secondary anemia

ANSWER THE FOLLOWING QUESTIONS ACCORDING TO THE CODE:

A: 1, 2, and 3 are correct
B: 1 and 3 are correct
C: 2 and 4 are correct
D: Only 4 is correct
E: All of the above are correct

714. Which of the following is(are) recommended treatment for internal hemorrhoids?
    1) injection therapy with a sclerosing solution
    2) rubber band ligation

3) hemorrhoidectomy

4) cryosurgery

715. A 35-year-old male limps into your office with an acute pain in the rectal area. He has had previous hemorrhoids, but they have never really caused him much trouble. He states the acute pain developed after he began sneezing when he came into contact with a cat (he is allergic to cats). On examination, there is a tense, blue, elevation beneath the skin of the external anal canal.

Which of the following statements regarding this patient's condition is (are) true?

1) this is most likely a thrombosed internal hemorrhoid

2) symptomatic treatment with sitz baths and analgesics are the most appropriate treatments in this situation

3) pain in this condition is unlikely to diminish for many days or weeks unless definitive therapy is undertaken

4) this condition is not a true hemorrhoid; rather it is thrombosis of the subcutaneous external hemorrhoidal veins of the anal canal

SELECT THE ONE BEST ANSWER TO THE FOLLOWING QUESTIONS:

716. A 51-year-old male presents with a 3-month history of bright red rectal bleeding. He also complains of constipation and a sensation of incomplete evacuation. The bleeding occurs with every bowel movement, and is sufficient to significantly color the toilet bowl water. It is sometimes mixed in with the stool.

On examination, there are no masses palpated in the abdomen. The rectal examination is normal. There are small internal hemorrhoids present on anoscopic examination.

Although each of the following diagnostic procedures may be indicated in the examination of the patient described above, which of the following is the most sensitive in ruling out significant colorectal pathology:

a) rigid sigmoidoscopy

b) flexible sigmoidoscopy

c) colonoscopy

d) single contrast barium enema

e) double contrast barium enema

717. Colorectal polyps are thought to be the origin of most colorectal cancers. Which of the following statements regarding colorectal polyps is false?

a) the larger the colorectal polyp, the greater the chance of malignancy

b) hyperplastic polyps have the highest malignant potential of all colorectal polyps

c) adenomatous polyps increase in incidence with each decade after age 30

d) routine removal of adenomas from the rectum reduces the incidence of subsequent rectal cancer

e) villous adenomas carry the highest malignant potential of all adenomas

718. Which of the following statements best describes the current evidence for occult blood screening as a measure to reduce the morbidity and mortality from colorectal cancer in patients over the age of 45?

a) there is good evidence to support the inclusion of fecal occult blood testing in the periodic health examination

b) there is fair evidence to support the inclusion of fecal occult blood testing in the periodic health examination

c) there is poor evidence to support the inclusion of fecal occult blood testing in the periodic health examination

d) there is fair evidence to support the exclusion of fecal occult blood testing from the periodic health examination

e) there is good evidence to support the exclusion of fecal occult blood testing from the periodic health examination

719. Which of the following statements best describes the use of sigmoidoscopy screening in patients over the age of 40 years as a measure to reduce the morbidity and mortality from colorectal cancer?

a) there is good evidence to support the inclusion of routine sigmoidoscopy in the periodic health examination

b) there is fair evidence to support the inclusion of routine sigmoidoscopy in the periodic health examination

c) there is poor evidence to support the inclusion of routine sigmoidoscopy in the periodic health examination

d) there is fair evidence to support the exclusion of routine sigmoidoscopy in the periodic health examination

ANSWER THE FOLLOWING QUESTIONS ACCORDING TO THE CODE:

A: 1, 2, and 3 are correct
B: 1 and 3 are correct
C: 2 and 4 are correct
D: Only 4 is correct
E: All of the above are correct

720. Which of the following statements regarding colorectal cancer is(are) true?
    1) dyspeptic symptoms may be the first manifestation of right-sided colon cancer
    2) in Western countries, cancer of the colon and rectum ranks second after cancer of the lung in incidence of new cases and death rates
    3) a dietary high in saturated fat has been proposed as a risk factor for colorectal cancer
    4) most colorectal cancers arise from adenomatous polyps

721. Which of the following statements regarding carcinoembyronic antigen (CEA) is(are) true:
    1) CEA is a useful screening test for colorectal cancer
    2) preoperative CEA levels correlate with postoperative recurrence rate
    3) CEA is a specific test for colorectal cancer
    4) failure of CEA to fall to normal levels after colonic resection implies a poor prognosis

722. Which of the following statements regarding the treatment of colorectal cancer is(are) true?
    1) numerous operative procedures exist for the treatment of colorectal cancer
    2) radiation therapy is assuming a greater role in the management of rectal cancer
    3) immunotherapy has not been shown to be of benefit in the treatment of colorectal cancer
    4) chemotherapy is assuming an increasingly important role in the treatment of colorectal cancer

ANSWERS

712. E. Although both the history and physical examination point to internal hemorrhoids as the most likely cause of the rectal bleeding, the minimum examination that is required is a flexible sigmoidoscopy. Whenever rectal bleeding occurs, even in the presence of an obviously benign lesion such as hemorrhoids, coexisting cancer must be ruled out.[1]

713. D. Hemorrhoids represent a normal anatomic state. Only when they become enlarged and symptomatic is treatment indicated.

Hemorrhoids are classified as either internal or external. Internal hemorrhoids are a plexus of superior hemorrhoidal veins above the mucocutaneous junction of the rectum. They occur in three primary positions: the right anterior, the right posterior, and the left lateral. External hemorrhoids occur below the mucocutaneous junction in the tissues beneath the anal epithelium in the anal canal and the skin of the perianal region. The plexuses of the internal and the external hemorrhoids anastomose freely and comprise the venous return of the lower rectum and anus.[1]

Although hemorrhoids may become symptomatic for many reasons, the most common reason is straining in the squatting position at the time of a bowel movement. This increases the venous pressure and distends the hemorrhoidal veins. This may create redundancy and enlargement of the vascular cushions, allowing for eventual bleeding or protrusion. Other important causative factors include chronic constipation, pregnancy, obesity, and a low fiber diet.[1]

Bleeding is usually the first symptom of internal hemorrhoids. It is bright red, unmixed with stool, and may vary in amount from streaking on the toilet tissue to amounts sufficient to color the toilet water. Recurrent hemorrhoidal bleeding may result in enough blood loss to cause a secondary anemia. With enlargement of the hemorrhoidal tissue, the hemorrhoids may begin to protrude (prolapse). This may progress to a stage where it is difficult or impossible to replace them back into the anal canal. Mucoid discharge and soiling of the undergarments are usually marked when the hemorrhoids are permanently prolapsed.[1]

Therapy will be assessed in a subsequent question; however, hemorrhoidal suppositories and rectal ointments have no known therapeutic value except for their anesthetic and astringent properties.[1]

714. E. Most patients with early (nonprotruding) hemorrhoids can be managed by simple local measures and dietary advice. A high fiber diet with an increased fluid intake, and the use of stool softeners is indicated in treatment.

Astringent compresses (containing witch hazel) and sitz baths provide symptomatic relief, but do not decrease the size of the hemorrhoids.

For prolapsing hemorrhoids, injection therapy with 5% phenol or rubber band ligation is indicated. An alternative is cryotherapy. Hemorrhoidectomy, which is currently performed much less frequently than previously, is reserved for patients who have failed to respond to the more conservative treatments, or which develop chronic bleeding and anemia.[1]

715. D. This patient has a thrombosed external (not internal) hemorrhoid. Although this lesion is called a hemorrhoid, it is not really a true hemorrhoid, but rather a thrombosis of the subcutaneous external hemorrhoidal veins of the anal canal. Characteristically, it is a painful, tense, bluish elevation beneath the skin or anoderm, varying in size from a few millimeters to several centimeters.[1]

An external thrombosed hemorrhoid usually follows a sudden increase in venous pressure such as that which occurs after heavy lifting, coughing, sneezing, straining at stool, or at parturition.

Pain is greatest at the onset of the condition and gradually subsides in 2–3 days as the edema resolves. The hemorrhoid may rupture, and resolve spontaneously. Symptomatic treatment including warm sitz baths, application of lubricants such as vaseline, bed rest, and mild analgesics are appropriate treatments if the hemorrhoid appears to be resolving. However, if the patient presents within the first 48 hours, obstruction can be relieved by evacuation of the thrombus or by complete excision under local anesthesia.[1]

716. C. The diagnostic procedure of choice in this patient is colonoscopy. The symptoms and signs are suggestive of a neoplasm of the colon or rectum and the most sensitive test for evaluation of the entire colon is colonoscopy. Although you might choose to start with a flexible sigmoidoscopy or a double contrast barium enema, the investigation is not complete without a colonoscopy, irrespective of whether or not a lesion is found with the first procedure performed.[4]

717. B. Colonic polyps or adenomas are common, and increase in incidence with each decade after age 30. They may be found in over 50% of asymptomatic patients. Generally, the larger the polyp, the greater the risk of malignancy.

Villous adenomas (compared to tubular and tubulovillous adenomas) carry the greatest risk of malignancy; hyperplastic polyps do not become malignant. Routine removal of adenomas from the rectum reduces the incidence of subsequent rectal cancer.[4]

718. C. According to the US Preventive Services Task Force, there is poor evidence to support the inclusion of fecal occult blood screening in the periodic health examination in patients over the age of 45 years.[2] In patients with a family history of colorectal cancer in a first-degree relative, a stronger argument can be made for routine screening.

719. C. According to the US Preventive Services Task Force, there is poor evidence to support the inclusion of sigmoidoscopy screening in the periodic health examination in patients over the age of 40 years.[3]

720. E. In Western countries, cancer of the colon and rectum ranks second after cancer of the lung in incidence of new cases and death rates.[4]

Signs and symptoms of right-sided colonic cancer include unexplained weakness or anemia, occult blood in the feces, dyspeptic symptoms, persistent right-sided abdominal symptoms, or a palpable abdominal mass.[4]

Signs and symptoms of left-sided colon cancer include a change in bowel habits (either diarrhea like or constipation), gross blood in the stool and obstructive symptoms.[4]

Signs and symptoms of rectal cancer include rectal bleeding, alteration in bowel habits, a sensation of incomplete evacuation, and sometimes a intrarectal palpable tumor.[4]

There is fair evidence that colon cancer is related to a diet high in saturated fat.[4]

As discussed previously, most colorectal cancers arise from adenomatous polyps.[4]

721. C. Carcinoembryonic antigen (CEA) has been found to be of value in the prognosis of colorectal cancer. Preoperative CEA levels correlate with postoperative recurrence rate. As well, failure of CEA to fall to normal levels after colonic resection implies a poor prognosis. CEA, however, is not a useful screening test nor a specific test for colorectal cancer. It may be elevated in other gastrointestinal cancers, other diseases, and cigarette smokers.[4]

722. A. Numerous operations exist for surgical treatment of colorectal cancer. Their description is beyond the scope of this book.

Radiation therapy (preoperative, intraoperative, and postoperative) is assuming a greater role in the management of rectal cancer.

Chemotherapy and immunotherapy have not yet been shown to be of any benefit in the treatment of colorectal cancer.[4]

SUMMARY OF THE DIAGNOSIS AND TREATMENT OF HEMORRHOIDS AND COLORECTAL CANCER

1. **Hemorrhoids:**
   Signs and symptoms: rectal bleeding, protrusion, discomfort, mucus discharge, sometimes secondary anemia
   Diagnosis: anoscopy, flexible sigmoidoscopy
   Treatment: nonprolapsing hemorrhoids: high fiber diet, fluids, sitz baths
   Prolapsing hemorrhoids: sclerotherapy, rubber band ligation, cryosurgery, hemorrhoidectomy

2. **Colorectal Cancer:**
   Signs and symptoms: rectal or occult bleeding, dyspepsia, abdominal discomfort, weakness, anemia, change in bowel habits, palpable abdominal mass, sensation of incomplete emptying
   Diagnosis: colonoscopy is the procedure of choice. Flexible sigmoidoscopy and air-contrast

barium enema are also useful in the diagnosis of colorectal cancer.

Screening: US Preventive Services Task Force does not recommend inclusion of fecal occult blood testing or sigmoidoscopy screening for the general population.

Treatment: surgical resection of tumor. Radiation therapy is assuming a greater importance in the management of rectal carcinoma.

References

1. Russell T. Anorectum. In: Way L, ed. Current surgical diagnosis and treatment. 8th Ed. Norwalk, Appleton & Lange, 1988: 633–638.

2. Knight K. Occult blood screening for colorectal cancer (including US Preventive Services Task Force Recommendations for fecal occult blood screening. JAMA 1989, 261(14):587--593.

3. US Preventive Services Task Force Recommendations on Sigmoidoscopic Screening. JAMA 1989, 261(14):594.

4. Schrock T. Large Intestine. In: Way L, ed. Current surgical diagnosis and treatment. 8th Ed. Norwalk: Appleton & Lange, 1988: 594–605.

PROBLEM 94: A 31-YEAR-OLD FEMALE WITH DIZZINESS, HEARING LOSS, TINNITUS, AND A FULL FEELING IN HER LEFT EAR

A 31-year-old female presents to your office with a sensation of episodic dizziness, ringing, hearing loss, and fulness in her left ear. The symptoms are often associated with nausea and vomiting. The symptoms appeared 6 months ago. The "dizziness" is described as a "sensation of the world spinning around her" and usually lasts for 6-8 hours. The other symptoms usually begin to disappear when the dizziness goes away. The last attack began 4 hours ago.

On examination, the patient has horizontal nystagmus. The slow phase of the nystagmus is to the left, and the rapid phase to the right. No other abnormalities are found on physical examination.

SELECT THE ONE BEST ANSWER TO THE FOLLOWING QUESTIONS:

723. The most likely diagnosis in this patient is:
    a) vestibular neuronitis
    b) acute labyrinthitis
    c) benign positional vertigo
    d) orthostatic hypotension
    e) Meniere's disease

724. The treatment protocol for the patient discussed in question 723 should include:
    a) discontinuation of caffeine
    b) discontinuation of alcohol
    c) hydrochlorothiazide
    d) a and b only
    e) all of the above

725. A 34-year-old female presents to your office with a 6 month history of "feeling dizzy." She says that she "feels dizzy" when she stands up. When asked

to describe this feeling of "dizziness," she states that it is a feeling of "lightheadedness," a feeling that she is "going to faint." This sensation lasts for 30–45 seconds and then passes away.

Her past history is significant for major depressive illness. She was placed on amitriptyline 6 months ago, and has gradually been improving. She has had no other significant illness.

On examination blood pressure is 120/80 mm Hg and drops to 100/70 mm Hg after assuming the upright position. There is no ataxia, no nystagmus, and her gait is normal. Examination of the cranial nerves is normal.

The most likely diagnosis in this patient is:
a) vestibular neuronitis
b) acute labyrinthitis
c) benign positional vertigo
d) orthostatic hypotension
e) Meniere's disease

726. The most appropriate treatment for the patient described in question 725 is:
a) an antiemetic
b) education and reassurance
c) hydrochlorothiazide
d) a change in the antidepressant
e) b and d

727. A 28-year-old male presents for assessment of "dizziness" that seems to occur when he rolls over from the lying position to either the right or to the left side. This dizziness also occurs when he is looking up (searching for stock on the shelfs of his store).

The episodes of "dizziness" are described as a sensation of the "world spinning around him." These episodes usually last for 10–15 seconds. They have been occurring for the past 6 months averaging 1–2 times per day.

The most likely diagnosis in this patient is:
a) vestibular neuronitis
b) acute labyrinthitis
c) benign positional vertigo
d) orthostatic hypotension
e) Meniere's disease

728. The treatment of choice for the patient discussed in question 727 is:
a) avoidance of alcohol and caffeine
b) hydrochlorothiazide
c) dimenhydrinate
d) reassurance and simple exercises
e) endolymphatic surgery

729. A 27-year-old female presents with a four day history of " unrelenting dizziness." The dizziness has been present for 4 days, and is associated with nausea and vomiting. There has been no hearing loss, no tinnitus, and no aural fulness. The patient had a cold a few days ago that appears to have cleared up completely.

On examination there is nystagmus present. The slow phase of the nystagmus is toward the left, and the rapid phase toward the right. There is also a significant ataxia present.

The most likely diagnosis in this patient is:
a) vestibular neuronitis
b) acute labyrinthitis
c) benign positional vertigo
d) orthostatic hypotension
e) Meniere's disease

730. The treatment of choice for the patient described in question 729 is:
a) avoidance of alcohol and caffeine
b) hydrochlorothiazide
c) endolymphatic surgery
d) reassurance and antiemetics
e) none of the above

731. A 23-year-old female presents with a 3-day history of severe "dizziness" associated with ataxia and right-sided hearing loss. She had an upper respiratory tract infection 1 week ago. At that time her right ear felt plugged.

On examination, there is fluid behind the right eardrum. There is horizontal nystagmus present with the slow component to the right, and the quick component to the left. Ataxia is present.

The most likely diagnosis in this patient is:
a) vestibular neuronitis
b) acute labyrinthitis
c) benign positional vertigo
d) orthostatic hypotension
e) Meniere's disease

732. The treatment of choice for the patient described in question 731 is:
a) avoidance of caffeine and alcohol
b) hydrochlorothiazide
c) endolymphatic surgery
d) rest, antiemetics, and antibiotics
e) none of the above

ANSWERS

723. E. This patient has Meniere's disease. The classical features of Meniere's disease are (1) recurrent episodes of vertigo; (2) fluctuating sensorineural hearing loss, particularly in the low frequencies; (3) tinnitus, which classically consists of buzzing; and (4) aural fulness in the affected ear.

Meniere's disease is associated with vertigo that typically lasts hours, not minutes or days. Low-tone sensorineural hearing loss occurs. The fluctuating hearing may not be related temporally to the vertigo. In many cases, the tinnitus and fulness become severe just before the vertigo attack begins.

To make the diagnosis of Meniere's disease, the characteristic pattern of vertigo lasting a matter of hours, as well as sensorineural hearing loss must be present. One additional factor (low-frequency hearing loss, aural fulness, or buzzing tinnitus) should also be present.[1] The other choices offered in the question will be discussed in subsequent questions.

724. E. Some patients with Meniere's disease appear to be sensitive to caffeine or alcohol. In these patients, caffeine and alcohol should obviously be avoided.

Meniere's disease is also known as endolymphatic hydrops. This suggests that a build-up of fluid in the endolymphatic system may be responsible for the development of the acute attack. Thus, the use of a mild diuretic such as hydrochlorothiazide is a reasonable treatment (especially for patients that are having frequent attacks).

The use of an antinauseant such as droperidol IM or chlorpromazine or dimenhydrinate IM or oral may be extremely effective for the acute attack.

Surgery is reserved for patients that do not respond to medical management.[1]

725. D. This patient has orthostatic hypotension. The case description in this patient illustrates the importance of obtaining an accurate history in the patient who complains of "feeling dizzy." In any patient who complains of "feeling dizzy," it is important to ask three questions: (1) Can you describe your dizziness? (is it more a sensation of vertigo or lightheadedness), (2) How long does it last—seconds, minutes, or hours?, and (3) Are there any accompanying symptoms such as deafness, fulness, or ringing. Orthostatic hypotension

is typically initiated after standing up suddenly, or in many cases, is experienced after the patient has been up for a long time, often in closed quarters or crowded shopping malls. The feeling described is that of a subjective dizziness and is closely related to a simple faint or a syncopal episode. It is often accompanied by nausea. It is not associated with any other neurologic sensations or ear symptoms.[1]

In this case, the orthostatic hypotension is almost certainly associated with the beginning of tricyclic antidepressant therapy 6 months ago.

726. E. The most appropriate treatment in this patient is to reassure the patient and explain how it can be minimized by slowly assuming the upright position.

As the orthostatic hypotension developed after the initiation of the tricyclic antidepressant, amitriptyline, it would be reasonable to switch to an antidepressant with fewer orthostatic effects. A good choice would be desipramine.

727. C. Benign postural vertigo is a disorder that consists of brief episodes (lasting anywhere from 2 to 10 seconds) usually caused by rolling over when supine toward either the right or left or sometimes by looking up, such as when searching for something on a shelf. The etiology may be related to trauma or may be idiopathic.[1]

728. D. The treatment of choice for the patient discussed in question 727 is reassurance and the prescription of simple exercise. The exercises involve assuming lateral positions: first with the head hanging to the right or left and then with the head hanging in the other direction, left or right. The patient is asked to move quickly into position and hold the position until the feeling of dizziness goes away or for 20 seconds, then to move quickly and hold in the other direction.

Performance of these exercises three or four times in a row three or four times a day often provides dramatic relief, but improvement in symptoms sometimes takes 10 days.

Even if the exercises are not prescribed, the condition tends to resolve with time (usually several weeks to a few months).[1]

729. A. This patient has a left vestibular neuronitis. This disorder is most likely caused by a viral infection (such as adenovirus) that following a respiratory tract infection, involves some portion of the vestibular system, with total sparing of the cochlea.

The disorder consists of severe vertigo with ataxia lasting several days. There is no hearing loss, no pain, no tinnitus, or no other symptoms. Recovery usually takes approximately 1 week.[1]

730. D. The treatment of choice for the patient described in question 729 is rest, reassurance, and antiemetics. Vestibular neuronitis will resolve within 1–2 weeks. Droperidol, chlorpromazine, or dimenhydrinate may be given for symptomatic relief of the vertigo, and rest and reassurance are all that is required in most cases.[1]

731. A. This patient has acute labyrinthitis. Acute labyrinthitis usually follows an upper respiratory tract infection that is accompanied by middle ear effusion. The disorder is thought to represent a chemical irritation of the inner ear from middle ear fluid. The features of acute labyrinthitis includes significant sensorineural hearing loss (with a conductive component if a middle ear effusion is present), and severe vertigo that lasts several days.[1]

732. D. The treatment of choice for acute labyrinthitis is rest, antiemetics, and antibiotics. Bacterial labyrinthitis may complicate serous labyrinthitis if antibiotics are not administered. Amoxicillin would be a good first line agent for antibiotic prophylaxis.[1]

SUMMARY OF DIAGNOSIS AND TREATMENT OF THE PATIENT COMPLAINING OF DIZZINESS

1. **Meniere's disease**: Vertigo (lasting hours not seconds or days) associated with hearing loss, tinnitus, and aural fulness. Treatment: avoidance of alcohol and caffeine may be helpful in some cases; hydrochlorothiazide may be used if attacks are frequent. Antiemetics provide symptomatic relief but should probably be avoided on a long-term basis.

2. **Acute labyrinthitis**: Vertigo (lasting for days) associated with significant hearing loss. Usually follows an upper respiratory tract infection in which there is a middle ear effusion. Treatment: rest, antiemetics, and prophylactic antibiotics.

3. **Vestibular neuronitis**: Vertigo (lasting for days) with no hearing loss, pain, or other symptoms. May also result from viral upper respiratory tract infection. Treatment: rest, reassurance, and antiemetics.

4. **Benign positional vertigo**: Vertigo (lasting for seconds) associated with rolling over toward the left or right when supine, or when looking up. Treatment: reassurance and simple exercises.

5. **Orthostatic hypotension**: Not true vertigo (rather a sensation of lightheadedness or faintness) on assuming the upright position. Often associated with antidepressant and antihypertensive medication. Treatment: reassurance, change in medication to one with fewer orthostatic side effects.

Reference

1. Blakely B, Swanson R. Otolaryngology for the House Officer. Baltimore: Williams & Wilkins, 1989: 35–50.

PROBLEM 95: AN 18-YEAR-OLD MALE WITH SKIN LESIONS ON HIS FOOT

An 18-year-old male presents to your office for assessment of numerous small skin lesions on the ball of his left foot. He has had these lesions for the past 3 months, but they have been increasing in number.

On examination, there are 18 small lesions, 2–3 mm in diameter. They are discrete, nonpruritic and hyperkeratotic. Superficial trimming of one of the lesions reveals small pinpoint-sized bleeding points.

SELECT THE ONE BEST ANSWER TO THE FOLLOWING QUESTIONS:

733. The most likely diagnosis in this patient is:
    a) condylomata acuminata
    b) flat warts
    c) plantar warts
    d) molluscum contagiosum
    e) common warts

734. The etiologic agent responsible for the condition described above is:

a) human wart virus
b) excessive moisture
c) human papilloma virus
d) human parvovirus
e) *Treponema pallidum*

b) local antibiotics
c) total nail avulsion
d) wedge resection
e) watch and wait; maybe it will go away

ANSWER THE FOLLOWING QUESTIONS ACCORDING TO THE CODE:

A: 1, 2, and 3 are correct
B: 1 and 3 are correct
C: 2 and 4 are correct
D: Only 4 is correct
E: All of the above are correct

735. Which of the following treatments is(are) useful in the management of human warts?
 1) cryosurgery
 2) carbon dioxide laser surgery
 3) chemical destruction
 4) surgical excision

736. Which of the following statements regarding cryotherapy for warts is (are) true?
 1) cryotherapy is most effective if limited to warts less than 5 mm in diameter
 2) repeated applications of liquid nitrogen may be required
 3) a normal rim of skin around the wart should be included in the freezing procedure
 4) cryotherapy may be ineffective in the treatment of plantar warts

737. Which of the following statements regarding ingrown toenails is (are) correct?
 1) an ingrown toenail usually presents as a tender, inflamed swelling at a corner of the toenail
 2) ingrown toenails occur almost exclusively in the first toe
 3) painful symptoms seldom occur if the nail is permitted to grow out beyond the end of the toe
 4) Misfitting shoes and improper nail trimming have been confirmed by scientific studies as the cause of most ingrown toenails

SELECT THE ONE BEST ANSWER TO THE FOLLOWING QUESTION:

738. The treatment of choice for an ingrown toenail is:
 a) hot compresses

ANSWERS

733. C. This patient has plantar warts. Plantar warts occur on the sole of the foot, are flat, extend deep into the thick skin, and on superficial trimming reveal small pinpoint-sized bleeding points.

 Plantar warts must be differentiated from callus formation. A callus does not reveal bleeding points on superficial trimming.

 Condyloma acuminata are single or multiple masses that appear in the anogenital areas and, less commonly, between the toes and at the corners of the mouth. They are also called moist warts.

 Flat warts are small flat tumors that are often barely visible but can occur in clusters of 10 to 30 or more. They are commonly seen on the forehead and the dorsum of the hand.

 Molloscum contagiosum is a viral infection of the skin characterized by the occurrence of one or more small skin tumors. These lesions may develop in the scratched areas of patients with atopic eczema. They are most common in children.

 Common warts are slightly raised papillary growths, varying in size from pinhead to large clusters of pea-sized tumors. These warts are most commonly seen on the hands.[1]

734. C. The etiologic agent responsible for human warts is the human papilloma virus.[1]

735. A. The primary forms of therapy for uncomplicated warts include cryosurgery with liquid nitrogen, electrocautery, carbon dioxide laser surgery, and chemical destruction. Surgical excision is not recommended for the treatment of human warts because of painful scar formation.[2]

736. E. Cryotherapy with liquid nitrogen is the most common treatment for warts. It is most effective if limited to warts less than 5 mm in diameter. It may, however, not be effective in the treatment of plantar warts. It often has to be repeated several times to totally eradicate the wart tissue. To maximize efficacy, a normal rim of skin around the wart should be included in the freezing procedure.[2]

737. A. An ingrown toenail usually presents as a tender, inflamed swelling at a corner of the toenail.

Ingrown toenails occur almost exclusively in the first toe. Painful symptoms seldom occur if the nail is permitted to grow out beyond the end of the toe.

Although misfitting shoes and improper nail trimming have always been thought to be the cause of ingrown toenails, there is little scientific data to support this.[3]

738. D. The treatment of choice for an ingrown toenail is wedge resection under a ring block with local anesthesia. Liquefied phenol may be applied to the sulcus under the cuticle where the nail was removed to destroy the matrix and prevent nail regrowth. Omitting phenol treatment minimizes the postoperative discomfort and permits regrowth of a full-width nail, but recurrence of nail ingrowth is then possible.[3]

SUMMARY OF THE TREATMENT OF WARTS AND INGROWN TOENAILS

1. **Warts**: Causative agent of warts: human papilloma virus.

Treatment of warts: cryotherapy, electrocautery, carbon dioxide laser, and chemical destruction. Surgical excision is not recommended. Treatment of warts may have to be repeated several times until all wart tissue has disappeared.

2. **Ingrown toenails**: Caused by distal corner of nail curling downwards and digging into the underlying skin. Usually occurs on the first toe.

Recommended treatment of ingrown toenails: wedge resection with or without phenol.

References

1. Lowy D, Androphy E. Warts. In: Fitzpatrick T, Eisen A, Wolff K, Freedberg I, Austen K, eds. Dermatology in general medicine. 3rd Ed. New York: McGraw-Hill, 1987: 2355–2364.

2. Taylor M. Successful treatment of warts. Postgrad Med 1988; 84(8):126–136.

3. Gillette R. Practical management of ingrown toenails. Postgrad Med 1988; 84(8):145–156.

PROBLEM 96: AN 82-YEAR-OLD MALE WITH NOCTURIA, HESITANCY, AND A SLOW URINARY STREAM

An 82-year-old male presents to the office with a 1-year history of nocturia × 5, hesitancy, slow stream, and terminal dribbling. The symptoms have been getting progressively worse. He is otherwise well, and has had no significant medical illnesses in his life.

On examination, the only abnormal finding is an enlarged prostate gland that is smooth in contour, firm, but with no irregularities or nodules.

SELECT THE ONE BEST ANSWER TO THE FOLLOWING QUESTIONS:

739. The most likely diagnosis in this patient is:
    a) benign prostatic hyperplasia
    b) carcinoma of the bladder
    c) prostatic carcinoma
    d) urethral stricture
    e) chronic prostatitis

740. The most important investigation to be undertaken for the patient described in question 739 is:
    a) urinalysis and culture
    b) intravenous pyelography
    c) renal ultrasound
    d) cystoscopy

    e) voiding cystourethrogram

741. The treatment of choice for the patient described in question 739 is:
    a) alpha-adrenergic blocking drugs
    b) periodic prostatic massage
    c) transurethral prostatectomy
    d) retropubic prostatectomy
    e) suprapubic prostatectomy

742. A 58-year-old male presents with a 3-month history of gradually worsening hesitancy of stream, urgency, nocturia, and terminal dribbling. He also complains of some lumbar and pelvic bone pain, which has been present for the last 3 weeks.

On examination, the prostate is enlarged and rock hard. There is some tenderness over the pelvic ischium on the left side and over the fourth and fifth lumbar vertebrae.

Which of the following statements regarding this patient's condition is false?

a) the patient most likely has a prostatic carcinoma
b) the primary treatment of this patient's disease is radiotherapy
c) this patient most likely has osseous metastases
d) evaluation of this patient should include a bone scan
e) combination chemotherapy may be indicated for the treatment of this condition in some cases

743. A 64-year-old male presents for a routine physical assessment. On physical examination, he is found to have a 1 cm nodule in the left lobe of the prostate. A biopsy reveals adenocarcinoma. A CT scan shows no pelvic lymphadenopathy and a bone scan is negative.

Which of the following statements regarding this patient is true?

a) no treatment should be undertaken at this time
b) radiotherapy to the pelvis with a boost to the prostate is the definite treatment of choice
c) radical prostatectomy produces a slightly higher survival rate in this stage than does radiotherapy
d) hormonal therapy is the treatment of choice in this patient at this time

744. Which of the following statements regarding the digital rectal examination as a screening test for prostatic cancer is(are) true?

a) rectal examination is the most efficient screening test for prostate cancer
b) there is conflicting data with regard to the sensitivity of digital rectal examination in detecting early prostatic cancer
c) mean survival time has been shown to be increased by early detection by rectal examination
d) a and b
e) all of the above

ANSWERS

739. A. The most likely diagnosis in this patient is benign prostatic hyperplasia. Hyperplasia of the prostate causes increased outflow resistance.

The symptoms of prostatism include nocturia, hesitancy, slow stream, terminal dribbling, and frequency. Residual urine volume is increased, and acute urinary retention may occur.

Differential diagnosis includes carcinoma of the prostate, neuropathic bladder, chronic prostatitis, and urethral stricture.[1]

740. D. The most important investigation to be undertaken for the patient described in question 739 is cystoscopy. This will exclude other causes of the symptoms described, will reveal the size of the prostate gland, and will reveal secondary vesical changes. Other investigations that should be considered include complete urinalysis and culture, excretory urograms or urinary tract ultrasound, and measurement of renal function.[1]

741. C. The treatment of choice for benign prostatic hyperplasia is transurethral prostatectomy.

Recently, alpha-adrenergic blocking drugs that relax the external urethral sphincter have been prescribed for the treatment of benign prostatic hyperplasia. Although these agents may provide short-term success, their side effects, including particularly orthostatic hypotension, have limited their success.

Other conservative measures that may be helpful include regular intercourse or masturbation to relieve prostatic congestion, and periodic prostatic massage.[1]

742. B. This patient most likely has a prostatic carcinoma with osseous bone metastases. Evaluation of this patient should include determination of serum acid phosphatase or prostate-specific antigen, a radionucleide bone scan, x-rays of the pelvis and lumbar areas, and either a CT or an MRI scan of the pelvis. If these investigations confirm stage D carcinoma of the prostate (pelvic lymph node metastases or distant metastases), the patient should receive hormonal therapy. Alternatively, some urologists feel that is appropriate to wait until the patient does become symptomatic. If hormonal treatment is elected, the treatment choices include orchidectomy, diethylstilbesterol, LHRH analogues, and antiandrogens (Androcur). Combination chemotherapy may be used in hormone-resistant cases. Palliative radiotherapy may be very beneficial in relieving metastatic bone pain.[1,2]

Palliative treatment of cancer is discussed in another section of this book.

743. C. This patient has stage B2 disease (a localized nodule 1–1.5 cm in diameter with no evidence of metastatic disease. Until recently, radiation therapy was the treatment of choice for stage B disease. However, radical prostatectomy with pelvic lymphadenectomy has recently been shown to produce a slightly higher long-term survival rate. With newer techniques, impotence can usually be avoided, and it would now seem that this is the treatment of choice.[1,2]

744. D. Rectal examination is the most efficient screening test for prostate cancer, but there is conflicting data with regard to its sensitivity in detection of early prostatic cancer. Mean survival time may not be increased by early detection, and this may be a case in which lead time bias (see section on epidemiology) may give a false impression of increased survival. The US Preventive Task Force on the Periodic Health Examination states "there is insufficient evidence to recommend for or against routine digital rectal examination as an effective screening test for prostate cancer in asymptomatic men."[3]

SUMMARY OF THE DIAGNOSIS AND MANAGEMENT OF BENIGN PROSTATIC HYPERPLASIA AND PROSTATIC CANCER

1. **Benign Prostatic Hyperplasia:**
   Symptoms: nocturia, hesitancy, slow stream, terminal dribbling, frequency. As the disease becomes more advanced, there may be a significant residual urine, acute urinary retention, and uremia
   Diagnosis: Cystoscopy is the main investigation

Treatment: Transurethral resection (TURP)

2. **Carcinoma of the prostate:** Carcinoma of the prostate is the second most common neoplasm and the third most common cause of death
   Symptoms: same as benign prostatic hyperplasia except abnormalities found on examination of the prostate. Stage B (localized disease), Stage C (periprostatic extension), and Stage D (pelvic lymph node involvement or distant metastases)
   Treatment: Stage A — no treatment
   Stage B — irradiation with or without pelvic lymphadenectomy may be the treatment of choice. Some centers use abdominal and prostatic radiation as treatment of choice.
   Stage C — irradiation with or without pelvic lymphadenectomy
   Stage D — asymptomatic—no treatment or hormone therapy; symptomatic—hormone therapy (orchidectomy, DES, antiandrogen, LHRH analogues). Combination chemotherapy may be used in hormone-resistant cases.

References

1. Williams R, Donovan J, Tanagho E. Urology. In: Way L, ed. Current surgical diagnosis and treatment. 8th ed. Norwalk: Appleton-Crofts, 1988: 842–843, 868–870.

2. Garnick M. Urologic cancer. In: Rubenstein E, Federman D, eds. Scientific American medicine. New York: Scientific American Medicine, 1988: 12(IX):1–6.

3. Guide to Clinical Preventive Services. An assessment of the US Preventive Services Task Force. Screening for prostate cancer. Baltimore: Williams & Wilkins, 1989: 63–65.

PROBLEM 97:   AN 8-YEAR-OLD FEMALE WITH A RED EYE

An 8-year-old female presents to your office with her mother for assessment of "red eyes." She has been sick for the past 3 days with a mild fever, nasal congestion, and a nonproductive cough. Her mother states that her eyes became red this morning.

On examination the child has a fever of 38° C. She has mild rhinorrhea and nasal congestion, and a nonproductive cough. The conjunctiva of both eyes are diffusely red, and there is a watery discharge present.

SELECT THE ONE BEST ANSWER TO THE FOLLOWING QUESTIONS:

745. The most likely diagnosis in this child is:
   a) bacterial conjunctivitis
   b) viral conjunctivitis

   c) allergic conjunctivitis
   d) autoimmune conjunctivitis
   e) none of the above

746. The most likely etiologic agent of the condition described in the patient above is:

a) pneumococcus
b) *Haemophilus influenzae*
c) adenovirus
d) rhinovirus
e) none of the above

747. A 17-year-old female presents to your office with a 1-day history of a red eye. She states her "right eye was difficult to open this morning because of the discharge." The right eye feels uncomfortable, although there is no significant pain.

On examination, she has significant injection of the right conjunctiva. There is a mucopurulent discharge present. No other abnormalities are found on physical examination.

The most likely diagnosis in the patient described above is:
a) bacterial conjunctivitis
b) viral conjunctivitis
c) allergic conjunctivitis
d) autoimmune conjunctivitis
e) none of the above

748. The most likely etiologic agent of the condition described in the patient in question 747 is:
a) pneumococcus
b) *Haemophilus influenzae*
c) *Staphylococcus aureus*
d) adenovirus
e) none of the above

749. A 29-year-old male presents to the office with bilateral red eyes. This condition came on quite suddenly 2 hours ago while he was visiting at a friend's home. He describes itching and a clear discharge from both eyes. The patient mentions one previous episode of the same condition, and interestingly enough, it also occurred while he was visiting the same friend.

On examination, the conjunctiva are diffusely injected and edematous. On eversion of the eyelids, there are large papillae present.

The most likely diagnosis in this patient is:
a) chemical conjunctivitis
b) toxic conjunctivitis
c) allergic conjunctivitis
d) bacterial conjunctivitis
e) none of the above

750. A 29-year-old female presents to the office for assessment of a red eye. She describes a tender, painful, and sore right eye that began yesterday. She has had no other symptoms.

On examination, the patient has a localized area of inflammation and injection in the area of the right conjunctiva. The inflammation appears to lie beneath the conjunctival surface.

The most likely diagnosis in this patient is:
a) localized bacterial conjunctivitis
b) acute iritis
c) acute angle closure glaucoma
d) acute episcleritis
e) none of the above

ANSWER THE FOLLOWING QUESTION ACCORDING TO THE CODE:

A: 1, 2, and 3 are correct
B: 1 and 3 are correct
C: 2 and 4 are correct
D: Only 4 is correct
E: All of the above are correct

751. A 35-year-old female presents with an acutely inflamed, painful, left eye. Her symptoms began 2 days ago. There is some visual blurring associated with her symptoms.

On examination, there is a diffusely inflamed left conjunctiva. On fluorescein staining, there is a dendritic ulcer seen in the center of the cornea.

Which of the following statements regarding corneal ulcers is(are) true?
1) the most likely cause of this patient's corneal ulcer is a herpetic infection
2) corneal ulcers may be caused by excessive contact lens wear
3) cycloplegic drops may be helpful in the management of this condition
4) normal visual acuity excludes a corneal ulcer

SELECT THE ONE BEST ANSWER TO THE FOLLOWING QUESTIONS

752. A 36-year-old male with ankylosing spondylitis presents to your office for assessment of a painful left red eye. His red eye is associated with pain and photophobia. There is no discharge present.

On examination, the left eye is red and the redness is most pronounced around the area of the cornea. The visual acuity in the left eye is decreased to 20/60.

The most likely diagnosis in this patient is:
a) bacterial conjunctivitis
b) viral conjunctivitis
c) acute iridocyclitis

d) acute episcleritis

e) acute angle closure glaucoma

753. A 61-year-old male presents with a 12-hour history of an extremely painful left red eye. The patient complains that his vision is blurred and he is seeing haloes around lights. He states that he has had similar, but milder, attacks in the past.

On examination, the eye is tender and inflammed. The cornea is hazy and the pupil is semidilated and fixed. On palpation, the left eye is significantly harder than the right.

The most likely diagnosis in this patient is:

a) bacterial conjunctivitis

b) viral conjunctivitis

c) acute iridocyclitis

d) acute episcleritis

e) acute angle closure glaucoma

754. A 20-year-old male presents with a localized, solidly bloody red eye. You make a diagnosis of subconjunctival hemorrhage. You should now:

a) hospitalize the patient for 7–10 days

b) refer the patient to an ophthalmologist for immediate surgery

c) begin oral amoxicillin

d) begin topical sulfacetamide

e) reassure the patient that it will resolve in 1–3 weeks on its own

ANSWERS

745. B. This child has viral conjunctivitis. Viral infection is the most frequent cause of conjunctivitis. The most common viral agent is adenovirus. Viral conjunctivitis is often preceded by an upper respiratory tract infection or flu-like illness. Conjunctival hyperemia, eyelid edema, and a serous or seropurulent discharge are usually present. Viral conjunctivitis, though self-limited, should be treated with the same agents recommended for bacterial conjunctivitis to prevent superinfection. The treatment of choice is 10–15% sulfacetamide or gentamicin drops q.i.d.

Viral conjunctivitis occurs in epidemics (pink eye). Viral conjunctivitis may persist for weeks.

Bacterial conjunctivitis and allergic conjunctivitis will be discussed in subsequent questions. Autoimmune conditions are sometimes associated with a red eye, but this tends to present as an episcleritis or scleritis, rather than a conjunctivitis.[1]

746. C. See critique of question 745.

747. A. This patient has a bacterial conjunctivitis. In bacterial conjunctivitis, the patient usually has discomfort and a purulent discharge in one eye that most often spreads to the other eye.

In bacterial conjunctivitis, the vision is normal after the discharge has been cleared away. There is usually uniform engorgement of all the conjunctival blood vessels. There is no staining of the cornea with fluorescein.

Bacterial conjunctivitis should be treated with an antibiotic drop such as sulfacetamide, chloramphenicol, or Garamycin. Initially, the drops may be used every hour or two; within 24 hours they may be decreased to q.i.d.[1]

748. C. The most common organism causing bacterial conjunctivitis is *S. aureus*. It is less frequently caused by *H. influenzae* or pneumococcus.

In both children and adults, conjunctivitis can also be caused by *Chlamydiae*. *Chlamydiae* is the most common cause of infantile conjunctivitis, and can be prevented by the administration of erythromycin drops at birth. In adults, chlamydiae conjunctivitis is usually associated with Reiter's syndrome.[1]

749. C. The most likely diagnosis in this patient is allergic conjunctivitis. The most common complaint with allergic conjunctivitis is itching. Both eyes are affected, and there is usually a clear discharge.

Examination reveals diffusely injected conjunctiva, which may be edematous (chemosis). The discharge is usually clear and stringy.

The treatment of choice for acute allergic conjunctivitis is either a corticosteroid drop or sodium cromoglycate drops. Because of the risk of steroid-induced cataracts and glaucoma, corticosteroid drops should be used cautiously, and only for short periods of time. Sodium cromoglycate drops, on the other hand, are without risk. Oral antihistamines may also be effective.

The most likely cause in the case presented in this question is contact with something in the friend's house (such as a cat).[1]

750. D. The patient has episcleritis. Episcleritis and scleritis differ from conjunctivitis in that they usually present as a localized area of inflammation. Although episcleritis and scleritis may occur secondary to autoimmune diseases such as rheu-

matoid arthritis, most cases of episcleritis are idiopathic. Episcleritis is almost always self-limiting; scleritis, on the other hand, may lead to serious complications such as eye perforation.

The patient with episcleritis usually presents with a sore, red eye that is often tender. Although there may be reflex lacrimation, there is usually no discharge present. Scleritis is much more painful than episcleritis, and the signs of inflammation are usually more prominent.

On examination, there is a localized area of inflammation that is tender to touch. The episcleral and scleral blood vessels are larger than the conjunctival blood vessels.

A patient with episcleritis should probably be referred to an ophthalmologist. The treatment of choice for episcleritis is corticosteroid eye drops. Any other disease should be identified.[1]

751. A. This patient's dentritic ulcer is most likely caused by a herpetic infection. Corneal ulcers may be caused by viral, bacterial, or fungal infections. These infections may be primary, or secondary to excessive contact lens wear, a corneal abrasion, or the use of corticosteroid eye drops.

The patient usually presents with an acutely painful eye, associated with conjunctival injection, discharge, and visual blurring. Visual acuity, however, depends on the location and size of the corneal ulcer; normal visual acuity does not exclude an ulcer. The discharge may be watery (reflex lacrimation), or purulent (bacterial). Conjunctival injection may be generalized or localized depending on the location of the ulcer.

Treatment consists of specific anti-infective therapy (idoxuridine for herpes simplex ulcer and topical antibiotics for ulcers suspected of being primarily or secondarily infected by bacteria), and cycloplegic drops to relieve pain due to ciliary muscle spasm. Topical corticosteroids are absolutely contraindicated in patients with a dentritic herpetic ulcer.[1]

A patient with a dentritic ulcer should probably be seen by an ophthalmologist.

752. C. This patient has an acute iridocyclitis or anterior uveitis. Patients at risk for anterior uveitis are those patients with a history of a seronegative arthropathy—particularly if they are positive for HLA-B27 (ankylosing spondylitis). Children with seronegative arthritis are also at high risk.

Symptoms include a painful, red eye; sometimes associated with photophobia and decreased visual acuity.

On examination the affected eye is red with the inflammation being particularly prominent over the area of the inflammed ciliary body (circumcorneal). The pupil is small because of spasm of the sphincter or irregular because of adhesions of the iris to the lens (posterior synechiae). Inflammatory cells may be seen on the back of the cornea (keratitic precipitates) or may settle to form a collection of cells in the anterior chamber of the eye (hypopyon).[1]

Treatment of anterior uveitis should include topical corticosteroids to reduce the inflammation and prevent adhesions within the eye. Mydriatics should be used to paralyze the ciliary body to relieve pain.[1]

As with episcleritis and dentritic ulcers, a patient with iridocyclitis should probably be seen by an ophthalmologist.

753. E. This patient has acute angle-closure glaucoma. Acute glaucoma should always be considered in a patient over the age of 50 years who presents with a painful red eye.

Acute glaucoma usually comes on rapidly. The most common symptom is severe pain in one eye, which may be accompanied by vomiting. The patient complains of impaired vision, and haloes around lights. This is due to edema of the cornea.

On examination, the eye is tender and inflammed. The cornea is hazy and the pupil is semidilated and fixed. Vision is impaired because of the edema of the cornea. On palpation, the involved eye feels significantly harder than the normal eye.

Intraocular pressure must be reduced immediately. Intravenous acetazolamide (Diamox) 500 mg should be given, and pilocarpine 4% should be instilled in the eye to constrict the pupil. This should be followed by either an iridectomy or a laser iridotomy to restore normal aqueous flow. The other eye should be treated prophylactically in a similar way.[1]

754. E. Rupture of a conjunctival vessel causes a localized, solidly bloody red eye. This hemorrhage is benign, although its appearance often alarms the patient. It requires no treatment and resolves spontaneously in 1–3 weeks.

SUMMARY OF THE DIAGNOSIS AND TREATMENT OF THE RED EYE

1. **Conjunctivitis:**
    Infectious conjunctivitis:
    a) adenovirus is the most common cause of conjunctivitis
    b) bacterial conjunctivitis is most commonly caused by *Staphylococcus*
    Symptoms:
    a) discharge: watery discharge with viral infection mucopurulent discharge with bacterial infection
    b) diffuse conjunctival injection, no visual impairment, normal corneal examination, normal pupils, normal intraocular pressure
    Treatment: gentamicin or sulfacetamide drops
    Allergic conjunctivitis:
    a) itching and clear discharge are main symptoms. Conjunctiva are diffusely injected and may be associated with swelling (chemosis).
    Treatment: sodium cromoglycate or corticosteroid eyedrops

2. **Episcleritis/scleritis:** Localized area of inflammation (as opposed to diffuse). The eye is often tender and sore.
    Treatment: Corticosteroid eye drops

3. **Corneal ulceration:**
    a) may be bacterial, viral, or fungal in origin or may be secondary to abrasion, contact lens wear, etc.
    b) visual acuity depends on the location and size of the ulcer. Conjunctival injection may be generalized or localized. Fluorescein must be used to stain cornea.

Treatment: Cycloplegic drops to relieve ciliary spasm. Idoxuridine for dentritic (herpetic) ulcer, antibiotic drops for suspected bacterial infection. Corticosteroid eye drops are absolutely contraindicated in herpetic ulcers.

4. **Iridocyclitis (anterior uveitis):**
    a) often associated with seronegative arthropathy.
    b) inflammation of the iris (iritis) and inflammation of the ciliary body (cyclitis) occur together.
    c) the inflammation of anterior uveitis is circumoral in location, and the pupil is usually small due to spasm.
    Treatment: Mydriatic to relieve ciliary spasm, corticosteroid drops to decrease inflammation

5. **Acute angle closure glaucoma:**
    a) acute, unilateral, painful red eye in patient over the age of 50.
    b) attack usually comes on quickly, characteristically in the evening.
    c) impaired vision due to corneal edema and haloes around lights are common.
    d) palpation reveals hard eye.
    Treatment: Intravenous acetazolamide (Diamox) 500 mg, and pilocarpine to constrict the pupil. This should be followed by iridectomy or laser iridotomy.

Reference

1. Elkington A, Khaw P. The red eye. Br Med J 1988; 296:1720–1724.

PROBLEM 98: A 25-YEAR-OLD MALE WITH FLANK PAIN

A 25-year-old male presents to the emergency room wih an abrupt onset of severe right sided flank pain. The pain radiates down the abdomen toward the groin and into the testicle, and is associated with hematuria, urinary frequency, urgency, and dysuria.

On examination, the patient has right costovertebral angle tenderness. The rest of the abdominal examination is normal. The patient is afebrile.

SELECT THE ONE BEST ANSWER TO THE FOLLOWING QUESTIONS:

755. The most likely diagnosis in this patient is:
    a) renal colic
    b) acute pyelonephritis
    c) acute pyelitis
    d) atypical appendicitis
    e) none of the above

756. The most common type of kidney stone is composed of:
a) calcium oxalate
b) mixed calcium oxalate/calcium phosphate
c) calcium phosphate
d) struvite
e) uric acid

757. Which of the following abnormalities are associated with calcium oxalate stones?
a) hypercalciuria
b) hyperuricosuria
c) hypocitnatruria
d) all of the above

758. The drug of choice for idiopathic hypercalciuria is:
a) cellulose sodium phosphate
b) orthophosphates
c) potassium citrate
d) a thiazide diuretic
e) pyridoxine

759. The most important component of the diagnostic work-up in a patient with a kidney stone is:
a) serum calcium/serum uric acid
b) serum creatinine
c) intravenous pyelogram
d) 24-hour urine for volume, calcium, uric acid, citrate, oxalate, sodium, creatinine, and pH
e) serum parathyroid hormone

ANSWER THE FOLLOWING QUESTIONS ACCORDING TO THE CODE:

A: 1, 2, and 3 are correct
B: 1 and 3 are correct
C: 2 and 4 are correct
D: Only 4 is correct
E: All of the above are correct

760. Which of the following statements regarding uric acid stones is(are) correct:
1) uric acid stones are formed in patients with a persistently acid urine
2) uric acid stones are formed in patients with a massively increased uric acid excretion (greater than 1000 mg/day)
3) initial treatment of uric acid stones is alkalinization of the urine
4) patients with recalcitrant uric acid stones may be treated with allopurinol

761. Which of the following statements regarding the treatment of nephrolithiasis is(are) true?
1) extracorporeal shock wave lithotripsy (ESWL) has become widely used for the treatment of renal stones
2) ureteral stones, unless large, are best managed by awaiting their spontaneous passage
3) ESWL has shown its greatest benefit in patients with stones less than 2 cm in diameter
4) ESWL and percutaneous nephrolithotomy are seldom used together

ANSWERS

755. A. This patient has renal colic. Renal colic is characterized by the sudden onset of severe flank pain that radiates down the abdomen toward the groin. It is usually associated with hematuria, urinary frequency, urgency, and dysuria, and is relieved immediately following stone passage.[1]

Acute pyelonephritis, which may be associated with similar symptoms, usually is accompanied by fever and chills.

The sudden onset of severe flank pain is not typical of appendiceal disease.

756. A. Calcium oxalate stones are the most common type of kidney stones; they comprise 60% of all stones. They are most commonly idiopathic. Other stones in order of frequency are mixed calcium oxalate and calcium phosphate, uric acid, struvite, and cystine.

757. D. Calcium oxalate stones may be associated with hypercalciuria, hyperuricosuria, and hypocitraturia. Hypercalciuria is the most common abnormality.[1]

758. D. Thiazide diuretics are the agents of choice for the treatment of idiopathic hypercalciuria. Thiazide diuretics work by lowering urine calcium excretion. Other measures that may be tried include increasing total daily fluid intake and decreasing total daily calcium.[1]

759. D. The basic laboratory evaluation of a patient with renal colic includes urinalysis, urine culture if clinically indicated, blood chemistry profile including serum calcium, phosphorus, uric acid, electrolytes, and creatinine, KUB, and intravenous pyelography. The most sensitive test, however, for the diagnosis of metabolic abnormalities associated with nephrolithiasis, is the 24-hour urine

collection. The 24-hour specimen should be analyzed for calcium, uric acid, citrate, oxalate, sodium, creatinine, and pH.[1]

When stone composition is unknown, urine should also be obtained for qualitative cystine screening. Patients who are hypercalcemic should have the serum parathyroid hormone assay performed.[1]

760. E. Uric acid stones, the second most common type of renal stone are formed in patients with a persistently acid urine and/or a very high uric acid excretion (exceeding 1,000 mg/day). The initial treatment of a patient with uric acid stones involves alkalinization of the urine with agents such as sodium bicarbonate or citrate. Patients with uric acid stones that do not respond to these measures should be treated with allopurinol. A decreased purine intake is also recommended.[1]

761. A. Extracorporeal shock wave lithotripsy (ESWL) has become widely used for the treatment of nephrolithiasis, and is based on the use of shock waves to break up kidney stones to facilitate passage through the ureter.

Lithotripsy is most effective for removal of stones that are less than 2 cm in diameter.

For patients with stones larger than 2 cm, a combination of ESWL and percutaneous lithotripsy tends to produce better results than ESWL alone. Initial percutaneous nephrolithotomy followed by ESWL and a "second look" percutaneous nephrolithotomy gives the best results.

For patients with large, infected, staghorn calculi, or complex anatomy or obstruction, open surgery is still the best treatment.

Ureteral stones are best managed by awaiting spontaneous passage. If spontaneous passage is unlikely or delayed, ESWL is best for stones in the upper two-thirds of the ureter, whereas endoscopic techniques remain best for lower ureteral stones. Ureteropelvic junction obstruction or other obstruction, or stones in calyceal diverticulae, are best managed by endourologic techniques.[1]

SUMMARY OF THE DIAGNOSIS AND MANAGEMENT OF KIDNEY STONES

1. **Classical symptoms of renal colic:** Sudden, severe, flank pain with radiation down the abdomen toward the groin and associated with hematuria, frequency, urgency, dysuria, and relief following stone passage.

2. **Types of stones:**
    Calcium oxalate:
    a) most frequent type of stone.
    b) usually idiopathic and associated with hypercalciuria, hyperuricuria, hypocitruria.
    c) can be prevented by thiazide diuretics; increased fluids and decreased calcium intake may also be effective.
    Uric acid:
    a) second most frequent type of stone.
    b) associated with persistently acid urine and massively increased urinary uric acid secretion (greater than 1,000 mg/day).
    c) prevention consists of alkalinization of urine with bicarbonate or citrate. Allopurinol may have to be used.
    Infective stones:
    a) caused by urea-splitting organisms—*Proteus* species.
    b) stone should be completely removed and antibiotic therapy prescribed.
    Cystine stones:
    a) occur with the inherited transport disorder, cystinuria.

3. **Treatment:**
    Ureteral stones: await spontaneous passage. If not forthcoming ESWL (upper two-thirds of ureter), endoscopic techniques (lower one-third of ureter). Renal stones: ESWL is the treatment of choice for stones less than 2 cm and located in the upper pole of the kidney. If stones greater than 1 cm are located in the lower pole of the kidney, a combination of ESWL and percutaneous nephrolithotomy is preferred.

Reference

1. Consensus Conference: Prevention and treatment of kidney stones. JAMA 1988; 260(7): 977–981.

Geriatric Medicine

PROBLEM 99: AN 85-YEAR-OLD FEMALE WHO HAS JUST MOVED INTO A NURSING HOME

You are called to see an 85-year-old patient who recently moved to a nursing home. She has been living alone in her own home since the death of her husband 6 years ago. In the last 6 months she has become increasingly disabled with congestive cardiac failure and osteoarthritis. She moved into the nursing home 3 months ago. During the past 4 weeks, she has lost 8 pounds, has not eaten, has lost interest in all social activities, and has been crying almost every day.

Her mood is worse in the morning. At times (especially when her mood is impaired) her short-term memory appears to be impaired. When she is not crying, her memory (both short-term and long-term) is normal.

SELECT THE ONE BEST ANSWER TO THE FOLLOWING QUESTIONS:

762. The most likely diagnosis in this patient is:
    a) depression
    b) Alzheimer's disease
    c) multi-infarct dementia
    d) hypothyroidism
    e) none of the above

763. Which of the following statements regarding the diagnosis above is false?
    a) the major variety of this condition is less frequent in older patients than in younger patients
    b) this patient has pseudodementia
    c) this condition is much more common in institutionalized elderly patients than in elderly patients in the community
    d) this condition may be related to physical illness
    e) this condition may be related to adjustment to life stresses

764. Which of the following investigations and assessments should be performed in the patient discussed in question 762?
    a) review of all medications
    b) complete blood count
    c) thyroid function studies
    d) a and b
    e) all of the above

765. Which of the following medications is recommended as an agent of first choice for elderly patients with the condition described above?
    a) imipramine
    b) clomipramine
    c) desipramine
    d) amitriptyline
    e) tranylcypromine

766. Which of the following statements regarding the condition described above is/are true?
    1) electroconvulsive therapy does not have any role to play in the treatment of the condition
    2) older patients appear to be less likely than younger patients to completely recover from the condition
    3) socialization, music therapy, and pet therapy do not have a role in the treatment of the condition
    4) cognitive and behavioral therapy may significantly improve the condition

ANSWERS

762. A. This patient is depressed. The criteria for major depressive illness[1] are summarized in another section of this book. However, special consideration to depression in the elderly.

    Depression in elderly patients is more likely to present with weight loss and less likely to present with feelings of worthlessness and guilt.[2] Elderly patients are no more likely than persons in midlife to report cognitive problems, although they do appear to have more difficulties with cognition during an episode of depression.[2]

    The other choices listed in the question are discussed in other sections of this book.

763. B. This patient does not have pseudodementia. Pseudodementia is a depression that presents as

cognitive impairment. It is not as common as previously thought. The much more common presentation is that of an older adult with mild to moderate dementia (in most cases senile dementia of the Alzheimer's type) who has a concomitant major depression.

Major depression is less prevalent among those aged 65 and older than in younger groups.[2]

The prevalence of major depression in elderly patients in the community is between 1 and 2%. The majority of depressed elderly patients, however, do not fit the DSM–III–R criteria, but rather have depressive symptoms that are associated with adjustment reactions (as in this patient who has just had to leave her own home), or with significant physical illness (as this patient also has).

In long-term care facilities, the prevalence of major depression is estimated to be 10–20%.[2]

764. E. The elderly patient who presents with depressive symptoms should have a complete history and physical examination performed. Part of the history should include a complete review of all medications (both prescribed and over the counter) that may contribute to depressive illness. Some of the most common pharmacologic agents that contribute to depression include antihypertensive agents such as propranolol and methyldopa, cimetidine, and sedative hypnotic drugs.

As well as the complete history and physical examination, certain laboratory investigations including a complete blood count (which may be followed by vitamin B_{12} and folate levels if so indicated by red blood cell indices), and thyroid function tests (particulary TSH) to exclude hypothyroidism.

765. A. If a tricyclic antidepressant is used to treat depression in the elderly it should have as favorable a side effect profile. Specifically, it should have a low incidence of postural hypotension, a low incidence of anticholinergic side effects, and a loss incidence of sedation. The antidepressant that best fits these criteria is desipramine.

766. C. Older patients are less likely than younger ones to completely recover from an episode of major depression. Even when improvement occurs, residual symptoms may persist.

Cognitive and behavioral therapies are effective in treating depression in elderly patients.

Attempts at increased socialization (especially in chronic care facilities), music therapy, pet therapy, and other therapies that serve to redirect the attention of the elderly patient appear to be effective in treating depression.

Electroconvulsive therapy may be the only effective therapy for severe depression in elderly patients, especially in patients with psychotic depression. ECT is well tolerated in geriatric patients and lacks the side effects associated with the tricyclic antidepressants.[2]

SUMMARY OF THE DIAGNOSIS AND TREATMENT OF DEPRESSION IN THE ELDERLY

1. Many elderly patients with depression do not fit the DSM–III–R criteria, but rather have depression associated with physical illness and adjustment to life stresses

2. Major depressive illness is especially common in chronic care institutions

3. **Symptoms:** Weight loss and decreased appetite is more common, feelings of guilt and worthlessness are less common than in younger patients

4. **Treatment:** Tricyclic depressants (particularly desipramine)

   Electroconvulsive therapy may be particularly effective in elderly patients.

References

1. American Psychiatric Association. Diagnostic and statistical manual of mental disorders. 3rd Ed. Revised (DSM–111–R). Washington, APA Press, 1987.

2. Blazer D. Depression in the elderly. N Engl J Med 1989; 320(3):164–166.

PROBLEM 100: A 78-YEAR-OLD FEMALE WITH INCREASING CONFUSION, IMPAIRMENT OF MEMORY, AND INABILITY TO LOOK AFTER HERSELF

A 78-year-old female is brought to your office by her daughter. She lives alone in an apartment and her daughter is concerned about her ability to carry on looking after herself. Her daughter tells you that she began to have difficulty with her memory 2 years ago, and since that time it has been a steady, downhill course. She is able to perform some of the activities of daily living such as dressing, bathing, and cleaning her apartment. However, when she cooks for herself she often leaves the burners on, and when she drives her car she often gets lost. She has had 4 motor vehicle accidents in the past 3 months. Her daughter became alarmed when she learned that her mother had gone to the bank the other day and withdrawn her entire $8000.00 savings account. Apparently, she wanted the entire amount in $1.00 bills and argued with the bank teller until her request was granted. The daughter states that the confusion has been getting worse, as has the impairment of memory. She also states that her mother's personality has changed; she has become much more agitated and aggressive.

SELECT THE ONE BEST ANSWER TO THE FOLLOWING QUESTIONS:

767. Based on this history, the most likely diagnosis in the mother is:
    a) Alzheimer's disease
    b) multi-infarct dementia
    c) major depressive illness
    d) hypothyroidism
    e) mixed dementia (Alzheimer's plus multi-infarct)

768. At this time you would:
    a) interview the patient, perform a physical examination and order appropriate laboratory investigations
    b) arrange for the patient to be admitted to a chronic care facility and placate the daughter
    c) prescribe diazepam for the daughter and haloperiodol for the patient
    d) refer the patient for immediate consultation with a geriatrician
    e) begin a trial of a tricyclic antidepressant in the patient

769. Which of the following statements concerning Alzheimer's disease is CORRECT?
    a) Alzheimer's disease is present to some degree in all persons over the age of 80 years
    b) Alzheimer's disease is a pathologic diagnosis
    c) Alzheimer's disease is a rapidly progressive dementia
    d) Alzheimer's disease is easy to differentiate from other dementias
    e) Alzheimer's disease usually has a sudden onset

770. Which of the following diseases is the MOST COMMON disease usually confused with Alzheimer's disease?
    a) hypothyroidism
    b) alcoholism
    c) congestive cardiac failure
    d) depression
    e) normal pressure hydrocephalus

771. In contrast to dementia, the cognitive impairment associated with depression often:
    a) comes on more slowly
    b) comes on more rapidly
    c) is usually only a minor impairment
    d) is not improved with tricyclic antidepressants
    e) none of the above

772. In contrast to dementia, patients with depression often:
    a) complain about their cognitive deficits
    b) deny that their cognitive deficits exist
    c) try to conceal their cognitive deficits
    d) usually try to answer questions even if they don't know the answers
    e) perform consistently on tasks of equal difficulty

ANSWER THE FOLLOWING QUESTIONS ACCORDING TO THE CODE:

A: 1, 2, and 3 are correct
B: 1 and 3 are correct
C: 2 and 4 are correct
D: Only 4 is correct
E: All of the above are correct

773. Reversible causes of confusion in the elderly include:
    1) drug intoxication
    2) hypothyroidism
    3) pernicious anemia
    4) hyponatremia

774. A cost-effective work-up of confusion in the elderly includes:
    1) complete blood count
    2) electrolytes
    3) blood glucose
    4) CT scan of the head

775. After a complete dementia work-up you are unsure whether a patient has Alzheimer's disease or a major depressive illness. At this point you should:
    1) reexamine the patient in 3 months time
    2) suggest a trial of ECT
    3) arrange for the patient to be admitted to a nursing home and begin supportive psychotherapy
    4) prescribe a trial of a tricyclic antidepressant

776. Which of the following are important aspects in the management of dementia?
    1) maintenance of a routine
    2) making the environment safe
    3) providing support for the family
    4) keeping external stimulation to a minimum

ANSWERS

767. A. The most likely diagnosis in this patient is dementia. The slow, insidious course of the decline is characteristic of Alzheimer's disease. Multi-infarct dementia tends to produce a "step-wise decline," with each step occurring at the time of a small infarct.

   Major depressive illness tends to come on rather abruptly. This is discussed in detail in another chapter. Hypothyroidism must always be considered as a reversible cause of dementia; in this case it is unlikely.

   Dementia is characterized by evidence of short- and long-term memory impairment with either impaired abstract thinking, impaired judgment, other disturbances of higher cortical function, or personality change.[1,2]

768. A. Alzheimer's disease is a diagnosis of exclusion. Before labeling a patient as having Alzheimer's disease a complete history, physical examination,

and laboratory evaluation should be done. It is inappropriate to arrange care in a chronic care facility and inappropriate to treat patients (even with an antidepressant) until a dementia work-up has been done.

   The cost effective work-up of dementia includes a complete history and physical examination (including a neuropsychiatric evaluation), a complete blood count, serum glucose, electrolytes, calcium, creatinine, and TSH. Other tests should only be done if there is a specific indication (example, B_{12} and folate if macrocytosis is present). A CT scan should only be performed if there is a specific clinical indication.[1]

769. B. Alzheimer's disease a diagnosis of exclusion; it is also a pathologic diagnosis that can only be firmly established at autopsy.

   Although the incidence of Alzheimer's disease increases with age it is not part of the normal aging process. Only 25% of patients over the age of 80 will show cognitive dysfunction characteristic of Alzheimer's disease.

   The onset and progression of Alzheimer's disease is slow and often unnoticed by both family and family physician.[1]

770. D. The disease most commonly confused with Alzheimer's disease is depression. Up to 15% of patients who are labeled with "Alzheimer's disease" actually have a major depressive illness. Many more patients with Alzheimer's disease have depression as a feature of the disease itself. Both misdiagnosed major depressive illness and the depression associated with Alzheimer's disease will respond to tricyclic antidepressants or MAO inhibitors.

771. B.

772. A. In contrast to dementia, the cognitive impairment associated with depression usually comes on rapidly. Also, in contrast to dementia, patients often complain about their cognitive deficits. They know that something is wrong. Other features that suggest depression include (1) a personal or family history of psychiatric illness, (2) depressive symptoms preceding cognitive changes, (3) feelings of hopelessness, guilt, and worthlessness, and (4) poor effort on psychologic testing.[1]

773. E. The reversible causes of dementia are included in the pneumonic DEMENTIA, which includes both reversible and irreversible causes

D= drugs (including alcohol)

E= emotional (depression)

M= metabolic (hyperglycemia, hyponatremia, hypercalcemia, acute renal failure, hepatic failure, vitamin B_{12} deficiency, hypothyroidism)

E= eyes/ears (visual and hearing problems)

N= neoplasms/normal pressure hydrocephalus

T= trauma (subdural hematoma)

I= infections (particularly pneumonia and urinary tract infection)

A= atherosclerotic vascular disease/Alzheimer's disease

Atherosclerotic vascular disease includes myocardial infarction, cerebrovascular accidents, pulmonary or systemic embolism, multi-infarct dementia

774. A. See critique of question 768.

775. D. You should begin a trial of a tricyclic antidepressant. See also the critique of question 771/772.

Desipramine is a good first line drug because of its low incidence of anticholinergic and orthostatic side effects.

776. E. The management of dementia involves both pharmacologic and behavioral methods. The four principles of behavioral management are (1) keeping external stimulation to a minimum, (2) maintaining a routine for the patient, (3) making the environment safe for the patient, and (4) supporting the family and offering respite care.[1]

SUMMARY OF THE DIAGNOSIS AND MANAGEMENT OF CONFUSION IN THE ELDERLY

1. **Differential Diagnosis**: Pneumonic Dementia

2. **Cost-effective work-up**: Complete history, physical examination, neuropsychiatric testing, complete blood count, plasma glucose, electrolytes, calcium, creatinine, TSH. Other tests only if indicated

3. If you are unsure whether the patient has Alzheimer's disease or depression, treat with a TCA for a month on an empiric basis.

4. **Treatment of dementia**: Keep external stimuli to a minimum, maintain a routine, make the environment safe, and support the family. If agitation, psychosis, or insomnia prescribe fluphenazine, haloperidol, or loxapine.

References

1. Chandler J. Geriatric psychiatry. Prim Care 1987; 14(4):761–771.

2. American Psychiatric Association. Diagnostic and statistical manual of mental disorders. 3rd Ed. Revised (DSM–111–R). Washington: APA Press, 1987; 107.

PROBLEM 101: AN 81-YEAR-OLD MALE WITH INCREASING CONFUSION AND SHORTNESS OF BREATH

An 81-year-old male is brought to the emergency department by his daughter. He was well until approximately 3 days ago. At that time, he became slightly confused. Apparently, for the last 3 days, he has been wandering aimlessly around the house and muttering incoherently. He has not been eating well, and has been sleeping restlessly. He became slightly short of breath last night.

On examination, the patient's blood pressure is 100/70 mm Hg. His pulse is 96 and regular. His respirations are 28/minute and slightly labored. Examination of the lung fields reveals a few bilateral rales, but no other abnormal findings.

Laboratory evaluation reveals a WBC of 11,000/mm^3. The chest x-ray reveals an incomplete consolidation in the right lower lobe.

Arterial blood gases reveal mild hypoxemia (PO_2–65 mm Hg) with a normal PCO_2 (40 mm Hg).

SELECT THE ONE BEST ANSWER TO THE FOLLOWING QUESTIONS:

777. The most likely diagnosis in this patient is:
    a) acute Alzheimer's disease with atelectasis of the right lower lobe
    b) viral pneumonia
    c) bacterial pneumonia
    d) congestive cardiac failure
    e) atypical pneumonia

778. In a community setting, the most common organism associated with the condition described above is:
    a) *Staphylococcus aureus*
    b) *Streptococcus pneumoniae*
    c) *Klebsiella pneumonia*
    d) *Legionella pneumophilia*
    e) no organism is associated with the condition

779. The treatment of choice for the patient discussed above is:
    a) penicillin G or ampicillin
    b) trimethoprim-sulfamethoxazole
    c) gentimicin
    d) cefazolin
    e) furosemide

780. A patient who is in hospital for the treatment of congestive cardiac failure develops a similar clinical presentation to the patient described above. Increasing confusion, increased respiratory rate, an elevated white blood cell count, and the chest x-ray findings described above are identical. The most likely organism associated with this condition in this patient is:
    a) *Staphylococcus aureus*
    b) *Streptococcus pneumoniae*
    c) a viral agent
    d) a gram-negative bacilli
    e) none of the above

781. The treatment of choice for the patient discussed in question 780 is(are):
    a) a third-generation cephalosporin and gentamicin
    b) ampicillin
    c) expanded spectrum penicillins
    d) a or c
    e) any of the above

ANSWER THE FOLLOWING QUESTIONS ACCORDING TO THE CODE:

A: 1, 2, and 3 are correct
B: 1 and 3 are correct
C: 2 and 4 are correct
D: Only 4 is correct
E: All of the above are correct

782. Which of the following is(are) risk factors for urinary tract infections in the elderly?
    1) advanced age
    2) decreased bladder emptying
    3) physiologic changes in the vagina and prostate
    4) decreased functional ability resulting from various disabilities

783. Which of the following statements regarding the diagnosis of urinary tract infections is/are correct?
    1) significant bacteriuria is defined as > 100,000 colony-forming units (CFU)/ml of a clean-voided urine specimen
    2) one culture with > 10^5 organisms/ml has a sensitivity of 80% in the diagnosis of urinary tract infection
    3) pyuria is defined as the presence of > 10 leukocytes/mm^3 in an unspun urine
    4) in acute urethral syndrome, fewer than 100 CFU/ml may be significant

784. Which of the following statements regarding asymptomatic bacteriuria in the elderly is(are) true?
    1) asymptomatic bacteriuria occurs in 20% of elderly women
    2) one urine culture is sufficient to make the diagnosis of asymptomatic bacteriuria
    3) even without treatment, approximately one-third of elderly patients who have asymptomatic bacteriuria will have bacteriuria 18 months later
    4) asymptomatic bacteriuria should be treated with antibiotic therapy in most cases

785. An 81-year-old female presents with a 5-day history of painful urination, increased frequency, urgency, and incontinence. She has had no other symptoms, including no costovertebral angle tenderness or other symptoms.

    On examination, her temperature is 37° C. Her blood pressure is 150/80 mm Hg, and her pulse is 84 and regular. No other abnormalities are found on physical examination.

Which of the following statements regarding this patient is(are) true?
1) this patient most likely has acute bacterial cystitis
2) the most likely organism responsible for this condition is *E. coli*.
3) the guidelines used for treating bacterial cystitis in younger patients also apply to elderly patients
4) elderly patients treated for 14 days have fewer recurrences than those patients treated with single-dose therapy

786. Which of the following statements regarding chronic prostatitis in males is(are) correct?
1) chronic prostatitis is the most common cause of relapsing urinary tract infection in elderly men
2) diagnosis is usually made by culturing prostatic secretions obtained by prostatic massage
3) the most common pathogenic organism is *E. coli*
4) with prolonged therapy, relapse is unlikely

787. A 75-year-old female presents with a 2-day history of fever, chills, confusion, dysuria, and diarrhea. There are no other symptoms present, including no costovertebral angle tenderness.

On examination, the patient's temperature is 38.5° C. Her blood pressure is 120/75 mm Hg, and her pulse is 96 and regular. There is slight abdominal tenderness, but no costovertebral angle tenderness present.

The most likely diagnosis in this patient is:
a) viral gastroenteritis
b) acute bacterial cystitis
c) acute pyelonephritis
d) bacterial gastroenteritis
e) none of the above

788. Which of the following statements regarding the use of antibiotics in patients with indwelling catheters is(are) true?
1) indwelling urinary catheters are the leading cause of nosocomial urinary tract infection
2) indwelling urinary catheters are the most common predisposing factor in hospital-acquired fatal gram-negative sepsis
3) by the time a urinary catheter has been in place for 2 weeks, 50% of catheterized patients have significant bacteriuria

4) antibiotic treatment should be instigated in patients with asymptomatic bacteriuria who have indwelling urinary catheters

ANSWERS

777. C. The most likely diagnosis in this patient is bacterial pneumonia.

The presentation of pneumonia in elders is usually much more subtle and nonspecific than in younger patients. As in this patient, confusion is a very common early sign. Other nonspecific early signs include disorientation and a change in interest level. As in other serious illnesses in elderly patients, a fall is often part of the presenting symptomatology.[1,2]

Findings on physical examination are also nonspecific. Signs of consolidation are not often found. Rales are common, but not very specific. An increased respiratory rate (as in this patient) may precede other signs and symptoms.[1,2]

No specific laboratory findings are usually found in elderly patients with pneumonia. An increased white blood cell count (> 10,000 cu mm) is commonly found, but this is neither sensitive nor specific for bacterial pneumonia. Hypoxemia is common.

In elderly patients with pneumonia, incomplete consolidation is the usual pattern noted on the chest x-ray.

Although viral pneumonia and atypical pneumonia are possibilities in this patient, bacterial pneumonia is more compatible with the clinical presentation, and x-ray findings.[1,2]

Congestive heart failure is not supported by the chest x-ray findings.

Acute Alzheimer's disease with atelectasis of the right lower lobe is a nondiagnosis.

778. B. The most common etiologic agent associated with community-acquired pneumonia is *Streptococcus pneumoniae*. *Haemophilus influenzae* and gram-negative bacilli are much less common unless there is associated COPD or another immune compromising condition.[1,2]

779. A. The treatment of choice for community-acquired pneumonia in the elderly is penicillin G or ampicillin. A first of second generation cephalosporin is also a reasonable alternative.[3]

780. D. The most likely etiologic agent associated with hospital-acquired pneumonia is a gram-negative

bacillus. The two most common organisms to cause nosocomial pneumonia are *Pseudomonas* and *Klebsiella* species.[1]

781. D. In hospitalized patients, exact diagnosis is often difficult because oral-pharyngeal colonization with gram-negative bacilli is greater. The therapy of choice is probably an extended spectrum penicillin such as piperacillin and an aminoglycoside. A third generation cephalosporin and an aminoglycoside is a good alternative.[3]

782. E. Urinary tract infections are second only to respiratory tract infections as causes of febrile illness in patients over the age of 65 years. The risk factors for urinary tract infections in the elderly include (1) advanced age; (2) decreased functional ability resulting from cardiovascular accidents, dementia, neurologic deficits, fecal incontinence, and other underlying chronic illness; (3) decreased bladder emptying resulting from neurogenic bladder, bladder-outlet obstruction (e.g., prostatic hypertrophy), and drugs with anticholinergic side effects; (4) nosocomial spread of organisms from hospitalized patients with asymptomatic bacteriuria, and the use of indwelling catheters; and (5) physiologic changes including decreased vaginal glycogen and increased vaginal pH in women, and decreased prostatic secretions and increased prostatic calculi in men.[4]

783. E. Significant bacteriuria is usually defined as the presence of greater than 100,000 colony-forming units (CFU/ml) of a clean-voided urine specimen.[4] One culture with > than 10^5 bacteria/ml accurately predicts infection 80% of the time.[4] Symptomatic infections (especially anterior urethral syndrome) can, however, occur with fewer than 100 CFU/ml.

Pyuria is defined as the presence of at least 5 to 10 leukocytes/HPF in the sediment of 10 ml of a centrifuged urine specimen, or more than 10 leukocytes/mm^3 in an unspun urine. Pyuria without bacteriuria (sterile pyuria) suggests causes other than acute infection, such as renal calculi, papillary necrosis secondary to obstruction or diabetes mellitus, chronic prostatitis, or tuberculosis.[4]

784. B. The overall prevalence of asymptomatic bacteriuria in noncatheterized, ambulatory patients is approximately 18% in women and 6% in men.[4]

The spontaneous cure rate in asymptomatic bacteriuria is high: approximately 33% of patients with asymptomatic bacteriuria will still have bacteriuria 18 months later. On the other hand, about 10% of nonbacteriuria elderly patients will become bacteriuric every 3 months.[4]

On microscopy, significant numbers of bacteria are usually evident in the urine, but pyuria is present in one-half of patients with asymptomatic bacteriuria.

Because cultures obtained from clean-voided specimens are often contaminated by organisms in the urethra or vagina, another culture one week later to confirm the diagnosis should be performed. If the same organism grows in the second culture, asymptomatic bacteriuria can be presumed to be present.[4]

The general consensus is that asymptomatic bacteriuria in the elderly should not be treated.[4] Treatment will result in the emergence of resistant organisms.

785. A. This patient has bacterial cystitis. Bacterial cystitis is suggested by the presence of > 10^5 CFU/ml in urine culture, and symptoms such as lower abdominal pain, dysuria, increased frequency of urination, or recent incontinence.[4]

The most likely organisms associated with acute bacterial cystitis include *E coli*, *Proteus*, *Klebsiella*, and *Pseudomonas*.

Ampicillin, trimethoprim-sulfamethoxazole, a cephalosporin, are all reasonable first choices for the treatment of gram-negative bacterial cystitis.[4] Single dose therapy with trimethoprim-sulfamethoxazole appears to be as effective as a full 10–14 day course.

786. A. Chronic bacterial prostatitis is the most common cause of relapsing urinary tract infections in elderly males.

The diagnosis of chronic bacterial prostatitis is established by culturing prostatic secretions obtained by prostatic massage.

The most common pathogen involved is *E.coli*, although *Klebsiella*, *Proteus*, and enterococci are also frequently involved.

The preferred antibiotic treatment is trimethoprim-sulfamethoxazole or a quinolone antibiotic such as ciprofloxacin or norfloxacin.[5] Relapses are common, even with prolonged therapy. Many patients are significantly helped by transurethral resection of the prostate.[4]

787. C. This patient has acute pyelonephritis. Patients who develop a syndrome of fever, chills, flank

pain, irritative voiding symptoms, bacteriuria likely have acute pyelonephritis. In elderly patients, however, the classical symptoms are not always present. Only 50% of elderly patients with pyelonephritis have costovertebral angle tenderness. Some even do not have fever. More than 20% of elderly patients present with gastrointestinal (as in this patient) or pulmonary symptoms.[4]

Bacteremia is much more common in elderly patients, and the urinary tract is the source of bacteremia in one-third of elderly patients admitted to the hospital with generalized sepsis. Thus, blood cultures are mandatory before initiating treatment. Septic shock occurs in up to 20% of elderly patients with acute pyelonephritis.

As with lower tract infections, the most common organisms involved are *E. coli, Klebsiella, Proteus* and *Pseudomonas*.[4]

The best initial antibiotic choice for suspected acute pyelonephritis is probably a combination of an extended spectrum penicillin such as piperacillin and an aminoglycoside, a third generation cephalosporin plus an aminoglycoside is a satisfactory alternative.

788. A. By 2 weeks, 50% of catheterized patients have significant bacteriuria, and after 1 month, virtually all patients have asymptomatic bacteriuria.

Indwelling urinary catheters are the leading cause of nosocomial urinary tract infections and the most common predisposing factor in hospital-acquired fatal gram-negative sepsis.

As discussed previously, patients with asymptomatic bacteriuria should not be treated with antibiotic therapy. This applies to patients with indwelling urinary catheters.[4,6]

SUMMARY OF THE DIAGNOSIS AND TREATMENT OF COMMON INFECTIONS IN THE ELDERLY

1. **Bacterial Pneumonia:**
   Etiology:
   a) community acquired: *Streptococcus pneumoniae* most common
   b) hospital acquired: gram-negative bacilli most common
   c) treatment:
      i) community acquired: ampicillin or penicillin
      ii) hospital-acquired: combination of extended spectrum penicillins and an aminoglycoside, or a third generation cephalosporin and an aminoglycoside.

2. **Urinary tract infection:**
   Bacterial cystitis:
   a) etiology: *E. coli, Proteus, Klebsiella, Pseudomonas*
   b) symptoms are usually the same as in younger individuals
   c) treatment: single dose of trimethoprim-sulfamethoxazole
   Chronic prostatitis:
   a) etiology: *E. coli, Klebsiella, Proteus*
   b) treatment: trimethoprim-sulfamethoxazole, ciprofloxacin, norfloxacin
   Pyelonephritis:
   a) presentation in elderly patients is less often classical. Only 50% of patients have costovertebral angle tenderness. Some patients present with confusion, gastrointestinal, and pulmonary symptoms as part of the clinical picture.
   b) etiology: *E. coli, Klebsiella, Proteus, Pseudomonas*
   c) treatment: Extended spectrum penicillin plus an aminoglycoside or a third-generation cephalosporin with an aminoglycoside.
   Asymptomatic bacteriuria: Common condition, especially in elderly women. Do not treat with antibiotics.

   Indwelling urinary catheters: Avoid whenever possible. All patients eventually develop bacteriuria. As with noncatheter associated asymptomatic bacteriuria, do not treat with antibiotics.

References

1. Meyers B. Serious infections in the elderly. Mount Sinai J Med 1987; 54(1):18–24.

2. Bentley D. Infectious diseases. In: Rossman I, ed. Clinical geriatrics. 3rd Ed. Philadelphia: JB Lippincott, 1987; 441–452.

3. Dunagan W, Powderly W. Antimicrobials and infectious diseases. In: Dunagan W, Ridner M, eds. Manual of medical therapeutics. 26th Ed. Boston: Little, Brown, 1989: 253–256.

4. Zilkosoki M, Smucker D, Mayhew H. Urinary tract infections in elderly patients. Postgrad Med 1988; 84(3):191–206.

5. Meares E. Prostatitis. In: Rakel R, ed. Conn's current therapy 1990. Philadelphia: WB Saunders, 1990: 633–635.

6. Kunin CM. Genitourinary infections in the patient at risk: extrinsic risk factors. Am J Med 1984; 76(5A):131–139.

PROBLEM 102: AN 80 YEAR-OLD-NURSING HOME RESIDENT WITH A BED SORE

You are called to a nursing home to see an 80 year-old-female with a fever of 40° C. The patient is disoriented and confused. The nurses said that they have had difficulty treating her pressure sores; especially one on her sacrum.

On examination, the patient's blood pressure is 110/80 mm Hg and her pulse is 72 and regular. Her temperature is 40° C. There is a large 10 X 5 cm decubitus ulcer present on her sacrum. The ulcer is oozing pus. You suspect septicemia.

SELECT THE ONE BEST ANSWER TO THE FOLLOWING QUESTIONS:

789. Which of the following statements concerning the prevention and etiology of pressure sores is FALSE?
   a) pressure sores are difficult to prevent in immobilized elderly patients
   b) good nutrition in the elderly will help prevent pressure sores
   c) anemia in the elderly predisposes to the formation of pressure sores
   d) incontinence in the elderly increases the risk of pressure sores by a factor of five
   e) patients who sit for long periods of time are just as likely to develop pressure sores as bedridden patients

790. Concerning the patient described in question 789, how long would it take the large ulcer described to develop from a small untreated ulcer?
   a) > 28 days
   b) 21–28 days
   c) 14–21 days
   d) 7–10 days
   e) 1–2 days

791. An elderly immobilized male is seen with a small 1 cm area of erthyema and bruising on his left heel. Which of the following is the MOST IMPORTANT aspect of treatment of a pressure sore at this stage?
   a) application of a full-thickness skin graft
   b) extensive debridement of the lesion and cleansing with an iodine-based solution
   c) application of a foam pad to protect the heel from further damage
   d) application of microscopic beads of dextran to the lesion
   e) elevation of the left leg by 30 degrees

ANSWER THE FOLLOWING QUESTIONS ACCORDING TO THE CODE:

A: 1, 2, and 3 are correct
B: 1 and 3 are correct
C: 2 and 4 are correct
D: Only 4 is correct
E: All of the above are correct

792. Which of the following anatomic sites is(are) common sites of ulcer formation?
   1)   sacrum
   2)   greater trochanter
   3)   lateral malleolus
   4)   medial malleolus

793. Pressure higher than normal capillary pressure exerted for a sufficient time may cause which of the following pathologic changes?
   1.   local edema
   2.   local thrombosis in small vessels and the microcirculation
   3.   occlusion of vessels by platelets
   4.   an aseptic mass of necrosis beneath the skin

794. Concerning the patient discussed in the problem, which of the following organisms are often associated with septic pressure sores?
   1)   *Bacteroides fragilis*
   2)   *Proteus mirabilis*
   3)   *Staphylococcus aureus*
   4)   *Pseudomonas*

ANSWERS

789. A. Pressure sores are a common problem in elderly, immobilized patients. Pressure sores form when a major part of body weight is transmitted between a bony prominence and a relatively hard surface

below, compressing the skin and adjacent soft tissues. The most vulnerable points are the sacrum, the heels, the greater trochanters, the knees, the iliac crest, and the shoulders. Both bedridden patients and patients who sit for prolonged periods with pressure on the ischial tuberosities are at risk.

A break in the skin, maceration of the skin, or incontinence increases the risk of pressure sores at least fivefold.

Good nutrition including a high protein diet will prevent anemia and hypoproteinemia, both risk factors for pressure sores.

Pressure sores can be prevented by (1) using old soft sheets or sheep skin, (2) rotating the patient every 1-2 hours, (3) checking all pressure points at least twice/day, (4) avoiding alcohol rubs, (5) avoiding complete bathing every day, (6) utilizing hydrotherapy and exercises, and (7) ensuring a high-protein, high-vitamin diet.[1,2]

790. E. Erythema may progress to ulceration quickly. A small ulcer can progress to a large one within 24–48 hours. The progression is due to local edema and/or infection, the former being the most important factor. As in the patient presented in question 1, severe infection can lead to septicemia, which must be recognized and treated with appropriate systemic antibiotic therapy.

791. C. Early lesions, as evidenced by erythema and mild bruising should be treated by the application of a foam pad to protect the area from further damage. Use of a hydrofloat device will help reverse the early changes and help fully developed lesions heal more quickly. Extensive debridement of the lesion and application of a full-thickness skin graft, and application of microscopic beads of dextran are not indicated for a lesion at the early stage described. Elevation of the leg to an angle of 30 degrees will not enhance the healing of the ulcer.

Definite ulcers should be treated by (1) relief of pressure, (2) debridement, (3) disinfection, and (4) support of tissue growth by hydrocolloid dressings or polyurethane film.[1,2]

792. A. Greater than 95% of ulcers develop in skin areas in the lower part of the body. The most common sites of ulcer formation are the sacrum, ischial tuberosity, greater trochanter, lateral malleolus,

and calcaneus. The medial malleolus is not a common site for ulcer formation.[2]

793. E. Pressure higher than normal capillary pressure exerted for a sufficient time causes edema, local thrombosis in small vessels and the microcirculation, and vacular endothelial damage that leads to occlusion of vessels by platelets. Tissue death may then result, and an aseptic mass of necrosis may develop beneath the skin.[1,2]

794. E. Septicemia and the possibility of septic shock are life-threatening complications of pressure sores. Pressure sores are colonized by both aerobes and anaerobes. The bacteria commonly associated with septic pressure sores include *Bacteroides fragilis*, *Proteus mirabilis*, *Staphylococcus aureus*, and *Pseudomonas*. Septic shock and death is often associated with *Bacteroides*. Other serious complications of pressure sores include osteomyelitis and spreading cellulitis.

SUMMARY OF THE MANAGEMENT OF PRESSURE SORES IN THE ELDERLY

1. **Common sites of pressure sores:** Sacrum, greater trochanter, ischial tuberosity, lateral malleolus, and calcaneus.

2. **Cornerstones of management:**
   a) relief of pressure
   b) debridement
   c) disinfection
   d) support of tissue growth.

3. Septicemia, cellulitis, and osteomyelitis should be treated with intravenous antibiotics; routine culturing of pressure sores is not encouraged.

References

1. Melcher R, Longe RL, Gelbart A. Pressure sores in the elderly: a systemic approach to management. Postgrad Med 1988; 83(1): 299–308.

2. Agnate J. Pressure sores. In: Patly M, ed. Principles and practice of geriatric medicine. Chichester, England: John Wiley & Sons, 1985: 899–905.

PROBLEM 103: AN 88-YEAR-OLD INSTITUTIONALIZED FEMALE WITH URINARY INCONTINENCE

You are called by a nursing home supervisor about an 88-year-old female with urinary incontinence. The nurse requests permission to insert an indwelling Foley catheter. When you question the nurse, she tells you that the patient has been incontinent for the past 6 days. She states that she hasn't got enough staff to keep cleaning up the bed.

SELECT THE ONE BEST ANSWER TO THE FOLLOWING QUESTIONS:

795. At this time, you should tell the nurse to:
    a) insert the Foley catheter and call you if there is any problem
    b) begin intermittent four-hourly catheterizations to avoid the necessity of a Foley catheter
    c) wait and see what happens over the next couple of weeks
    d) order some routine blood work to try and elicit a cause for the incontinence
    e) wait until you come up to the nursing home to examine the patient; you will be up this evening

796. Which of the following statements regarding urinary incontinence in the elderly is false?
    a) 50% of elderly patients in nursing homes have established urinary incontinence
    b) 5–15 % of elderly patients in the community have urinary incontinence
    c) women are twice as likely to have urinary incontinence as men
    d) humiliation and embarrassment suffered by the patient are important consequences of urinary incontinence
    e) none of the above statements are false

797. The most common type of urinary incontinence in elderly patients is:
    a) urge incontinence
    b) stress incontinence
    c) complex incontinence
    d) overflow incontinence
    e) functional incontinence

ANSWER THE FOLLOWING QUESTIONS ACCORDING TO THE CODE:

A: 1, 2, and 3 are correct
B: 1 and 3 are correct
C: 2 and 4 are correct
D: Only 4 is correct
E: All of the above are correct

798. Which of the following statements regarding incontinence in the elderly is(are) true?
    1) stress incontinence is usually manifested by the loss of small amounts of urine with increases in intra-abdominal pressure
    2) overflow incontinence occurs through bladder overdistention
    3) prostatic obstruction is a common cause of overflow incontinence
    4) functional incontinence is characterized by an involuntary loss of urine despite normal bladder and urethral functioning.

799. Which of the following is(are) contributory factors in urinary continence in the elderly?
    1) a loss of ability of the kidney to concentrate urine
    2) a decreased bladder capacity
    3) decreased urethral closing pressure following menopause
    4) decreased mobility

800. Which of the following drugs has(have) been implicated in the pathogenesis of urinary incontinence in the elderly?
    1) diuretics
    2) neuroleptics
    3) hypnotics and sedatives
    4) antibiotics

801. Which of the following nonpharmacologic treatment(s) may be effectively used in the treatment of urinary incontinence in the elderly?
    1) bladder exercises
    2) clean intermittent catheterization
    3) bedside commodes and urinals
    4) periurethral injection of polytetrafluoroethylene paste

802. Which of the following pharmacologic treatment(s) may be indicated in the therapy of urinary incontinence?
    1) Pro-Banthine for urge incontinence
    2) imipramine for urge incontinence
    3) intravaginal cream for stress incontinence

4) calcium-channel blockers for urge incontinence

ANSWERS

795. E. In an elderly patient who has just become incontinent, it is inappropriate to insert a Foley catheter or to do anything else until you have made an attempt to establish the cause. The pathophysiology of urinary incontinence in the elderly population is complex, even among patients with dementia. Elderly patients deserve the same investigation of etiology as you would perform in a younger individual.

796. E. Fifty percent of elderly patients in nursing homes, and 5–15% of elderly patients in the community have urinary incontinence.

Women are twice as likely as men to have urinary incontinence.

Humiliation and embarrassment are important consequences of urinary incontinence in elderly patients. This embarrassment leads to social isolation, and subsequent anxiety and depression. Incontinence is the second leading cause of admission to nursing homes.

In North America, it is estimated that the total health care costs associated with urinary incontinence are over $8 billion dollars per year.[1,2]

Physical consequences, such as predisposition to skin irritations, infections and pressure sores, are also a major problem.

797. A. The most common type of urinary incontinence in the elderly is urge incontinence. Urge incontinence (detrusor hyperreflexia) is characterized by leakage of urine due to strong and sudden sensations of bladder urgency. Patients with urge incontinence may also experience frequency, urgency, and nocturia. Urge incontinence is also called unstable bladder, uninhibited bladder, and hyperreflexic bladder. Many conditions may predispose to urge incontinence; these include (1) stroke, (2) Parkinson's disease, (3) Alzheimer's disease, (4) spine cord injury or tumor, (5) multiple sclerosis, (6) prostatic hypertrophy, and (7) interstitial cystitis. Urge incontinence may also be present in individuals in whom no neurologic or genitourinary abnormality is present.[1]

798. E. Stress incontinence (urethral incompetence) is characterized by loss of small amounts of urine secondary to increases in intrabdominal pressure.

Stress incontinence is most commonly associated with pelvic floor weakening through childbirth, obesity, injury, menopause and aging, and sphincter damage.

Overflow incontinence occurs with bladder overdistention. Overdistention results in a constant leakage of small amounts of urine or "dribbling" when a physiologic situation in which the intravesicular pressure exceeds the intraurethral resistance. Bladder overdistention is usually caused by an anatomic obstruction by an enlarged prostate, urethral stricture, or by fecal impaction. A hypotonic bladder secondary to diabetes mellitus, syphilis, spinal cord compression, or from anticholinergic medication may also cause overflow incontinence.

Complex incontinence refers to incontinence that has both urge and stress components.

Functional incontinence refers to involuntary loss of urine despite normal bladder and urethral functioning. This is most commonly seen with severe dementia and closed head injuries.[1,2]

799. E. Many factors are associated with the development and maintenance of urinary incontinence in the elderly. These include (1) a loss of ability of the kidney to concentrate urine, (2) a decreased bladder capacity, (3) decreased urethral closing pressure following menopause, (4) decreased mobility, (5) decreased vision, (6) depression and secondary inattention to bladder cues, and (7) an inadequate environmental setting.[1,2]

The importance of drugs in elder incontinence is discussed in a subsequent question.

800. A. Drugs are a very common cause of elder incontinence. The major drugs that have been implicated in the pathogenesis of urinary incontinence include diuretics, hypnotics, sedatives and tranquillizers, ethanol, muscle relaxants, and neuroleptics.[2]

801. E. Treatment of urinary incontinence should begin with nonpharmacologic treatment. Drugs that may be associated with incontinence should be eliminated. Toilets, commodes, and urinals should be made as accessible as possible. Absorbent bed pads, protective undergarments, external collecting devices such as condoms or Texas catheters, skin protectants, and deodorants should be used whenever possible.

Bladder retraining exercises (gradually increasing the period of time between voidings) should be encouraged.[3] Kegel exercises, which are perineal muscle exercises designed to increase urethral resistance, should be promoted in patients with stress incontinence.

Nonobstructive overflow incontinence may be treated by intermittent catheterizations. Indwelling urinary catheters should be used only when all other treatment measures have proven unsuccessful. Indwelling urinary catheters are a major source of urinary tract infections, and lead to increased morbidity and mortality in elderly patients.

Surgical procedures to correct prolapse and to increase outlet resistance and enhance sphincter action are useful in women with stress incontinence. Surgery in males may involve synthetic prosthesis implantation for treatment of traumatic sphincter, prostate resection, or electronic implants to treat male sphincter incompetence.

A new procedure, injection of polytetrafluoroethylene paste to narrow the urethral opening and increase urethral resistance, may be effective in up to 75% of patients.[2] Support groups and self-help programs are important adjuvants, not only in treating the actual incontinence, but also in facilitating psychologic therapy for the problem.

802. E. Urge incontinence may be successfully treated with anticholinergic and antispasmodic agents such as oxybutynin, Pro-Banthine, and imipramine. Recently, three new classes of drugs have been suggested for treatment of urge incontinence. These drugs are the prostaglandin inhibitors, the calcium-channel blockers, and the beta-adrenergic agonists. Extensive use of these medications will have to await further study.

Stress incontinence in women may be treated with intravaginal estrogen cream or with alpha-adrenergic agonists such as phenylpropanolamine.

Overflow incontinence (when not caused by a mechanism obstruction) may be treated with a cholinergic agent such as bethanechol or alpha-adrenergic blocking drugs such as phenoxybenzamine, clonidine, and prazosin.[2]

SUMMARY OF THE DIAGNOSIS AND MANAGEMENT OF URINARY INCONTINENCE IN THE ELDERLY

1. Incontinence affects 50% of institutionalized elderly and 10–15% of elderly in the community

2. **Types of incontinence:**
    a) urge incontinence
    b) stress incontinence
    c) overflow incontinence
    d) functional incontinence
    e) complex incontinence

3. Assess and treat contributing factors (including drugs and systemic infections) before initiating specific therapy for the incontinence

4. Utilize nonpharmacologic therapy whenever possible

5. **Pharmacologic therapy:**
    a) urge incontinence: anticholinergics, antispasmodics, imipramine. New agents under investigation include prostaglandin inhibitors, calcium-channel blockers, and beta-adrenergic agonists
    b) stress incontinence: local estrogen, phenylpropanolamine
    c) overflow incontinence: cholinergic agents, alpha-adrenergic blockers

References

1. Resnick N , Yalla S, Laurino E. The pathophysiology of urinary incontinence among institutionalized elderly persons. N Engl J Med 1989; 320(1): 1–7.

2. Romanowski G, et al. Urinary incontinence in the elderly: etiology and treatment. Drug Intell Clin Pharm 1988; 22: 525–533.

3. Frank S. The genitourinary system. In: Taylor R, ed. Family medicine, principles and practice. 3rd Ed. New York: Springer-Verlag, 1988: 294.

PROBLEM 104: A 70-YEAR-OLD MALE WITH HYPERTENSION

A 70-year-old male, previously healthy, presents for a routine physical examination. He was last seen by a physician 15 years ago. His blood pressure is recorded at 180/105 mm Hg. A complete history reveals no other cardiovascular risk factors. A complete physical examination reveals no evidence of end organ damage or secondary causes of hypertension. Basic laboratory evaluations including complete blood count, urinalysis, serum potassium, calcium, creatinine, fasting blood sugar, plasma cholesterol, serum uric acid, and electrocardiography are normal.

The patient is on a fixed income and is trying to keep up with payments for his wife's nursing home care.

SELECT THE ONE BEST ANSWER TO THE FOLLOWING QUESTIONS:

803. Based on the history and physical examination, you would now:
    a) begin therapy with a thiazide diuretic
    b) begin therapy with a calcium-channel blocker
    c) begin therapy with a angiotension converting enzyme inhibitor
    d) begin therapy with a beta blocker
    e) none of the above

804. The patient described in question 803 returns for follow-up. His blood pressure remains elevated (175/105 mm Hg). You would now:
    a) prescribe a thiazide diuretic
    b) prescribe a calcium-channel blocker
    c) prescribe a beta blocker
    d) prescribe an angiotension converting enzyme inhibitor
    e) prescribe a vasodilator

805. Appropriate therapy is prescribed for the patient and he returns in 1 month for follow-up. His blood pressure is now 170/100 mm Hg. His serum potassium level has decreased from 4.0 mEq/L to 3.0 mEq/L. At this time, it would be most reasonable to add:
    a) a thiazide diuretic
    b) a beta blocker
    c) a calcium-channel blocker
    d) an angiotension converting enzyme inhibitor
    e) a vasodilator

806. A 75-year-old male with angina pectoris is found on physical examination to have a blood pressure of 170/100 mm Hg. His angina is being controlled with isorsorbide dinitrate 30 mg q.i.d.
    This reading is repeated on several occasions and found to be the same. At this time the most reasonable treatment for his blood pressure would be:
    a) a calcium-channel blocker
    b) a beta blocker

c) athiazide diuretic
    d) an ACE inhibitor
    e) either a or b

807. A 72-year-old female with a previous myocardial infarction and mild congestive cardiac failure (controlled with furosemide 40 mg od) presents for a routine assessment. She is found to have a blood pressure of 180/100 mm Hg. This reading is repeated on two further occasions. Considering her congestive cardiac failure, the most appropriate treatment for her hypertension would be:
    a) an ACE inhibitor
    b) a calcium-channel blocker
    c) a beta blocker
    d) a thiazide diuretic
    e) none of the above

808. A 72-year-old male with a 20 year history of noninsulin dependant diabetes is found to have a blood pressure of 170/105 mm Hg. He has no history of angina pectoris or other significant vascular disease. His blood pressure is repeated on two further occasions. Laboratory evaluation reveals microalbuminuria. At this time, the most appropriate treatment for this patient's blood pressure would be:
    a) a thiazide diuretic
    b) a beta blocker
    c) a calcium-channel blocker
    d) an ACE inhibitor
    e) a vasodilator

ANSWER THE FOLLOWING QUESTION ACCORDING TO THE CODE:

A: 1, 2, and 3 are correct
B: 1 and 3 are correct
C: 2 and 4 are correct
D: Only 4 is correct
E: All of the above are correct

809. Which of the following statements regarding hypertension in the elderly is/are TRUE?

1) the treatment of hypertension in patients older than age 75 has not been shown to be effective
2) patients with isolated systolic hypertension have demonstrated significant reductions in cardiovascular and cerebrovascular mortality
3) elderly hypertensives should all be treated with a stepped care approach, regardless of concurrent illness
4) overall cardiovascular and cerebrovascular mortality are decreased by the effective treatment of diastolic hypertension in the elderly

ANSWERS

803. E. None of the above. The patient's blood pressure should be measured on at least two further occasions before you label him as being hypertensive. These readings should all be taken after at least 5 minutes of rest. In addition, the patient should be counseled regarding the importance of sodium restriction, alcohol restriction, and weight control.[1]

804. A. A thiazide diuretic is the least expensive medication, and where cost is a consideration, should certainly be thought of as the drug of first choice. As discussed in another section of this book, first line drugs include the thiazide diuretics, the beta blockers, the calcium-channel blockers and the angiotension enzyme converting inhibitors. Beta blockers are somewhat less effective in elderly patients than in younger patients and calcium-channel blockers and angiotensin converting enzyme inhibitors are expensive. Hydrochlorothiazide, in a dosage of 25 mg/day, should control blood pressure in at least 50% of patients.[1]

805. D. Although the addition of either a betablocker or a calcium-channel blocker would enhance control of the patient's blood pressure, the drug of choice is probably an ACE inhibitor. The addition of an ACE inhibitor in this case will not only increase the efficacy of blood pressure control but will also blunt the metabolic side effects produced by diuretics. Hypokalemia, hyperuricemia, hyperglycemia, and hyperlipidemia may be significantly ameliorated or normalized completely by the addition of an ACE inhibitor to a thiazide diuretic.

Increasing the dose of hydrochlorothiazide (even with the addition of a potassium-sparing agent) is probably not the therapeutic maneuver of choice. The probability of hyperuricemia, hyperglycemia, and hyperlipidemia will be increased, and the efficacy of blood pressure control is unlikely to be significantly affected by increasing the dose of hydrochlorothiazide.[1-3]

806. E. This patient's blood pressure would be best managed with either a betablocker or a calcium-channel blocker. Addition of either of these drugs will enhance control of angina pectoris as well as controling his hypertenion.[1,2]

807. A. This patient should be treated with an ACE inhibitor. ACE inhibition will decrease the preload and afterload associated with congestive cardiac failure as well as effectively treating the patient's blood pressure.

Beta blockers are contraindicated in congestive cardiac failure and a thiazide diuretic will probably increase metabolic side effects that may have already occurred with furosemide. Although a calcium-channel blocker will effectively control hypertension, it will not have a significant beneficial effect on the patient's congestive cardiac failure.[1,3]

808. D. This patient should be treated with an ACE inhibitor. ACE inhibitors have become the preferred antihypertensives for patients with diabetes mellitus. Also, this patient has microalbuminuria, which may be the first manifestation of diabetic nephropathy.

Thiazide diuretics increase hyperglycemia and are relatively contraindicated in diabetics. If they are combined with an ACE inhibitor, however, they may well be the drugs of second choice.

Most beta blockers can effect plasma lipids adversely. As well, they blunt the response of the sympathetic nervous system to hypoglycemia.

A calcium-channel blocker could be used in this patient. However, it would be a second choice to the ACE inhibitor.[1,3]

809. D. Geriatric patients with a diastolic blood pressure of 90 mm Hg or greater do benefit from treatment of their hypertension.

Definitive data on isolated systolic hypertension in the elderly is not yet solid. The findings of the Systolic Hypertension in the Elderly Study, which will be published in 1991, should provide the answer to this question.

The treatment of geriatric hypertension should be based on the presence or absence of concurrent illnessess, and should take into account any other significant factors, not the least of which is cost of medication.

SUMMARY OF THE TREATMENT OF GERIATRIC HYPERTENSION

1. Geriatric patients with a diastolic blood pressure of 90 mm Hg or greater do benefit from treatment of their blood pressure.

2. The benefit of treating isolated systolic hypertension is not yet established. In the interim, a cautious lowering of systolic pressure into the 150–160 mm Hg range seems reasonable.

3. An individualized approach to treating geriatric hypertension:
   a) no concurrent illness:
   1st: thiazide diuretic
   2nd: ACE inhibitor
   b) hypertension with angina pectoris
   1st/ 2nd: calcium-channel blocker/beta blocker
   c) hypertension with congestive cardiac failure
   1st: ACE inhibitor
   2nd: thiazide diuretic
   d) hypertension with diabetes mellitus
   1st: ACE inhibitor
   2nd: thiazide diuretic
   e) hypertension with asthma or COPD
   1st: calcium-channel blocker
   2nd: thiazide diuretic
   f) hypertension with peripheral vascular disease
   1st: calcium-channel blocker
   2nd: ACE inhibitor
   g) Isolated systolic hypertension
   1st: thiazide diuretic
   2nd: ACE inhibitor/calcium-channel blocker

References

1. The 1988 Report of the Joint National Consensus Committee on Detection, Evaluation, and Treatment of High Blood Pressure. Arch Intern Med 1988; 148: 1023–1038.

2. Moser M. Diuretics and alternative drugs in geriatric hypertension. Geriatrics 1987; 42(2): 39–49.

3. M'Buyamba-Kabangu J R. ACE-inhibitors in the treatment of elderly hypertensives. Geriatrics 1987; 42(6): 45–49.

PROBLEM 105: A 75-YEAR-OLD FEMALE WITH A BAGFUL OF PILLS

A 75-year-old female presents to your office with her daughter. Her daughter complains that her mother began seeing "pink rats coming out of the walls" 3 days ago. The daughter brings in her mother's medications in a bag. The daughter had taken her mother to her local physician 1 week ago. At that time the doctor instituted a number of medications including pills for her blood pressure, her heart, her arthritis, her stomach, her depression, and her insomnia. The daughter states that her mother had been feeling fairly well before the visit to her physician, but had complained to the doctor of a few minor ailments. He had placed her on hydrochlorothiazide, propranolol, digoxin, ibuprofen, cimetidine, Maalox, amitriptyline, and triazolam. Knowing that medications in the elderly can often produce significant side effects you conclude that there probably is a connection between the pink rats and a medication.

On examination, the patient is agitated and confused. She points to the ceiling and yells "pink rats, pink rats." Her blood pressure is 100/70 mm Hg, and her pulse is 54 and regular. She has a bruise on her head from a fall 3 days ago. Examination of the cardiovascular system reveals a normal S1 and S2 with a grade III/VI systolic murmur heard along the left sternal edge. There are no other abnormalities found on physical examination.

SELECT THE ONE BEST ANSWER TO THE FOLLOWING QUESTIONS:

810. The most likely cause of this patient's visual hallucinations is:
   a) propranolol
   b) hydrochlorothiazide
   c) ibuprofen
   d) cimetidine
   e) digoxin

811. Considering the rapid introduction of multiple medications that took place last week, the most appropriate course of action at this time would be to:
   a) discontinue the digoxin
   b) discontinue the hydrochlorothiazide

c) discontinue the propranolol

d) discontinue the triazolam

e) discontinue everything, observe, and re-evaluate the patient

812. Which of the following drug combinations is the most likely combination to result in a drug-drug interaction in the elderly?

a) cimetidine and propranolol

b) digoxin and a diuretic

c) ibuprofen and captopril

d) triazolam and amitriptyline

e) haloperidol and digoxin

813. The most common side effect of antihypertensive medication in the elderly is:

a) confusion

b) orthostatic hypotension

c) dizziness

d) fatigue

e) skin rash

814. Which of the following are the three most common drug classes usually associated with adverse drug reactions in the elderly?

a) cardiovascular drugs, psychotropics, and antibiotics

b) cardiovascular drugs, psychotropics, and analgesics

c) gastrointestinal drugs, psychotropics, and analgesics

d) gastrointestinal drugs, psychotropics, and antibiotics

e) gastrointestinal drugs, psychotropics, and analgesics

ANSWER THE FOLLOWING QUESTIONS ACCORDING TO THE CODE:

A: 1, 2, and 3 are correct

B: 1 and 3 are correct

C: 2 and 4 are correct

D: Only 4 is correct

E: All of the above are correct

815. Which of the following is/are important risk factors for undesirable side effects of medication in the elderly?

1) multiple drugs

2) multiple physicians

3) multiple pharmacies

4) living alone

816. Which of the following is/are important variables in increasing the incidence of adverse drug reactions in the elderly?

1) altered free concentration of drug in serum

2) altered volume of distribution

3) altered renal drug clearance

4) altered tissue sensitivity

817. Which of the following is(are) examples of adverse drug reactions in the elderly?

1) drug side effects

2) drug toxicity

3) drug-disease interaction

4) drug-drug interaction

818. Some drugs are excreted virtually unchanged by the kidney. The dosages of these drugs must be carefully titrated in any elderly patient with renal impairment. Drugs in this category include:

1) cimetidine

2) gentamicin

3) lithium

4) diazepam

819. Which of the following is(are) true regarding the use of antipsychotic drugs in the elderly?

1) antipsychotic drugs are often prescribed for behaviors that nursing home staff find objectionable

2) double-blind, randomized, controled trials have established the efficacy of antipsychotic drugs in Alzheimer's disease

3) tardive dyskinesia is a frequent side effect of antipsychotic drug use in the elderly

4) the noninstitutionalized elderly are just as likely to receive antipsychotic drugs as the institutionalized elderly

820. Which of the following is(are) valid rules for prescribing drugs for elderly patients?

1) dose carefully: start low and go slow

2) consider nondrug alternatives in therapy

3) establish a priority order regarding the drugs to be used

4) treat all symptoms whenever possible

ANSWERS

810. A. The most common iatrogenic cause of hallucinations in elderly patients is propranolol. Many patients who are started on this medication develop visual or auditory hallucinations. Unfortunately,

many of these patients are then started on anti-psychotics to treat the hallucinations.

811. E. The most appropriate course of action at this time would be to discontinue everything. The patient had been placed on multiple medications during her last visit for uncertain reasons. The visual hallucinations should clear rapidly after the propranolol is discontinued, and the confusion will probably also clear after the assortment of other medications is discontinued.

812. B. Patients who develop adverse drug reactions (ADRs) are more likely to be taking six or more drugs than those who do not experience ADRs. The most commonly identified combination likely to result in a drug-drug interaction was a digitalis preparation along with a diuretic.[1]

813. B. Antihypertensive medication produces many side effects in the elderly. The most significant side effect is orthostatic hypotension. Orthostatic hypotension is due to impaired cardiovascular homeostasis and may result in dizziness, falls, and hip fractures. Therefore, any patient on antihypertensive medication should have their blood pressure taken in both the sitting and the standing position. Confusion, fatigue, and impotence are other common side effects.[1]

814. B. The three most common drug classes associated with ADRs in the elderly are cardiovascular drugs, psychotropics, and analgesics (especially the non-steroidal anti-inflammatory drugs). Unfortunately, many of the drugs used in the treatment of geriatric patients are prescribed for symptoms related to the effects and the diseases of aging, not to treat a specific or to maintain or restore function.[1,2]

815. E. Many factors increase the risk of undesirable drug effects in the elderly. They are (1) a physician with no knowledge of pharmacogeriatrics; (2) multiple drugs; (3) history of a tendency to adverse drug reactions; (4) concurrent diseases, especially renal disease and severe liver insufficiency; (5) impairments: mental, visual, auditory, locomotive; (6) late senescence: very limited homeostasis; (7) self-medication; (8) multiple physicians; (9) multiple pharmacies; (10) lower lean body mass; (11) living alone; (12) lack of community support services; and (13) socioeconomic problems resulting in inadequate follow-up.[3]

816. E. Many physiologic and social variables increase the incidence of adverse drug reactions in the elderly. They include (1) number of drugs, (2) compliance, (3) absorption of drug, (4) concentration of free drug in the serum, (5) volume of distribution, (6) tissue sensitivity, (7) metabolic clearance, (8) renal drug clearance, (9) general homeostasis, and (10) concentration of serum albumin.[1-3]

817. E. An adverse drug reaction is defined as any unintended or undesired effect of a drug in a patient.[1] This effect, or clinical manifestation, may include abnormal laboratory tests, symptoms, or signs. ADRs can be divided into (1) side effects (dry mouth-tricyclic antidepressants, hypokalemia-diuretics); (2) drug toxicity (daytime sedation-hypnotics, diarrhea-laxatives, syncope-antihypertensive agents); (3) drug-disease interaction (benzodiazepines and drugs with anticholinergic properties may exacerbate Alzheimer's disease); (4) drug-drug interaction (digoxin and diuretics); and (5) secondary effects (haloperidol causing drug-induced parkinsonism).[1]

818. A. The kidney is the major source of elimination of many commonly prescribed drugs. Drugs that undergo extensive renal clearance and that are therefore likely to accumulate in the elderly include (1) digoxin, (2) gentamicin and other aminoglycosides, (3) lithium, (4) cimetidine, (5) co-trimoxazole, (6) disopyramide, (7) nadolol, (8) procainamide, and (9) sulfonamides.

The longer-acting benzodiazepines such as diazepam and flurazepam are metabolized by hepatic oxidation are examples of drugs that accumulate rapidly in any elderly patient with hepatic disfunction.[1-3]

819. B. Psychotropic drugs are commonly prescribed for geriatric patients. Indications for the use of these drugs are not well established. In nursing home situations, psychotropic drugs are often prescribed for behaviors that staff members find objectionable, and the patient may remain on the drug(s) for long periods of time. The institutionalized elderly are ten times as likely to receive antipsychotic agents as age-matched noninstitutionalized controls.[4]

Double-blind, randomized, controlled trials have not established the efficacy of antipyschotic drugs in Alzheimer's disease. Tardive dyskinesia, rigidity, and excessive sedation are frequent side effects of antipyschotic drug use.[2]

820. A. The following are a good set of rules for prescribing medication in geriatric patients:[3]
1) Recognize that there is no drug to treat senescence.
2) Recognize that mere prolongation of life is not a valid reason for using medications that decrease the quality of life.
3) Make sure that the effects of treatment are better than no treatment.
4) Establish a priority order for treatment.
5) Keep the number of drugs administered concurrently to a minimum.
6) Know your patient well. Consider renal and hepatic impairment. Consider what else (including over the counter medications) is being taken, and who else is prescribing.
7) Consider nonpharmacologic therapy.
8) If you decide to prescribe a drug, know it well. Consider using a few drugs often rather than a lot of drugs infrequently.
9) Select the dose carefully: "Start low and go slow".
10) Anticipate and minimize adverse reactions by considering side-effect profiles.
11) Determine whether or not the patient needs help using the medication.
12) Educate the patient and family.
13) Continually reevaluate whether or not your patient needs a specific drug.

SUMMARY OF ADVERSE DRUG REACTIONS IN THE ELDERLY

1. Adverse drug reactions are at least twice as common in elderly patients as in younger patients

2. Most common types of adverse drug reactions:
a) side effects
b) drug toxicity
c) drug-disease interaction
d) drug-drug interaction

3. Most common drugs associated with adverse drug reactions in the elderly are:
a) cardiovascular drugs
b) psychotropic drugs and analgesics (especially nonsteroidal anti-inflammatory agents).

4. Keep the number of drugs prescribed to elderly patients to a minimum.

5. Only prescribe medications to elderly patients when the benefits clearly outweigh the risks

6. Schedule a "medication review" on a regular basis (at least every 3 months).

References

1. Hershey L. Avoiding adverse drug reactions in the elderly. Mount Sinai J Med 1988; 55(3): 244–250.

2. O'Brien J, Kursch J. Healthy prescribing for the elderly. How to minimize adverse drug effects and prevent 'dementia in a bottle.' Postgrad Med 1987; 82(6): 147–157.

3. Davison W. Pharmacology of aging — prescribing and the "treatment of aging." In: Brockelhurst JC, ed. Textbook of geriatric medicine and gerontology. 3rd Ed. Edinburgh: Churchill-Livingstone, 1985: 157–161.

4. Ray W, Federspiel C, Schaffner W. A study of antipsychotic drug use in nursing homes: epidemiologic evidence suggesting disease. Am J Public Health 1980; 70(5): 485–491.

PROBLEM 106: A 75-YEAR-OLD DEPRESSED MALE WITH A SLOW SHUFFLING GAIT AND RIGIDITY

A 75-year-old male is brought into the office by his wife. She states that he has just been "staring into space for the last 2 months." He has been unable to move around the house without falling over. Also, his movements appear to be very slow. According to his wife, he has also been very depressed.

On examination, the patient has a slow, shuffling, gait, and walks stooped over. His lying blood pressure is 140/90 mm Hg. His standing blood pressure is 100/70 mm Hg. He has marked rigidity of his upper and lower extremities.

No tremor or other abnormalities are found on examination.

SELECT THE ONE BEST ANSWER TO THE FOLLOWING QUESTIONS:

821. The most likely diagnosis in this patient is:
    a) Alzheimer's disease
    b) major depressive illness with psychomotor retardation
    c) orthostatic hypotension secondary to old age
    d) Parkinson's disease
    e) olivopontocerebellar atrophy

822. The most common presenting symptom of the condition described above is:
    a) orthostatic hypotension
    b) depression
    c) gait disturbance
    d) tremor
    e) rigidity

823. The lesion associated with the disease described above is located in a certain anatomic area of the brain. In which area of the brain is the lesion?
    a) the caudate nucleus
    b) the hypothalamus
    c) the substantia nigra
    d) the putamen
    e) the globus pallidus

824. The condition described above is associated with a deficit of particular brain neurotransmitter. What is that neurotransmitter?
    a) acetylcholine
    b) serotonin
    c) gamma-aminobutyric acid
    d) dopamine
    e) norephinephrine

825. Which of the following medications IS NOT a cause of some of the symptoms described in the case above?
    a) diazepam
    b) haloperidol
    c) largactil
    d) perphenazine
    e) reserpine

826. Which of the following statements regarding the condition discussed above is FALSE?
    a) there is marked heterogeneity in this disease
    b) there are at least two major subgroups of this condition

c) patients who present with marked postural instability have a better prognosis than those who present with tremor
    d) personality changes usually occur in early stages of the disease
    e) significant depression and dementia appear in one-third to one-half of patients with the condition

827. The drug of choice for treatment of severe symptoms of the condition discussed above is:
    a) amantadine
    b) trihexyphenidyl
    c) hydroxyzine
    d) levodopa
    e) bromocriptine

ANSWER THE FOLLOWING QUESTIONS ACCORDING TO THE CODE:

A: 1, 2, and 3 are correct
B: 1 and 3 are correct
C: 2 and 4 are correct
D: Only 4 is correct
E: All of the above are correct

828. Which of the following may be indicated in the treatment of the condition discussed above if the symptoms are mild and not significantly impairing functioning?
    1) amantadine
    2) trihexyphenidyl
    3) tricyclic antidepressants
    4) no therapy

829. Which of the following statements about benign essential tremor is/are CORRECT?
    1) it is commonly familial
    2) a nodding head tremor and tremulousness of speech are often observed
    3) it predominantly affects the hands
    4) it is a resting tremor

830. Treatment of benign essential tremor may include which of the following agents?
    1) propranolol
    2) diazepam
    3) alcohol
    4) levodopa-carbidopa

ANSWERS

821. D. This patient has Parkinson's disease. The most common presenting symptoms in Parkinson's disease include tremor, bradykinesia, rigidity, impaired postural reflexes, gait disturbance, autonomic dysfunction (causing orthostatic hypotension), and depression. A "masked facies" expression is typical of the disease.[1,2]

Other presenting symptoms can be constipation, vague aches and pains, paresthesias, decreased smell sensation, vestibular symptoms, pedal edema, fatigue, and weight loss.[1,2]

The other choices listed in the question do not explain the constellation of presenting symptoms.

822. D. The most common presenting symptom of Parkinson's disease is tremor at rest. This symptom is seen in 70 % of patients with the disease.[1,2] It may initially be confined to one hand, but it usually extends to involve all limbs.

823. C. The principal pathologic feature in Parkinson's disease is degeneration of the substantia nigra. Degenerative changes are also found in other brain stem nuclei.[2]

824. D. Parkinson's disease is associated with a depletion of dopamine in the nigrostriatal pathway.[2]

825. A. The most common classes of drugs producing Parkinsonism are the antipsychotics including both the phenothiazines and butyrophenones. Examples of these drugs include haloperidol, largactil and perphenazine. The antihypertensive agent reserpine that was formerly extensively used is also a potential cause. Diazepam is not associated with the production of parkinsonism symptoms.[1,2]

826. C. There is marked heterogeneity in Parkinson's disease. There are at least two major subtypes of the disease. In one group of patients, tremor is the predominant clinical symptom. In the other, postural instability and gait difficulty (PIGD) are the predominant symptoms. There was some overlap, but most patients fit well into one subgroup or the other. Patients with tremor predominant Parkinson's disease have slower progression of disease, and have few problems with bradykinesia. They are also less likely to develop significant mental symptoms.

Personality changes usually occur in the early stages, and patients often become withdrawn, apathetic, and dependent on their spouses. Significant depression occurs in one-half of patients, and dementia occurs in one-third of patients. As mentioned earlier, these personality and mental changes are more common in patients who present with the PIGD subtype of Parkinson's disease.[1]

827. D. The drug of choice for severe Parkinson's disease is levodopa (L-Dopa). Levodopa provides a precursor for dopamine synthesis in the basal ganglia. The drug is usually administered in combination with carbidopa, a decarboxylase inhibitor. Treatment must be individualized; it is desirable to "start low and go slow."[2]

Levodopa tends to lose its effect after several years. If this occurs, therapy with a new agent, deprenyl, may be tried.[3] Alternatively, bromocriptine may be initiated.

828. E. The first decision that should be made by the clinician treating a patient with Parkinson's disease is whether or not the symptoms justify treatment. If the symptoms are relatively mild and not significantly impairing functioning, then it may be reasonable to withhold treatment. Alternatively, mild medications such as trihexyphenidyl, amantadine, and the tricyclic antidepressants may be used.[1,2]

829. A. Benign essential tremor, is the most common disorder of movement encountered in clinical practice. It often has a hereditary pattern; it is then known as familial tremor. It is often aggrevated by stress and excessive caffeine intake. It predominantly affects the hands; the trunk and legs are infrequently involved. A nodding head tremor and tremulousness of speech are often observed. The tremor is characteristically an action tremor.[2]

830. A. The treatment of choice for benign essential tremor is propranolol. Other choices include alcohol or diazepam levodopa-carbidopa is not indicated for the treatment of benign essential tremor.[2]

SUMMARY OF THE DIAGNOSIS AND MANAGEMENT OF PARKINSON'S DISEASE AND ESSENTIAL TREMOR

I. **Parkinson's disease:**
   1. **Major symptoms:** Resting tremor, bradykinesia, rigidity, impaired postural reflexes, gait disturbance, autonomic dysfunction, depression

2. There are two major subtypes of Parkinson's disease: that group of patient exhibiting tremor as the major sign and that group exhibiting postural instability and gait disturbance as the major signs (PIGD). Progression of the disease is usually more rapid in the latter group; neurobehavioral changes are also more common in the later group.

3. **Treatment of Parkinson's disease:**

   A. Minor symptoms (not significantly impairing function): no pharmacologic treatment, amantadine, trihexyphenidyl, tricyclic antidepressants

   B. Functions significantly impairing function: levodopa/carbidopa, deprenyl, bromocriptine

4. **Benign essential tremor:** Benign essential tremor is an action tremor, most often seen in the extremities and sometimes associated with head nodding and tremulousness of speech. It is often familial. Drug treatment: propranolol, alcohol, diazepam

References

1. Jankovic J. Parkinson's disease: recent advances in therapy. Southern Med J 1988; 81(8): 1021–1027.

2. Cutler R. Degenerative and heritary diseases. In: Rubenstein E, Federman D, eds. Scientific American medicine. New York: Scientific American, 1988; 11 (IV): 1–13.

3. The Parkinson Study Group. Effect of deprenyl on the progression of disability in early Parkinson's disease. N Engl J Med 1989; 321: 1364–1371.

Epidemiology and Public Health

PROBLEM 107: A 19-YEAR-OLD MEDICAL STUDENT WHO DISLIKES EPIDEMIOLOGY

A 19-year-old medical student presents to your office in a state of acute anxiety. He intensely dislikes epidemiology and has an examination to prepare for. He is experiencing sweating and palpitations. In an effort to treat the symptoms you decide to spend some time discussing basic epidemiologic principles with him. You begin with a discussion of a 2×2 table relating patients with and without disease to positive and negative test results. (Numbers represent number of patients)

Table 1 is an example of a 2 × 2 table.

TABLE 1 Disease X

	Present	Absent
Test Y Positive	30	50
Test Y Negative	10	80

SELECT THE ONE BEST ANSWER TO THE FOLLOWING QUESTIONS:

Questions 831–836 refer to the 2×2 table shown above:

831. The sensitivity of test Y for disease X is:
   a) 25%
   b) 37.5%
   c) 75%
   d) 62.5%
   e) 11%

832. The specificity of test Y for disease X is:
   a) 25%
   b) 37.5%
   c) 75%
   d) 61.5%
   e) 11%

833. The positive predictive value of test Y in the diagnosis of disease X is:
   a) 37.5%
   b) 25%
   c) 75%
   d) 61.5%
   e) 11%

834. The negative predictive value of test Y in the diagnosis of disease X is:
   a) 37.5%
   b) 89%
   c) 25%
   d) 75%
   e) 61.5%

835. The likelihood ratio for test Y in disease X is:
   a) 0.39
   b) 1.95
   c) 3.80
   d) 0.79
   e) 1.51

836. The prevalence of disease X in this population is:
   a) 15.5%
   b) 23.5%
   c) 40.0%
   d) 10.5%
   e) 18.4%

Consider the following data that illustrates the prevalence of disease A in various populations.

Based on this information about disease prevalence, and assuming that the sensitivity of test B for disease A is 80%, and the specificity of test B for disease A is 90%, answer questions 837–839.

837. The positive predictive value of test A in the diagnosis of disease B in the general population is:
   a) 0.4%
   b) 1.3%

Table 2   Prevalence of disease A in certain populations

Setting	Prevalence Cases/100,000
General population	50
Women, age 50 or older	500
Women, age 65 and older with a suspicious finding on clinical examination	40,000

   c)   5.4%
   d)   15.7%
   e)   39.6%

838. The positive predictive value of test B for disease A in women age 50 and older is:
   a)   0.4%
   b)   3.9%
   c)   10.7%
   d)   23.6%
   e)   52.7%

839. The positive predictive value of test B in the diagnosis of disease A in women greater than 65 years with a suspicious finding of clinical examination is:
   a)   0.4%
   b)   5.6%
   c)   34.7%
   d)   84.2%
   e)   93.0%

840. If the positive predictive value of a test for a given disorder in a given population is 4%, how many true positives are there in a sample of 100 positive test results?
   a)   4
   b)   10
   c)   40
   d)   96
   e)   none of the above

841. The design of clinical studies greatly influences how much trust you can put in the results. Which of the following lists the study designs in order of strength (from strongest to weakest)?
   a)   cohort study, case-control study, randomized-controlled trial, case study
   b)   case-control study, cohort study, randomized-controlled trial, case study
   c)   randomized-controlled trial, case-control study, cohort study, case study
   d)   randomized-controlled trial, cohort study, case-control study, case study
   e)   randomized-controlled trial, case-control study, case study, cohort study

ANSWER THE FOLLOWING QUESTION ACCORDING TO THE CODE:

A: 1, 2, and 3 are correct
B: 1 and 3 are correct
C: 2 and 4 are correct
D: Only 4 is correct
E: All of the above are correct

842. A prominent physician writes an article in a world famous medical journal describing the etiology of hypertension in patients over the age of 50 years. In his research, the incidence of renovascular hypertension is 15%. He advises all physicians to investigate all patients over the age of 50 years for renovascular hypertension before prescribing therapy.

   Which of the following statements regarding this physician's claim is/are true?
1) we should follow his advice and begin more intensive investigation of all patients over the age of 50 years
2) we are probably missing a significant number of patients with renovascular hypertension in our practices
3) this physician's practice is likely to be quite similar to our own
4) this is probably an example of referral filter bias

ANSWERS

831. C

832. D

833. A

834. B

835. B

836. B

The following 2×2 Table will illustrate the answers to questions 831–836.

Table 3 Disease X

	Present	*Absent*
Test Y Positive	30(a)	50(b)
Test Y Negative	10(c)	80(d)

Sensitivity is defined as the proportion of people with the disease that have a positive test result.[1] A sensitive test will rarely miss patients with the disease. In the 2×2 table above, sensitivity is defined as the number of true positives/ the number of true positives + the number of false negatives.

$$\text{SENSITIVITY} = \frac{a}{a+c} = \frac{30}{40} = 75\%$$

Specificity is defined as the proportion of people without the disease who have a negative test result.[2] A specific test will rarely misclassify people without the disease as diseased. In the 2×2 table above, specificity is defined as the number of true negatives / the number of true negatives + the number of false positives

$$\text{SPECIFICITY} = \frac{d}{b+d} = \frac{80}{130} = 61.5\%$$

A sensitive test (i.e, one that is usually positive in the presence of disease) should be chosen when there is an important penalty for missing a disease.[1] Specific tests are useful to confirm (or "rule in") a diagnosis that has been suggested by other data. A highly specific test is rarely positive in the absence of disease. Highly specific tests are particularly needed when false positive results can harm the patient physically, emotionally, or financially.[1]

There is always a trade off between sensitivity and specificity. Generally, if a disease has a low prevalence choose a more specific test; if a disease has a high prevalence choose a more sensitive test.

Positive predictive value is defined as the probability of disease in a patient with a positive (abnormal) test result.[1] In the 2×2 table shown above:

$$\text{POSITIVE PREDICTIVE VALUE} = \frac{a}{a+b} = \frac{30}{80} = 37.5\%$$

Negative predictive value is defined as the probability of not having the disease when the rest result is negative (normal).[1] In the 2×2 table shown above:

$$\text{NEGATIVE PREDICTIVE VALUE} = \frac{d}{c+d} = \frac{80}{90} = 89\%$$

The likelihood ratio of a positive test result is probability of that test result in the presence of disease divided by the probability of the result in the absence of disease.[1] In the 2×2 table shown above:

$$\text{LIKELIHOOD RATIO (+)} = \frac{\frac{a}{a+c}}{\frac{b}{b+d}} = 1.95$$

The prevalence of a condition is the fraction (proportion) of a group possessing a clinical condition at a given point in time.[1] Prevalence is measured by surveying a defined population containing people with and without the condition of interest, at a given point in time.[1] Prevalence can be equated to "pretest probability of disease." In the 2×2 table shown above, prevalence is defined as:

$$\text{PREVALENCE} = \frac{a+c}{a+b+c+d} = 23.5\%$$

As prevalence falls, positive predictive value must fall along with it, and negative predictive value must rise.

837. A.

838. B.

839. D.

The respective positive predictive values for test B in the diagnosis of disease A in the general population, women greater than 50, and women older than 65 with a suspicious finding on clinical examination are 0.4%, 3.9%, and 84.2% respectively.

To perform these calculations the following steps are recommended:[2]

1. Identify the sensitivity and specificity of the sign symptom, or diagnostic test that you plan to use. Many are already published. If you are not sure, consider asking a consultant with special expertise in the area.

2. Using a 2×2 table, set your total = an even number (consider 1000 as a reasonable number) Therefore, a + b + c + d = 1000

3. Now, using whatever information you have about the patient before you apply this diagnostic test, estimate his or her pretest probability (prevalence) of the target disorder. Next, put appropriate numbers at the bottom of the columns (a + c) and (b + d). The easiest way to do this is to express your pretest probability (or prevalence) as a decimal three places to the right. This result is (a + c), and 1000 minus this result is (b + d).

4. Now you can start to fill in the cells of the 2×2 table. Multiply sensitivity (expressed as a decimal) by (a + c) and put the result in cell a. You can then calculate cell c by simple subtraction.

5. Similarly, multiply specificity (expressed as a decimal) by (b + d) and put the result in cell d. Calculate cell b by subtraction.

6. You can now calculate positive and negative predictive values for the test with the prevalence (pretest probability) used.

Table 4 Calculations involved in a general 2 × 2 Table

| | Target Disorder | |
	Present	Absent
Test Positive	CELL A Sensitivity $\times (a+c)$	CELL B $(b+d)-d$
Test Negative	CELL C $(a+c)-a$	CELL D Specificity $\times (b+d)$

Total = a + b + c + d

For example, to calculate the positive predictive value for test B in the diagnosis of disease in women greater than 65 years with a suspicious finding on clinical examination:

Prevalence = 40,000 cases/100,000 = 400/1000
Setting the total number equal to 1000:
a + c / a + b + c + d = 400/1000
Therefore, a + c = 400 and b + d = 600
Therefore, CELL A = SENSITIVITY × 400
= 0.8 x 400 = 320
Therefore, CELL C = 400-320 = 80
Similarly, CELL D = SPECIFICITY × 600

= 0.9 × 600 = 540
Therefore, CELL B = 600-540 = 60
POSITIVE PREDICTIVE VALUE = a/ a + b
= 320 / 320 + 60 = 84.2%

Similar calculations can be made for the general population (prevalence 50/ 100,000) and for women greater than 50 years (prevalence 500/100,000).

840. A. If the positive predictive value of a test for a given disorder in a given population is 4%, then only 4 of 100 positive test results will be true positives; the remainder will be false positives. Further testing (often invasive) and anxiety will be inflicted on the 96% of the population with a positive test result but without disease.

Thus, careful consideration should be given to the positive predictive value of any test for any disease in a given population before ordering the test.

841. D. Evidence from a randomized-controlled trial is the soundest evidence we can ever obtain about causation. Patients are randomly assigned to one treatment group or the other. The design is even stronger if both patient and investigator are blind to the experiment (double blind).[1,2]

The next most powerful study method (the cohort study) involves the assembly of a group of people, none of whom has experienced the outcome of interest. On entry into the study, people in the cohort are classified according to those characteristics that might be related to outcome. These people are then observed over time to see which of them experience the outcome of interest.[1,2]

The third type of evidence that we can obtain is from a case-control study. In a case-control study, the investigator gathers "cases" of patients who already have suffered some adverse event and "controls" who have not. Both the "cases" and the "controls" are questioned, or alternatively their records are examined to determine whether they received the intervention of interest.[1,2]

A case study is the description of a case with no formal study of the possible link between the factor of interest and the outcome. Case studies often lead to more formal research.[1,2]

842. D. Referral filter bias refers to the fact that patients who are referred to and treated at tertiary care centers form a much different population from patients who are seen in primary care settings. The physician who published this article obviously has

a much greater incidence of secondary hypertension in his practice because of its referral nature.[2]

SUMMARY OF BASIC PRINCIPLES OF CLINICAL EPIDEMIOLOGY

1. **Sensitivity:** the proportion of people with a disease that have a positive test (the true positive rate)

2. **Specificity:** the proportion of people without a disease that have a negative test (the true negative rate)

3. **Positive predictive value:** the probability of disease in a patient with a positive test result

4. **Negative predictive value:** the probability of not having the disease in a patient with a negative test result

5. **Likelihood ratio of a positive test result:** is the probability of that test result in the presence of

disease divided by the probability of the result in the absence of disease.

6. **Prevalence:** is the fraction (proportion) of a group possessing a clinical condition at a given point in time

7. **Quality of evidence:**
   Type 1: Randomized-controlled trial
   Type 2: Cohort study
   Type 3: Case-control study
   Type 4: Case study

References

1. Fletcher R, Fletcher S, Wagner E. Clinical epidemiology: the essentials. 2nd Ed. Baltimore, MD: Williams & Wilkins, 1988.

2. Sackett D, Haynes R, Tugwell P. Clinical epidemiology: a basic science for clinical medicine. Boston: Little, Brown, 1985.

PROBLEM 108: A 24-YEAR-OLD MALE WITH GENERALIZED LYMPHADENOPATHY, FEVER, AND A COUGH

A 24-year-old male presents to your office with a 2-month history of a dry, nonproductive cough that has been associated with significant shortness of breath. He has felt tired and has had an intermittent fever for the past 6 weeks.

On examination he looks pale. He has significant cervical, axillary, and inguinal lymphadenopathy. No other abnormalities are found.

He states that he is bisexual. He has a wife and one child but also has two other male partners.

His chest x-ray shows a significant bilateral infiltrate. His HIV serology is positive.

SELECT THE ONE BEST ANSWER TO THE FOLLOWING QUESTIONS:

843. The most likely diagnosis in this patient is:
    a) AIDS- related complex
    b) AIDS
    c) HIV- positive status with underlying pneumonia
    d) generalized lymphadenopathy syndrome
    e) none of the above

844. The most likely cause of this patient's cough is:
    a) viral pneumonia
    b) *Streptococcal pneumonia*
    c) *Klebsiella* pneumonia
    d) *Mycoplasma* pneumonia
    e) none of the above

845. The treatment of choice for this patient's respiratory tract infection is:
    a) tetracycline
    b) ampicillin
    c) trimethoprim-sulfamethoxazole
    d) cephalexin
    e) none of the above

846. The most common malignancy associated with the condition described above is:
    a) Kaposi's sarcoma
    b) non-Hodgkin's lymphoma
    c) primary lymphoma of the brain
    d) acute lymphoblastic leukemia
    e) Hodgkin's disease

ANSWER THE FOLLOWING QUESTIONS ACCORDING TO THE CODE:

A: 1, 2, and 3 are correct
B: 1 and 3 are correct
C: 2 and 4 are correct
D: Only 4 is correct
E: All of the above are correct

847. Which of the following statements regarding testing for the condition discussed above is/are true?
   1) more than 90% of individuals with the disease harbor antibodies to the virus
   2) more than 95% of asymptomatic carriers of the virus are antibody positive
   3) the antibody test for this disorder usually becomes positive 1 to 3 months after infection with the agent
   4) culture for the agent concerned is highly sensitive

848. Which of the following is/are risk factors for the condition discussed above?
   1) homosexual orientation
   2) bisexual orientation
   3) intravenous drug abuse
   4) school or work contact with an infected person

849. Which of the following statements regarding the treatment of the condition described above is/are true?
   1) trimethoprim-sulfamethoxazole may be a useful prophylactic agent
   2) most immunizations are contraindicated in patients with this condition
   3) azidothymidine is the first drug available that specifically treats the infection
   4) few complications have been noted with azidothymidine treatment

ANSWERS

843. B. This patient most likely has acquired immunodeficiency syndrome. Acquired immunodeficiency syndrome (AIDS) refers to the occurrence of a life-threatening opportunistic infection or Kaposi's sarcoma, or both, in patients who have not received immunosuppressive drugs and who had no apparent immunosuppressing disease.[1]

The syndrome is caused by human immunodeficiency virus (HIV). The subclassification of HIV disease is reviewed elsewhere.[2]

844. E. The most likely cause of this patient's cough and chest x-ray findings is *P. carinii* pneumonia. *P. carinii* pneumonia is the initial clinical disorder in approximately 50% of cases of AIDS.[1] Pneumocystis pneumonia usually presents in AIDS patients as a nonproductive cough and/or dyspnea. Interstitial pneumonitis is seen on chest x-ray.

845. C. The treatment of choice in this patient is IV trimethoprim-sulfamethoxazole.[3]

846. A. The most common malignancy associated with AIDS is Kaposi's sarcoma. Approximately 30% of AIDS patients present with Kaposi's sarcoma.[1] Kaposi's sarcoma in AIDS patients frequently involves multiple organs and lymph nodes.[1] Other common malignancies associated with AIDS are non-Hodgkin's lymphoma (small, noncleaved lymphoma or immunoblastic sarcoma) and primary lymphoma of the brain.

847. A. The major diagnostic advance recently has been the development of tests for measuring antibody to HIV. More than 90% of individuals with AIDS harbor antibodies to the virus, and more than 95% of asymptomatic carriers of the virus are antibody positive.[1] For practical purposes, anyone who is antibody positive should be assumed to have transmissable virus in his or her blood and body secretions. A positive ELISA test (enzyme-linked immunosorbent assay) should be confirmed with a Western blot test. In contrast to the diagnostic utility of antibody testing, cultures of HIV have a high false negative rate (30–70%).

Typically, ELISA antibody tests become positive 1 to 3 months after infection with HIV.[1]

848. A. Four population groups account for the majority of AIDS cases in the United States. The four risk groups are homosexual or bisexual men, intravenous drug users, recipients of blood transfusions before 1983, and hemophiliacs.[1] The number of heterosexuals who have been exposed to bisexual men and who are developing AIDS is increasing.

The transmission of HIV by routes other than intimate contact, transfusion of blood products, or communal intravenous drug abuse is virtually unknown. Thus, household, school, or work contacts of patients with HIV infection who are not the children or sexual partners of such patients are at minimal or no risk of infection.[1]

849. B. Therapy for patients with AIDS can be divided into two categories: treatment aimed at the HIV infection itself and treatment aimed at the secondary infections and malignant disorders associated with HIV infection.[1]

Azidothymidine (zidovudine) is the only drug proven effective for treatment of HIV infection.[1] Serious side effects including anemia and granulocytopenia may, however, require discontinuation of the drug.

Trimethoprim-sulfamethoxazole has been shown to be a useful prophylactic agent in the prevention of *P. carinii* pneumonia.

Immunizations are not contraindicated in patients with AIDS.

SUMMARY OF THE DIAGNOSIS AND MANAGEMENT OF ACQUIRED IMMUNODEFICIENCY SYNDROME

1. **Definition of AIDS**: the occurrence of a life-threatening opportunistic infection of Kaposi's sarcoma, or both, in patients who have not received immunosuppressive drugs and who have no apparent immunosuppressing disease.

2. **Diagnosis**: ELISA antibody testing; confirmation by Western blot

3. **High risk groups**:
   a) homosexual or bisexual males
   b) intravenous group abusers
   c) recipients of blood transfusions before 1983
   d) hemophiliacs.

4. **Usual presentation**: Pneumocystis carinii pneumonia (50%), Kaposi's sarcoma (30%), both (7%)

5. **Treatment and prophylaxis**: Consider prophylaxis with trimethoprim-sulfamethoxazole against *P. carinii* pneumonia; the same drug effective in treatment. Azidothymidine is first drug that directly treats HIV infection.

References

1. Rubin R. Acquired immunodeficiency syndrome. In: Federman D, Rubenstein E, eds. Scientific American medicine. New York: Scientific American, 1988, 7(XI): 1–19.

2. Centers for Disease Control. Classification system for human T-lymphotropic virus type III/lymphadenopathy-associated virus infections. MMWR 1986; 35: 334.

3. Dunagan W, Powderly W. Sexual transmitted diseases. In: Dunagan W, Ridner M, eds. Manual of medical therapeutics, 26th Ed. Boston: Little, Brown, 1989; 275.

4. The Medical Letter on Drugs and Therapeutics. Drugs for HIV infection. Med Let 1990; 31(811): 11–13.

PROBLEM 109: A 51-YEAR-OLD MALE WHO IS PLANNING ON TRAVELING TO AFRICA

A 51-year-old male presents to you office for a periodic health assessment. He is planning on traveling to equatorial Africa in the near future and wishes to discuss immunizations and prophylaxis against malaria. You offer him advice on all the necessary immunizations and prophylaxis against malaria.

ANSWER THE FOLLOWING QUESTIONS ACCORDING TO THE CODE:

A: 1, 2, and 3 are correct
B: 1 and 3 are correct
C: 2 and 4 are correct
D: Only 4 is correct
E: All of the above are correct

850. Which of the following immunizations is/are recommended for this patient before beginning his travel to Africa?
   1) hepatitis B
   2) poliomyelitis
   3) smallpox
   4) yellow fever

851. Which of the following statements regarding prophylaxis against malaria for this patient is/are true?

1) prophylaxis with chloroquine should begin when travel begins and continue until the week of return to North America
2) prophylaxis with chloroquine may be insufficient to prevent malaria
3) chloroquine is usually given three times/week for 2 weeks before travel, during the time away, and for 2 weeks after return from travel
4) chloroquine resistant *P. falciparum* malaria is best prevented with Fansidar (sulfasoxine-pyrimethamine) or doxycycline

852. An operating room nurse presents to your office to discuss immunization against hepatitis B. She was planning on receiving the vaccine but has been told by a co-worker that there is a small possibility of the transmission of the AIDS virus through hepatitis B vaccine.

Which of the following statements regarding vaccination against hepatitis B in this patient is/are true?
1) the AIDS virus is not transmitted through hepatitis B vaccine
2) three doses of the vaccine should be administered to ensure seroconversion
3) this nurse is at risk of acquiring hepatitis B through her occupation and should be immunized
4) inactivated hepatitis B virus vaccine is the only vaccine available for immunization against hepatitis B

853. Pneumococcal vaccine is an effective agent for prophylaxis against pneumococcal pneumonia. Which of the following is/are indications for the administration of pneumococcal vaccine?
1) chronic cardiorespiratory disease
2) chronic renal disease
3) chronic alcoholism
4) Hodgkin's disease

854. A 27-year-old female presents to your office requesting a prescription for the prevention of "travelers' diarrhea." She is leaving for a holiday in Mexico in 3 days time.

Which of the following statements regarding travelers' diarrhea is/are true?
1) the most commonly identified etiologic agent is enterotoxigenic *E. coli*
2) the patient should be instructed to avoid eating fresh fruit and vegetables, and from drinking water that has not been boiled

3) trimethoprim-sulfamethoxazole can be used either prophylactically or as treatment for the acute condition
4) parasites and bacteria other than *E. coli* seldom cause travelers' diarrhea

SELECT THE ONE BEST ANSWER TO THE FOLLOWING QUESTIONS:

855. A 43-year-old farmer presents to your local emergency department after having punctured his foot on a rusty pitchfork while cleaning out a pig barn. You consider tetanus immunization. The patient states that he is unsure of when and if he was immunized.

Which of the following regimens for protection against tetanus should be administered to this patient?
a) a single dose of tetanus toxoid
b) two doses of tetanus toxoid
c) three doses of tetanus toxoid
d) three doses of tetanus toxoid and a single dose of tetanus immunoglobulin
e) three doses of tetanus toxoid and three doses of tetanus immunoglobulin

856. Diptheria and tetanus boosters should be a routine part of preventive health care in adults. How often should these boosters be administered?
a) every year
b) every 2 years
c) every 3 years
d) every 5 years
e) every 10 years

ANSWERS

850. C. Individuals traveling to South America, Africa, and some areas of Asia should receive immunization against yellow fever and polio before their departure. In addition, they should receive prophylaxis against hepatitis A, possible immunization against meningococcal disease, and a tetanus-diphtheria booster. Hepatitis B vaccination is only necessary in high-risk situations. Immunization against typhus and smallpox is no longer recommended. Routine immunization against cholera is also not recommended.[1,3]

851. C. Chloroquine is the drug of choice for malaria prophylaxis. Chloroquine phosphate 500 mg (300 mg of chloroquine base) should be taken once

weekly beginning 1 to 2 weeks prior to travel and continuing during the stay and for six weeks after departure from malarial areas.

There is a high risk of acquiring chloroquine-resistant *P. falciparum* (CRPF) in the areas of East Africa that tourists often visit. In these areas, in addition to chloroquine, Fansidar (sulfasoxine-pyrimethamine) should be considered for prophylaxis.[2]

852. A. Inactivated hepatitis B vaccine is extremely effective. Approximately 90 % of immunocompetent vaccine recepents develop protective antibody titers that persist for at least 3 years. Three doses are required, and full protection lasts for at least 3 years.

Inactivated hepatitis B vaccine is also extremely safe. The inactivation process by which the vaccine is prepared will kill all known infectious agents, including AIDS.

A new vaccine, produced by DNA recombinant technology is now available. In comparative trials, the recombinant DNA and the inactivated hepatitis B vaccines have proven equally effective. As the recombinant DNA vaccine becomes more widely available and clinical experience increases, it will replace the older, inactivated vaccine.

Inactivated and recombinant DNA hepatitis B vaccines are very cost-effective in high-risk groups. Groups at high risk for hepatitis B include homosexual men, uses of illicit injectable drugs, prison inmates, residents of institutions for the mentally retarded, and sexual and household contacts of hepatitis B carriers, and hemodialysis patients.[2] Hepatitis B vaccine is also indicated in health care workers that are in frequent contact with blood, blood products and body fluids.

Postexposure prophylaxis to prevent hepatitis B (hepatitis B immunoglobulin) should be considered in three circumstances; perinatal exposure of an infant born to a carrier, accidental percutaneous or permucosal exposure to blood positive for HBsAg, or sexual exposure to a hepatitis B carrier.[2]

853. E. A single dose of pneumococcal vaccine is recommended in the following patients: those with asplenia, splenic dysfunction, sickle cell disease, hepatic cirrhosis, chronic cardiorespiratory disease, chronic alcoholism, chronic renal disease, Hodgkin's disease, and conditions associated with immunosuppression.[3] Since mortality from bacteremic pneumococcal disease increase with age,

elderly patients with or without chronic illnesses should be considered for immunization.[3]

854. A. The most commonly identified etiologic agent is enterotoxigenic *Escherichia coli*. Other common agents include *Giardia lamblia, Entamoeba histolytica, Salmonella* and *Shigella*.

Several agents, including doxycycline, bismuth subsalicylcate (Pepto-Bismol), trimethoprim, trimethoprim-sulfamethoxazole, and ciprofloxacin have been used as preventive and therapeutic agents for travelers' diarrhea.[1]

Patients should be instructed to avoid eating fresh fruit and vegetables, and from drinking water that has not been boiled.[1]

855. D. Because this wound is classifed as a "dirty wound," the patient should receive both tetanus toxoid and a single dose of tetanus immunoglobulin. Because his primary immunization is unsure three doses of tetanus toxoid should be administered. Two doses can be administered 1 month apart and a third dose 6–12 months later. Tetanus immunoglobulin should be administered intramuscularly (250 units).[3]

856. E. Adults should be given a booster dose of Td (tetanus-diphtheria) every 10 years unless there are contraindications to the administration of tetanus toxoid.[3]

SUMMARY OF COMMON ADULT IMMUNIZATIONS, INCLUDING ADVICE FOR THE INTERNATIONAL TRAVELER

1. **International travel (immunizations):** Yellow fever, cholera, poliomyelitis, tetanus-diptheria, meningococcal vaccine, hepatitis A prophylaxis, and typhoid vaccine should be considered depending on the destination of the travel

2. **Malaria prophylaxis:** Chloroquine 500 mg/week for 1–2 weeks before travel, during travel, and for 6 weeks after. Fansidar or doxycycline should be carried in areas of CRPF and taken if symptoms develop

3. **Diphtheria/tetanus booster:** Recommended every 10 years

4. Consider tetanus immunoglobulin in dirty wound if immunization history unknown.

5. Consider hepatitis B immunization for high-risk individuals.

6. Consider pneumococcal immunization for high-risk individuals.

7. **Travelers disease:** Most commonly caused by enterotoxigenic *E.coli*. Prophylaxis with trimethoprim-sulfamethoxale, doxycycline or Pepto-Bismol. Treatment with trimethoprim, trimethoprim-sulfamethoxazole, ciprofloxacin; or symptomatic treatment with oral fluids, loperamide, or Pepto-Bismol

References

1. Weller P. Health advice for international travelers. In: Federman D, Rubenstein E, eds. Scientific American medicine. New York: Scientific American Medicine, 1988, IV: 1–7.

2. Simon H. Immunizations and chemotherapy for viral infections. In: Federman D, Rubenstein E, eds. Scientific American medicine. New York: Scientific American Medicine, 1988, 7(XXIII): 1–19.

3. Canadian immunization guide. 3rd Ed. Health and Welfare Canada, Government of Canada, 1989.

PROBLEM 110: A 30-YEAR-OLD MALE WHO PRESENTS TO YOUR OFFICE REQUESTING A "COMPLETE LABORATORY WORK-UP"

A 30-year-old male patient presents to your office requesting a"complete laboratory work-up." He has been told that there are "blood tests for everything these days" and requests the "once over."

His history and physical examination are unremarkable. He has had no previous significant illness and appears to be in excellent health.

SELECT THE ONE BEST ANSWER TO THE FOLLOWING QUESTIONS:

857. On the basis of the patient's request and your history and physical examination you would now:
    a) order a complete battery of investigations in order to get rid of the patient
    b) order selected investigations
    c) suggest that the patient see another physician
    d) discuss the advantages and disadvantages of screening for various conditions with the patient
    e) none of the above

858. The measure of the ability of a test to discriminate betwen normal and diseased states is known as:
    a) the sensitivity of the test
    b) the specificity of the test
    c) the likelihood ratio of the test
    d) the positive predictive value of the test
    e) the negative predictive value of the test

ANSWER THE FOLLOWING QUESTIONS ACCORDING TO THE CODE:

A: 1, 2, and 3 are correct
B: 1 and 3 are correct
C: 2 and 4 are correct
D: Only 4 is correct
E: All of the above are correct

859. Which of the following is/are reasons for ordering a laboratory or radiologic investigation?
    1) screening (case finding)
    2) confirmation of clinical findings
    3) disease treatment and follow-up
    4) patient and doctor reassurance

860. Which of the following is/are important questions to consider before deciding on whether or not to implement a screening program for a specific disease?
    1) does the current burden of suffering warrant screening?
    2) has the program's effectiveness been demonstrated in a clinical trial
    3) can the health care system cope with the screening program?
    4) will people who screen positive accept advice and intervention for the condition?

861. Which of the following screening tests is/are recommended for inclusion in routine preventive health care?

1) counseling and education of patients about tobacco use
2) Pap smear
3) mammogram after age 50 years
4) sigmoidoscopy after age 40 years

ANSWERS

857. D. Laboratory testing is increasing at an alarming rate. While an individual test is not expensive, when taken together laboratory tests are responsible for an ever increasing percentage of the health care budget.[1]

There is no evidence that physicians' increased use of laboratory tests has improved the care of their patients.[1] In one study, only 5% of laboratory data was actually used in patient diagnosis and treatment.[2]

We must begin to educate ourselves and our patients regarding the appropriateness and often inappropriateness of laboratory testing. Furthermore, we must critically evaluate the reason for performing each test on epidemiologic grounds.

858. C. The likelihood ratio (LR) is a measure of the ability of a test to discriminate between normal and diseased states. The LR is the likelihood of finding a positive test result in a person with, rather than without, disease. The higher the LR, the more likely that the disease is present if the test is positive.[1]

859. E. Screening (case finding), confirmation of clinical findings, disease treatment and follow-up, and patient and doctor reassurance are all valid reasons for ordering a laboratory or radiologic investigation.[1]

860. E. In deciding whether a screening program does more harm than good questions you should ask should include: (1) Has the program's effectiveness been demonstrated in a clinical trial? (2) Are there effective treatments or preventive measures for the disorder? (3) Does the current burden of suffering warrant screening? (4) Is there a good screening test available? (5) Can the health care system cope with the screening program? and (6) Will people who screen positive accept advice and intervention for the condition?[3]

If a screening test is to be performed, the following criteria should be met: (1) the condition should have a significant effect on the quality or quantity of life, (2) treatment must be available for the condition, (3) the condition should have an asymptomatic period during which detection and treatment significantly reduce morbidity or mortality, (4) treatment in the asymptomatic period should result in an outcome that is superior to delaying treatment until symptoms appear, (5) tests to detect the condition in the asymptomatic period must be readily available, accepted by patients, and not excessively costly, and (6) there must be a high enough incidence of the condition to justify screening.[3]

861. A. Counseling and education of patients regarding tobacco use, regular Pap smears, and mammograms every 1–2 years after age 50 are recommended by the US Preventive Services Task Force. Sigmoidoscopy and fecal occult blood screening are not recommended.[4]

SUMMARY OF AN APPROACH TO DIAGNOSTIC TESTING AND SCREENING

1. Realize that the ordering of a "battery of diagnostic tests" on a "routine" basis is not cost-effective.

2. Carefully consider guidelines and criteria for screening tests before ordering them.

3. Try and establish prevalence, sensitivity, specificity, likelihood ratio and positive predictive value of a test before ordering it.

4. Consider screening recommendations of The US Preventive Services Task Force[4] before screening a patient for a given condition.

References

1. Birtwhistle RV. Diagnostic testing in family practice. Can Fam Physician 1988; 34: 327–331.

2. Dixon RH, Laszlo J. Utilization of clinical chemical services by medical housestaff: an analysis. Arch Intern Med 1974; 134: 1064–1067.

3. Sackett D, Haynes R, Tugwell P. Clinical epidemiology: a basic science for clinical medicine. 1st Ed. Boston: Little, Brown, 1985.

4. Guide to Clinical Preventive Services. An assessment of the effectiveness of 169 interventions. US Preventive Services Task Force. Baltimore: Williams & Wilkins, 1989.

PROBLEM 111: A 65-YEAR-OLD MALE WITH INFLUENZA

A 65-year-old male presents to your office with a 4-day history of fever, muscle aches, headache, and cough. You suspect an influenza infection.

SELECT THE ONE BEST ANSWER TO THE FOLLOWING QUESTIONS.

862. Which of the following symptoms of influenza is usually the last symptom to appear?
    a) cough
    b) headache
    c) myalgia
    d) fever
    e) malaise

863. The major cause of death from influenza is:
    a) viral meningitis
    b) staphylococcal pneumonia
    c) pneumococcal pneumonia
    d) acute viral encephalopathy
    e) dehydration

864. The primary mode of transmission of influenza is:
    a) oral-fecal contamination
    b) direct skin contact
    c) sneezing
    d) coughing
    e) c and d

ANSWER THE FOLLOWING QUESTIONS ACCORDING TO THE CODE:

A: 1, 2, and 3 are correct
B: 1 and 3 are correct
C: 2 and 4 are correct
D: Only 4 is correct
E: All of the above are correct

865. Which of the following persons should receive high priority for immunization against influenza?
    1) adults with chronic cardiac or pulmonary disorders
    2) children with recurrent or continuing pulmonary disorders
    3) residents of nursing home or other chronic care facilities
    4) persons who provide community service

866. Which of the following statements regarding amantadine therapy in the prevention of influenza is/are correct?

1) amantadine can be used in the influenza season as an adjunct to immunization
2) amantadine can be used as a supplement to preseason vaccination in immunodeficient persons
3) amantadine is usually given in a single daily dose of 200 mg
4) amantadine can reduce the spread of influenza in nursing homes or chronic care facilities once an outbreak has begun

ANSWERS

862. A. The most common initial symptom is severe generalized or frontal headache, often accompanied by retroorbital pain. Other early symptoms include diffuse myalgias, fever, and chills. Respiratory symptoms, particularly cough, appear later in the course of the illness.[1]

   The term "flu" is used loosely by both physicians and patients. True influenza has a very specific set of symptoms that can usually be used to differientiate it clinically from other viral infections in adults.

   In children, the signs and symptoms of influenza are more subtle; it may simply appear as another upper respiratory tract infection.[1]

863. C. The most common cause of death from influenza is secondary pneumococcal pneumonia. This illustrates the importance of administering pneumococcal vaccine to patients with chronic disease, immunocompromised patients and the elderly.[1] Other causes of death include staphylococcal pneumonia and a direct effect of the virus itself. Viral meningitis and acute viral encephalopathy are uncommon complications of influenza. Dehydration can be a contributing factor in death from any infection.

864. E. The influenza virus is transmitted through respiratory secretions and thus is easily spread to susceptible persons. Sneezing, coughing and close contact while talking are thought to be the main modes of transference.[1]

865. A. Influenza vaccine is about 70% effective in preventing the disease. Patients who should

receive high priority for the administration of the vaccine include (1) adults with chronic cardiovascular or pulmonary disorders that have required regular medical follow-up or hospitalizations during the preceding year; (2) children with (a) continuing or recurrent pulmonary disorders such as asthma or bronchopulmonary dysplasia, or (b) hemodynamically significant heart disease; and (3) residents of nursing homes and other chronic care facilities.[1]

866. E. Amantadine is the only drug approved in the United States for specific prophylaxis and treatment of influenza A virus.

Amantadine can be used during the influenza season as an adjunct to late vaccination, as a supplement to preseason vaccination in immunodeficient persons, and as chemoprophylaxis in the absence of vaccination. Amantadine can also be used to reduce the spread of virus and minimize disruption of patient care both in the home and in the institutional setting. It can be prescribed as prophylaxis for healthy unvaccinated persons who simply want to avoid illness during an outbreak.[1]

Amantadine is 70–90% effective in preventing influenza A infections. It is also the treatment of choice once influenza A is contracted. When given 24–48 hours after the onset of infection, amantadine reduces both the severity and duration of symptoms.

The standard dose of amantadine is 200 mg daily. Elderly patients should probably receive 100 mg.

To minimize spread in hospitals, nursing homes, and other chronic-care institutions, amantadine should be administered to all residents, vaccinated or not, as soon as possible after an outbreak has begun, and should be continued until the outbreak is over.[1]

SUMMARY OF THE DIAGNOSIS AND TREATMENT OF INFLUENZA

1. **Diagnosis:** Headache, myalgia, and fever followed by the onset of respiratory symptoms

2. **Epidemic period:** October to December

3. **Prevention:**

Immunization: Protects against influenza A and B (only strains present in vaccine) should be given to priority patients.

Amantadine: Protects only against influenza A. Amantadine can be used to prevent disease in high-risk situations (nursing home and chronic care residents) and to ameliorate disease in those contacting it if given early enough

Reference

1. Douglas RG Jr. Influenza prevention and treatment. The primary care physician's role. Postgrad Med 1988; 83(5): 207–214.

PROBLEM 112: A 24-YEAR-OLD MALE WITH A URETHRAL DISCHARGE

A 24-year-old male presents to your office with a 4-day history of burning on urination. Two days ago he developed a purulent, creamy, profuse urethral discharge. He has no other symptoms. He has never had similar symptoms.

SELECT THE ONE BEST ANSWER TO THE FOLLOWING QUESTIONS:

867. The most likely diagnosis in this patient is:
    a) *C. trachomatis* urethritis
    b) *N. gonorrhoeae* urethritis
    c) nonspecific urethritis
    d) *E. coli* urethritis
    e) none of the above

868. On careful questioning, it becomes apparent that the patient described in queston 867 has had three heterosexual contacts in the past 2 weeks. Which of the following statements regarding these heterosexual contacts is FALSE?
    a) contact tracing should be initiated by the physician or the local public health department
    b) dysuria, frequency, and urgency are common symptoms in females
    c) few female patients with the infection are asymptomatic
    d) pelvic inflammatory disease is a major complication of the infection

e) the oral contraceptive pill is protective against the infection

869. A smear of the urethral discharge is taken from the patient described in question 867. A gram-stain is performed on that smear. What would most likely be seen on the gram-stain?
   a) nothing
   b) numerous WBCs, no bacteria
   c) numerous WBCs with intracellular gram-positive diplococci
   d) numerous WBCs with intracellular gram-negative diplococci
   e) numerous WBCs with intracellular gram-negative bacilli

870. The drug(s) of choice for the patient described in question 867 is(are):
   a) amoxicillin 3.0 g plus probenecid 1.0 g
   b) ceftriaxone 250 mg IM
   c) doxycycline 100 mg b.i.d.
   d) a plus c
   e) a or b plus c

871. Which of the following is(are) complications of the disorder discussed above?
   a) arthritis
   b) tenosynovitis
   c) bacteremia
   d) a and b
   e) a, b, and c

872. A 24-year-old male presents with a mucoid urethral discharge. This has been preceded by a 2-day history of urgency and frequency. He has had no other symptoms.

   The most likely diagnosis in this patient is:
   a) *C. trachomatis* urethritis
   b) *N. gonorrhoeae* urethritis
   c) nonspecific urethritis
   d) *E. coli* urethritis
   e) none of the above

873. The treatment of choice for the patient described in question 872 is:
   a) tetracycline or doxycycline
   b) amoxicillin
   c) ceftriaxone
   d) sulfamethoxazole
   e) clindamycin

874. A 24-year-old female presents with a 2-day history of dysuria, accompanied by painful genital lesions

that have coalesced to form ulcers. The patient also describes systemic symptoms including fever, malaise, myalgias, and headache. The patient has never had similar symptoms.

   Which one of the following statements regarding this patient is FALSE?
   a) this patient most likely has a herpes simplex Type II viral infection
   b) this patient is unlikely to experience a recurrence of these symptoms at a later date
   c) the duration of viral shedding can be reduced by acyclovir
   d) the time to heal the lesions can be reduced by acyclovir
   e) severe or frequent recurrences can be treated with acyclovir tablets prophylactically

875. A 25-year-old female presents with " growths" in the vulva region. On examination, you find multiple verrucous lesions in the area of the posterior introitus and on the labia majora and labia minora.

   Which of the following statements regarding this patient is FALSE?
   a) the most likely diagnosis is condyloma acuminatum
   b) these lesions are caused by human papilloma virus
   c) this patient is not at increased risk for cervical carcinoma in situ
   d) patients with this disease should be screened for other sexually transmitted diseases
   e) there is an association between this disease and laryngeal papillomas in the newborn

876. The treatment that has been reported to provide the highest cure rate in the patient described in question 875 is:
   a) podophyllin resin
   b) trichloroacetic acid
   c) surgical removal
   d) cryosurgery
   e) 5-fluorouracil cream

ANSWERS

867. B. This patient has gonorrhea. Gonorrhea is the most prevalent reportable communicable disease in North America, with an estimated 3 million cases annually. It is caused by *Neisseria gonorrhoeae*, and is transmitted solely by sexual intercourse.[1]

   Initial symptoms consist of burning on urination and a serous or milky discharge. This is usually followed by a change to a yellow, creamy discharge and significant urethral pain. Gonococcal urethritis may become chronic and spread to the prostate gland, the epididymis, and the periurethral glands. Urethral strictures are not uncommon.[1]

Gonococcal proctitis and pharyngitis are common in homosexual men.

The other major sexually transmitted urethritis in males is caused by *C. trachomatis*. It will be discussed in a subsequent section. *E. coli* is a major cause of urinary tract infection, but this infection usually resides in the bladder or kidney. Nonspecific urethritis is really a nondiagnosis.

868. C. Contact tracing is mandatory. This can be initiated by the physician and followed by the local public health department.

In females, gonococcal infection may present with dysuria, frequency, urgency, pelvic pain, and urethral or cervical discharge. Most often, however, the infection is asymptomatic, with only slightly increased vaginal discharge and moderate cervicitis. This may become a chronic cervicitis with the potential of spread to other contacts. Gonococcal cervicitis may progress to pelvic inflammatory disease with subsequent sterility.[1]

The oral contraceptive pill can prevent gonococcal pelvic inflammatory disease. It is estimated that 51,000 hospitalizations and 100 deaths are prevented annually in the United States because of the protect effect of the oral contraceptive pill.[2]

869. D. The most likely finding is numerous WBCs with intracellular gram-negative diplococci. The discharge should be cultured in both sexes, and from all potential sites of infection.[1]

870. E. The treatment of choice for gonorrhea is either amoxicillin/probenecid (3.0 g/1.0 g) or ceftriaxone 250 IM plus doxycycline 100 mg b.i.d. Ceftriaxone has emerged as a drug of choice in areas where penicillin-resistant gonorrhea has been isolated. Doxycycline is considered as a standard part of the treatment because of the high incidence of combined gonococcal/nongonococcal (mainly chlamydial) infections.[3]

871. E. Systemic complications of gonorrhea include bacteremia, arthritis, tenosynovitis, and perihepatitis.[1]

872. A. This patient most likely has *C. trachomatis* urethritis. It is the most common cause of non-

gonococcal urethritis (NGU). Symptoms in men include dysuria, frequency, and mucoid to purulent urethral discharge. Some men have asymptomatic infections. Female partners of men with chlamydial NGU are likely to have chlamydial mucopurulent cervicitis.

The second most common etiologic agent in NGU is *Ureaplasma urealyticum*.

Men with typical clinical symptoms are presumed to have NGU when their urethral (gram-stained) smear shows white blood cells with no gram-negative diplococci, and/or their rapid antigen-detection test is positive. As well, cultures for *N. gonorrhoeae* should confirm the absence of this organism.[1]

873. A. When the etiology is *C. trachomatis, U. urealyticum*, or unknown, the treatment of choice is tetracycline or doxycycline, given for 10 days.

874. B. This patient has a primary genital herpes infection.

The most common symptom is painful genital lesions. With primary infection, the multiple vesicles that are initially present coalesce to form intensively painful ulcers. Most lesions are found on the vulva and vaginal mucosa.[4] Other symptoms include fever, malaise, myalgias, and headache. Dysuria and vaginal discharge are also common.[4] Recurrences are common; the severity of the primary disease symptoms bears no relationship to the chance of acquiring recurrent disease.

The diagnosis of genital herpes should always be confirmed by culture.

The treatment of choice for primary herpes simplex genital virus infection is acyclovir. Acyclovir has been shown to shorten the duration of viral shedding and to shorten the time to healing.[4]

Patients with severe or frequent recurrences can be treated with acyclovir prophylactically. General supportive measures including povidone iodine will often provide relief. Bacterial superinfection can be treated with a topical antibiotic such as fusidic acid ointment or cream.

875. C. This patient has condyloma acuminatum. This is caused by human papilloma virus.

Condyloma lesions may appear on the introitus, the labia majora, the labia minora, the perianal area, and the urethra.[4]

Patients with condyloma are four times more likely to develop cervical carcinoma in situ. Therefore, these women should have frequent Pap smears (yearly). If any abnormalities are found, colposcopy should be performed.[4]

Patients with condyloma acuminatum should also be carefully screened for other sexually transmitted diseases.[4]

An association has also been demonstrated between condyloma acuminatum and laryngeal papillomas of the newborn.[4]

876. D. The treatment that has reported the highest rate of cure in condyloma acuminatum is cryosurgery. Cure rates with this form of therapy approach 90%.

Other treatment options include podophyllin resin, trichloroacetic acid, carbon dioxide laser removal, and 5-fluorouracil.[4]

SUMMARY OF THE DIAGNOSIS AND TREATMENT OF SELECTED SEXUALLY TRANSMITTED DISEASES

1. *N. gonorrhoeae:*

Diagnosis: Males—dysuria, frequency, purulent, creamy urethral discharge. Females—most often asymptomatic, although local symptoms and mucopurulent cervicitis do occur

Laboratory diagnosis: Urethral/cervical/rectal/pharyngeal swab to demonstrate gram-negative intraceullular diplococci. If no diplococci seen, culture

Treatment: ceftriaxone 250 mg IM or amoxicillin 3.0 g/probenecid 1.0 g orally or ampicillin 3.5 g/probenecid 1.0 g orally, plus, doxycycline 100 mg b.i.d. for 7 days or tetracycline 500 mg q.i.d. for 7 days

2. *Chlamydia trachomatis:*

Diagnosis: Males—dysuria, frequency, thin or mucoid urethral discharge. Females—most often asymptomatic, although local symptoms and mucopurulent cervicitis do occur

Laboratory diagnosis: rapid antigen tests (e.g., Chlamydiazyme: highly sensitive)

Screening: Consider screening women for chlamydia if they have two of the following risk factors:

1) age <25 years old
2) nonbarrier method of contraception
3) multiple sexual partners
4) new partner within last 2 months
   Treatment: tetracycline 500 mg q.i.d. × 7 days, or doxycycline 100 mg b.i.d. × 7 days

3. **Herpes simplex virus type II:**

Diagnosis: Painful genital ulcers plus systemic symptoms

Laboratory diagnosis: Culture necessary to confirm

Treatment: Acyclovir 200 mg five times/day orally or acyclovir ointment q.i.d. will reduce viral shedding and decrease healing time in primary infection. Severe or frequent recurrences: acyclovir 200 mg t.i.d.

4. **Condyloma acuminatum:**

Diagnosis: typically warty lesions. Cervical lesions visible only on colposcopy. Caused by human papilloma virus and associated with in situ carcinoma of the cervix

Treatment: Cryosurgery is probably the treatment of choice for dysplasias caused by condyloma acuminatum.

References

1. Grossman M, Jawetz E. Gonorrhea/chlamydial infections. In: Krupp M, Schroeder S, Tierney L, McPhee S, eds. Current medical diagnosis and treatment 1989. Norwalk, CT: Appleton & Lange, 1989; 920–925.

2. Ory HW. The noncontraceptive health benefits from oral contraceptive use. Fam Plann Perspect 1982; 14: 182–184.

3. 1988 Canadian guidelines for the treatment of sexually transmitted diseases in neonates, children, adolescents, and adults. Canada Diseases Weekly Report. Vol. 14S2, April 1988. Health and Welfare Canada.

4. Nesse R. Office management of sexually transmitted disease and management of pelvic inflammatory disease in the ambulatory patient. Prim Care 1988; 15(3): 489–507.

Emergency Medicine

PROBLEM 113: A 55-YEAR-OLD MALE FOUND COLLAPSED IN THE STREET

A 55-year-old male was found collapsed in the street by a passerby. The passerby began one-man CPR and called the ambulance. The ambulance brings him into the emergency department where you are the casualty officer in charge. Basic cardiac life support is continuing, but advanced cardiac life support has not been started.

SELECT THE ONE BEST ANSWER TO THE FOLLOWING QUESTIONS:

877. A "quick-look" paddles is performed on the patient described above and shows ventricular fibrillation. Your first step should be:
    a) defibrillate with 200 joules at once
    b) administer sodium bicarbonate 50 mEq IV bolus, epinephrine 10 cc 1: 10000 solution followed by countershock
    c) administer sodium bicarbonate 500 mEq IV bolus, calcium chloride 5 ml 10% solution IV bolus, and then countershock
    d) defibrillate with 400 joules at once
    e) administer atropine 1.0 mg IV bolus and epinephrine 10 cc 1:10000 solution and wait for the response

878. The antiarrhythmic of choice in the management of ventricular arrhythmias is:
    a) bretylium
    b) lidocaine
    c) procainamide
    d) verapamil
    e) amrinone

879. The patient described in question 869 is successfully converted to sinus rhythm. Unfortunately, on the way to the coronary care unit he arrests again. The rhythm strip reveals asystole. CPR is begun again. Which of the following is the next step in this patient's treatment?
    a) administration of epinephrine 1: 10,000—1.0 mg IV push
    b) administration of calcium chloride—10 cc 10% solution-IV push
    c) administration of sodium bicarbonate 1 mEq/kg IV push

    d) administration of isoproterenol 2–20 µg/kg/min
    e) administration of lidocaine 75 mg IV push

880. With appropriate treatment the patient reverts to sinus rhythm and is stablized in the coronary care unit. Unfortunately, 2 hours later his rhythm strip shows a ventricular tachycardia. At this time his blood pressure is 100/60 and he has a palpable pulse. What is the most appropriate management at this time?
    a) lidocaine—75 mg IV bolus
    b) synchronized DC countershock
    c) procainamide—100 mg/min IV
    d) bretylium 15 mg/kg IV
    e) verapamil 5 mg IV

881. Two hours after sinus rhythm is restored after the complication discussed in question 880 the rhythm strip once again reveals ventricular tachycardia. At this time his blood pressure is 40 mm Hg systolic and his pulse is not palpable. What is the most appropriate management at this time?
    a) lidocaine—75 mg IV bolus
    b) procainamide—20 mg/min
    c) bretylium 5 mg IV bolus
    d) verapamil 5 mg IV bolus
    e) none of the above

882. Sinus rhythm is restored in the patient and he appears to be doing well. Unfortunately, he develops a second degree AV block (Mobitz Type II). His pulse is 40 beats/minute and his blood pressure drops to 70/40 mm Hg. What is the most appropriate treatment in the patient at this time?
    a) observation only
    b) isoproterenol 2–10 µg/min
    c) atropine 0.5–1.0 mg

d) epinephrine 0.5–1.0 mg
e) none of the above

883. The definitive therapy for this patient at this time is:
   a) a constant infusion of isoproterenol 2–20 μg/min
   b) a constant infusion of lidocaine 2–4 mg/min
   c) a constant infusion of procainamide 2–4 mg/min
   d) a transvenous pacemaker
   e) none of the above

884. CPR is in progress on a 70-kg man who collapsed in the street. He was brought into the emergency department by the ambulance and advanced cardiac life support is begun. A blood gas sample is drawn and the following results are obtained:
   pH—7.10
   PCO_2—60 mm Hg
   PO_2—75 mm Hg
   HCO_3—15 mEq/L
   This represents:
   a) metabolic acidosis with respiratory alkalosis
   b) respiratory acidosis with metabolic alkalosis
   c) pure metabolic acidosis
   d) pure respiratory acidosis
   e) mixed respiratory and metabolic acidosis

885. The appropriate treatment of the patient described in question 884 at this time is:
   a) sodium bicarbonate 1 mEq/kg
   b) sodium bicarbonate 0.5 mEq/kg
   c) increased ventilation
   d) both a and c
   e) both b and c

886. A 53-year-old male presents to your emergency room with a 2-hour history of a "rapid heart beat," nausea, and dizziness. A 12-lead ECG shows atrial flutter with variable A-V conduction. As you are taking his history he becomes disoriented. Blood pressure is measured at 40 mm Hg systolic. What is the most appropriate treatment for this patient at this time?
   a) epinephrine 1.0 mg IV
   b) isoproterenol 2–20 μg/min IV
   c) defibrillate with 300 joules
   d) cardiovert with 300 joules
   e) cardiovert with 75–100 joules

ANSWERS

877. A. The first step in the treatment of ventricular fibrillation is defibrillation with an energy of 200 joules. If the first attempt is not successful, two further defibrillations (200–300 and 360 joules) should follow before pharmacologic therapy is initiated. If defibrillation is not successful, IV access should be established, epinephrine given, intubation performed, and antiarrhythmic drugs administered. The role of sodium bicarbonate in the management of cardiac arrest is now limited. Atropine is indicated in the management of asystole, not ventricular fibrillation. Calcium chloride is no longer recommended in the management of any arrhythmia or dysrhythmia.[1,2]

878. B. The antiarrhythmic agent of choice is lidocaine. Lidocaine should be administered in a dosage of 1 mg/kg IV push up to a maximum of 3 mg/kg. In addition, a lidocaine infusion in a dosage of 2–4 mg/kg should be started in a patient with a ventricular arrhythmia.

   Bretylium and procainamide are equally good second line agents. Bretylium is administered in a dosage of 5 mg/kg IV and repeated at 15–30 min intervals in a dosage of 10 mg/kg to a maximum dose of 30 mg/kg. Procainamide is administered in a dosage of 50 mg every 5 minutes until one of the following is observed: (1) the arrhythmia is suppressed; (2) hypotension ensues; (3) the QRS complex is widened by 50% of its original width; or (4) a total of 1 g of drug has been injected. Bretylium and procainamide levels can be maintained by IV infusion in a dosage of 2–4 mg/min.

   Verapamil is indicated in the treatment of supraventricular arrhythmias. Amrinone is a rapid-acting inotropic agent that is useful in the treatment of patients with severe congestive heart failure refractory to diuretics, vasodilators, and conventional inotropic agents.[1,2]

879. A. The next step in the management of this patient is the administration of epinephrine 1:10000—1.0 mg IV push. This should be repeated every 5 minutes. If intubation has not been performed it should be. Atropine in a dosage of 1.0 mg IV push should be given as well, and repeated every 5 minutes. If the patient's arrest has been unwitnessed, sodium bicarbonate may be considered if the patient does not respond to previous measures. The only other possible treatment is cardiac

pacing, but this is really a treatment of last resort.[1,2]

880. A. The treatment of choice for patients with ventricular tachycardia who are hemodynamically stable is lidocaine 1 mg/kg. This can be repeated in a dosage of 0.5 mg/kg every 8 minutes until the ventricular tachycardia resolves or until a total of 3 mg/kg has been given. The second line drug in this case is procainamide in a dosage of 20 mg/min until the ventricular tachycardia resolves, or up to 1000 mg.

DC countershock is recommended only in hemodynamically unstable patients. Bretylium can be used, but is recommended for use after procainamide in stable ventricular tachycardia. Verapamil is used in the treatment of supraventricular, not ventricular arrhythmias.[1,2]

881. E. None of the above. When hemodynamically unstable ventricular tachycardia is diagnosed (pulseless or hypotensive) the treatment of choice is synchronized cardioversion. The initial energy recommended is 50 joules. This should be followed by repetitive shocks of 100 joules, 200 joules, and up to 360 joules. If recurrent, lidocaine should be given as an IV bolus and cardioversion again performed (at the energy level that was previously successful).[1,2]

882. C.

883. D. Second degree heart block (Mobitz Type II) occurs below the level of the AV node either at the bundle of His (uncommon) or bundle branch level (more common). It is usually associated with an organic lesion in the conduction pathway. It often progresses to third degree block. Initial treatment is aimed at increasing the heart rate. Thus, atropine 0.5–1.0 mg is the drug of choice. The maximum dose of atropine is 2.0 mg. If signs or symptoms persist, an external pacemaker can be placed or an isoproterenol infusion begun in a dosage of 2–10 μg/min. Epinephrine or observation are not appropriate treatments for this patient. The definitive treatment in this patient is a transvenous pacemaker.[1,2]

884. E.

885. C. Most patients who are undergoing cardiopulmonary resuscitation have a mixed respiratory and metabolic acidosis. Normal PCO_2 is 40 mm Hg.

The patient in this case has a markedly elevated PCO_2 of 60 mm Hg. and thus is being hypoventilated. The patient's bicarbonate level of 15 mEq/L is below the normal range of 21–28 mEq/L and thus he has a metabolic acidosis as well.

Recent recommendations, however, suggest that bicarbonate should be used with caution. Although cardiac function is depressed by acidosis, the determining factor is intracellular pH, not extracellular pH as is measured by arterial blood gases. Hypoxia, not acidosis, accounts for most of the cardiac depression. Respiratory acidosis, however, produces immediate and profound depression. Thus, increasing ventilation should be used as the primary means of correcting acidosis.

By contrast, the use of bicarbonate has long been known to present the risks of alkalosis, hypernatremia, and hyperosmolarity. All of these conditions are easily and commonly brought about by the typical ACLS-recommended doses and are predictors of an unsuccessful outcome.[1,2]

886. E. The treatment of choice for acute unstable atrial flutter is synchronized cardioversion. If the patient is unstable, synchronized cardioversion is the treatment of choice. The initial energy chosen should be 75–100 joules. If unsuccessful it should be followed by cardioversion at 200 and 360 joules. If the patient is stable vagal maneuvers, followed by verapamil if vagal maneuvers are unsuccessful.[1,2]

SUMMARY OF THE TREATMENT OF THE CARDIAC ARREST PATIENT

1. **Ventricular fibrillation:**
   a) defibrillation 200–300–360 joules
   b) epinephrine 0.5–1.0 mg IV push (repeat q 5 min)
   c) defibrillate again
   d) lidocaine 1.0 mg/kg IV push
   e) second line antiarrhythmic (procainamide/bretylium)

2. **Asystole:**
   a) epinephrine 0.5–1.0 mg IV push (repeat q 5 min)
   b) atropine 1.0 mg IV push (repeat in 5 min)
   c) consider bicarbonate
   d) consider pacing

3. **Ventricular tachycardia:**
   Stable ventricular tachycardia:

a) lidocaine 1.0 mg/kg (repeat at dosage of 0.5 mg/kg every 8 minutes until ventricular tachycardia resolves)

b) procainamide 20 mg/min until VT resolves or up to 1000 mg

c) cardiovert as in unstable patients

Unstable ventricular tachycardia:

a) consider sedation

b) cardiovert 50–100–200–360 joules if recurrent, add lidocaine and cardiovert again starting at energy level previously successful; then procainamide or bretylium

4. **Heart block (second degree Mobitz II and third degree):**
   a) atropine 0.5–1.0 mg IV (maxiumum 2.0 mg)
   b) isoproterenol 2–10 µg/min/external pacemaker
   c) transvenous pacemaker

5. **Supraventricular tachycardia:**
   Stable:
   a) vagal maneuvers
   b) verapamil 5 mg IV (10 mg IV if not successful [maximum 30 mg])
   c) cardioversion, digoxin, beta blockers, pacing as indicated
   Unstable:
   a) synchronized cardioversion 75–100, 200, 360

References

1. Standards and guidelines for cardiopulmonary resuscitation and emergency cardiac care. JAMA 1986; 251(21): 2843–2989.

2. Swanson R, Ramsden V. Emergency cardiac care: an update. Can Fam Physician 1988; 34: 689–699.

PROBLEM 114: A 34-YEAR-OLD MALE WHO HAS BEEN INJURED IN A MOTOR VEHICLE ACCIDENT

A 34-year-old male is brought into the emergency room after being injured in a head-on motor vehicle accident. He is unconscious and is markedly short of breath. He is brought in on a spine board.

On examination, he is unresponsive to verbal commands but responds to deep pain. His pupils are equal and reactive to light and accommodation. Blood pressure is 90/60 mm Hg. His pulse rate is 108/minute. His respiratory rate is 60/minute and labored. There is no air entry over the right side of the chest. The trachea is deviated to the left. There is a large contusion over the right side of the chest.

SELECT THE ONE BEST ANSWER TO THE FOLLOWING QUESTIONS:

887. At this time, your first priority should be:
   a) carry on with the rest of the complete assessment of the patient
   b) establish an intravenous infusion
   c) send the patient to x-ray for a stat chest x-ray
   d) send the patient for a lateral x-ray of the cervical spine
   e) none of the above

888. Your first priority has been completed. The patient's level of consciousness is improving. He is beginning to moan. Air entry is equal and bilateral, and the respiratory rate is 24/minute. His blood pressure is now 70/50 mm Hg. On examination of his abdomen, he moans as you palpate his left upper quadrant.

The most likely cause of his abdominal pain is:
   a) liver laceration
   b) duodenal rupture
   c) renal hematoma
   d) splenic rupture
   e) pancreatic tear

889. After having made the diagnosis in question 888, you should:
   a) schedule a CT scan of the abdomen
   b) perform peritoneal lavage
   c) reassess the patient in one-half hour
   d) move on to the examination of the rest of the patient
   e) none of the above

890. A 23-year-old female injured in a motor vehicle accident is brought into the emergency department. She is alert and oriented, but is in significant respiratory distress.

On examination, the respiratory rate is 32/minute. Her blood pressure is 100/70 mm Hg. Her pulse rate is 96 and regular.

On examination, the left side of the rib cage moves inward during inspiration and outward during expiration. The rest of the physical examination is within normal limits.

The most likely diagnosis in this patient is:
a) flail chest
b) simple rib fractures
c) pneumothorax
d) costochondral seperation
e) none of the above

891. The treatment of choice for the patient described in question 890 is:
a) observation only
b) surgical intervention
c) endotracheal intubation
d) chest tube insertion
e) none of the above

892. A 31-year-old male is brought into emergency after having been involved in a car-motorcycle accident.

On examination, he is drowsy but conscious. His respiratory rate is 32/minute. His blood pressure is 70/50 mm Hg. His heart sounds are muffled. He has significant elevation of jugular venous pressure. He has a large contusion over the sternal area. There is a laceration seen over the precordial region. No other significant abnormalities are noted on primary survey.

The most likely diagnosis in this patient is:
a) myocardial contusion
b) pericardial tamponade
c) aortic rupture
d) pulmonary contusion
e) pneumothorax

893. The treatment of choice in the patient described in question 892 is:
a) regular observation
b) increased rate of crystalloid infusion
c) crystalloid plus blood
d) pericardiocentesis
e) chest tube insertion

894. The first priority upon arrival at the scene of an accident with a multiply injured patient is to:
a) clear the oropharynx and establish an airway
b) check pulse
c) check blood pressure
d) check the mobility of the cervical spine
e) stop obvious external hemorrhage

ANSWER THE FOLLOWING QUESTIONS ACCORDING TO THE CODE:

A: 1, 2, and 3 are correct
B: 1 and 3 are correct
C: 2 and 4 are correct
D: Only 4 is correct
E: All of the above are correct

895. A patient is brought into emergency following a fight. He was stabbed in the abdomen, and appears to be in shock. His airway has been cleared and there is good air entry bilaterally. His pulse is 108 and regular, and blood pressure is 100/70 mm Hg. You wish to establish secure intravenous access. Which of the following veins should be considered first choice sites for the establishment of multiple, large-bore catheters?
1) femoral vein
2) internal jugular vein
3) antecubital vein
4) subclavian vein

896. The intravenous access is established for the patient described in question 895. Which of the following maneuvers may also be indicated in this patient?
1) obtaining arterial blood gas samples
2) insertion of a urinary catheter
3) insertion of a nasogastric tube
4) continuous cardiac monitoring

ANSWERS

887. E. None of the above. This patient has a tension pneumothorax that may be rapidly fatal.

A tension pneumothorax requires immediate decompression and the placement of a chest tube. An immediate thoracostomy should be performed through an incision between the fifth and sixth ribs in the anterior axillary line. Alternatively, a tension pneumothorax can be decompressed by making an incision and inserting a finger or a clamp into the pleural space.[1,2]

Many patients with tension pneumothoraces have died while an x-ray of the chest is awaited or performed.

888. D. This patient also has a ruptured spleen.

Splenic rupture is the commonest injury resulting from blunt abdominal trauma. The symptoms of ruptured spleen include abdominal pain, which may be generalized or localized. Radiation to the left shoulder is common. Splenic rupture is often associated with left lower rib fractures.[3,4]

889. E. This patient needs an immediate laparotomy. In cases where the blood pressure is stable, a peritoneal lavage or a CT scan can be performed to document the extent of the abdominal injuries. In this case, the patient may exsanguinate while the diagnostic study is being performed. Similarly, if a reassessment of the abdomen is left for one-half hour, the patient may well be dead.[3,4]

890. A. This patient has a flail chest. A flail chest results when multiple rib fractures produce a mechanically unstable chest. There is paradoxical movement of the flail segment on respiration (inward movement with inspiration).

Patients with flail chest present with dyspnea, respiratory distress, and rib pain and tenderness. Hyperventilation may initially compensate, but fatigue secondary to increased effort of breathing eventually occurs. Respiratory failure follows if the flail chest is untreated.[1,2]

891. C. The treatment of choice for flail chest is endotracheal intubation. Supplemental oxygen should be given until intubation is complete. Analgesia with intravenous morphine should also be administered to relieve pain and anxiety.

External supports such as rib taping etc. are not indicated.

The patient should be monitored in an intensive care unit.[1,2]

892. B. This patient has a pericardial tamponade.

Pericardial tamponade results in increased resistance to ventricular filling, and a decrease in cardiac output. Hypotension and shock result.[1,2]

There is usually evidence of penetrating chest trauma or penetrating injury of the upper abdomen or back. The diagnostic triad of the muffled heart sounds, hypotension, and increased jugular venous pressure is usually present unless there is hypovolemia secondary to other injuries.[1,2]

Although myocardial contusion and pulmonary contusion may also be present, the primary diagnosis is pericardial tamponade.

893. D. This treatment of choice in this patient is pericardiocentesis. An alternative is emergency left anterolateral thoracotomy and pericardiotomy.

Adequate fluid replacement with crystalloid solutions will temporarily sustain ventricular filling pressure. Inotropic agents including dopamine and isoproterenol will temporarily increase the blood pressure.

Respiratory support should be continued with supplemental oxygen at 5–10 L/min prior to pericardiotomy.[1,2]

894. A. The first priority at the arrival at the scene of an accident with a multiply injured patient is to clear the oropharynx and establish an airway. Once the airway is established, ventilation should be begun. Supplemental oxygen should be used in a conscious, breathing patient; in an unconscious patient or a patient who is not breathing this should be followed by endotracheal or nasotracheal intubation. The nasotracheal route is preferred in patients suspected of having cervical spine injuries.[5] Cricothyroidotomy can be attempted in life-threatening situations where intubation is impossible.

The second priority is to check cardiac activity (feel for pulse). If an obvious external hemorrhage is apparent, it should be dealt with at this time.[5]

Following this, a clinical assessment for shock should take place.

The mobility of the cervical spine should not be assessed; a cervical spine injury should be assumed to be present until proven otherwise.

895. B. Shock in the traumatized patient is usually due to hypovolemia from hemorrhage, cardiac tamponade, or tension pneumothorax. Therefore, multiple large-bore catheters (> 16 guage) should be used. The subclavian and internal jugular veins should initially be avoided due to their flaccidity in shock.

Intravenous infusion of crystalloid solution (up to 2 L) should be given to support intravascular volume before blood is given.[5]

896. E. After intravenous access is established, blood should be drawn for hematocrit, typing and crossmatch. As well, arterial blood gases should be drawn.

An ECG should be obtained, and continuous cardiac monitoring should be begun.

A urinary catheter should be inserted in all patients with shock to monitor the effectiveness of resuscitation. The only contraindications to the insertion of a urethral catheter is obvious injury to the external genitalia, obvious blood at the urethral meatus, or difficulty in passing the catheter.

A nasogastric tube should also be inserted in any patient with abdominal or chest trauma.[5]

SUMMARY OF THE DIAGNOSIS AND MANAGEMENT OF MAJOR TRAUMA

1. **On the scene managment:** ABCs
   A= airway: clear airway
   B= breathing: begin ventilation
   C= circulation: pulse check, stop major hemorrhage, check blood pressure
   S= stabilize cervical spine

2. **Emergency management:**
   a) establish intravenous access (two #16 guage catheters) and begin infusion of crystalloid solutions
   b) perform primary survey: rule out tension pneumothorax, flail chest, hemothorax, major abdominal trauma
   c) consider orotracheal intubation
   d) reassess circulation
   e) perform neurologic assessment
   f) totally expose patient to avoid missing any injuries
   g) insert urinary catheter
   h) insert nasogastric tube as indicated
   i) begin continuous ECG monitoring
   k) perform secondary survey: reassess all previous injuries
   l) perform x-rays: cervical spine, chest, A-P pelvis

COMMON ERRORS IN TRAUMA STABILIZATION

1. Inadequate airway management
2. Inadequate shock therapy
3. Inadequate C-spine mobilization
4. Failure to recognize or decompress pneumothorax
5. Distraction by visually impressive but not life-threatening injuries (maxillofacial trauma, compound fractures)
6. Delay in transfer (unnecessary suturing or x-ray survey)
7. Failure to accompany patient to trauma center

References

1. Wilson R, Steiger Z. Thoracic trauma. In: Tintinalli J, Krome R, Ruiz E, eds. Emergency medicine, a comprehensive study guide. 2nd Ed. New York: McGraw-Hill, 1988; 850–863.

2. Trunkey D, Cheitlin M. Chest Trauma. In: Mills J, Ho M, Salber P, Trunkey D, eds. Current emergency diagnosis and treatment. 2nd Ed. Los Altos, CA: Lange Medical Publications, 1985; 41–50.

3. Ney A. Andersen R. Abdominal trauma. In: Tintinalli J, Krome R, Ruiz E, eds. Emergency medicine, a comprehensive study guide. 2nd Ed. New York: McGraw-Hill, 1988; 864–871.

4. Trunkey D. Abdominal trauma. In: Mills J, Ho M, Salber P, Trunkey D, eds. Current emergency diagnosis and treatment. 2nd Ed. Los Altos, CA: Lange Medical Publications, 1985; 249–259.

5. Ruiz E, Mayron R. Initial approach to the trauma patient. In: Tintinalli J, Krome R, Ruiz E, eds. Emergency medicine, a comprehensive study guide. 2nd Ed. New York: McGraw-Hill, 1988; 825–828.

PROBLEM 115: A 65-YEAR-OLD FEMALE WHO SLIPPED AND FELL ON HER OUTSTRETCHED HAND

A 65-year-old female is brought into the emergency department by her daughter after having fallen on her outstretched hand. She complains of pain in the right wrist.

On examination, there is a deformity in the area of the right wrist. The wrist has the appearance of a "dinner-fork." There is significant tenderness over the distal radius. Pulses and sensation in the right wrist are normal.

SELECT THE ONE BEST ANSWER TO THE FOLLOWING QUESTIONS:

897. The most likely diagnosis in this patient is:

a) fracture of the distal ulna with dislocation of the radial head
b) fracture of the carpal scaphoid
c) fracture of the radial styloid

d) Colles' fracture
e) fracture of the shaft of the radius with dislocation of the ulnar head

898. The treatment of choice for the patient described in question 897 is:
a) internal reduction and immobilization
b) internal reduction and fixation
c) external reduction and immobilization
d) external reduction and fixation
e) none of the above

899. An 18-year-old basketball player is brought into emergency after having fallen on his outstretched hand in a league game.

On examination, there is slight tenderness and swelling just below the distal radius. No other abnormalities are found. X-ray examination of the wrist and hand is normal.

The most likely diagnosis in this patient is:
a) second degree wrist sprain
b) avulsion fracture of the distal radius
c) fractured scaphoid
d) fractured triquetrum
e) none of the above

900. The treatment of choice for the patient discussed in question 899 at this time is:
a) active physiotherapy
b) passive physiotherapy
c) ice, compression, and elevation of the extremity
d) surgical exploration of the wrist
e) none of the above

901. A 25-year-old male is brought into the emergency department after being thrown from his motorcycle. He complains of severe pain in the area of his right ankle.

On examination, there is swelling of the entire right ankle, with a more prominent swelling on the lateral side. There is point tenderness over the area of the lateral malleolus. There does not appear to be any other abnormality or any deformity seen.

The most likely diagnosis in this patient is:
a) second degree ankle sprain
b) third degree ankle sprain
c) fractured distal tibia
d) fractured lateral malleolus
e) fractured tallus

902. The treatment of choice for the patient described in question 901 is:

a) internal reduction and fixation
b) external reduction and fixation
c) active physiotherapy
d) ice, compression, and elevation
e) a walking plaster boot

ANSWER THE FOLLOWING QUESTIONS ACCORDING TO THE CODE:

A: 1, 2, and 3 are correct
B: 1 and 3 are correct
C: 2 and 4 are correct
D: Only 4 is correct
E: All of the above are correct

903. Which of the following statements regarding acute compartment syndrome is(are) correct?
1) it is caused by increasing pressure in a closed fascial space
2) the fascial compartments of the leg and the forearm are most commonly involved
3) Volkmann's contracture is a complication of the syndrome
4) it may be caused by vigorous exercise

904. The emergency treatment of orthopedic injuries includes which of the following?
1) assessment and searching for multiple injuries
2) assessment of arterial injury in the involved region
3) correction of deformites
4) splinting or immobilization of each injured area

ANSWERS

897. D. Colles' fracture, a fracture of the distal radius, is the most common fracture seen in emergency departments today. It occurs most commonly in elderly patients, especially women. It is often associated with osteoporosis.

Colles' fracture is almost always caused by a fall on the outstretched hand.

The typical displacement is reflected in a characteristic clinical appearance that has been termed the "dinner-fork" deformity.

The clinical history and deformity are not compatible with the other fractures listed in the question.[1,2]

898. C. The treatment of choice for the patient described in question 897 is external reduction under

regional or general anesthesia, and immobilization with a plaster cast.[1,2]

899. C. This patient has a fractured scaphoid bone. It is common in young adults. The most common cause is a fall on the outstretched hand.

Fracture of the scaphoid should be suspected in any injury to the wrist in men unless a specific diagnosis of another type of injury is obvious. Fractures of the scaphoid bone are often overlooked, either because of failure to x-ray the wrist or failure to detect the fracture in an x-ray.[1,2]

In many cases, as in this patient, pain from the injury is not marked and the patient can continue to use the hand. A patient will often regard the injury as a sprain and not even consult his physician.

The most common physical finding is tenderness in scaphoid region (the anatomic snuff box). Swelling is usually minimal. The only other possible diagnosis based on the history, physical examination, and x-ray findings is a wrist sprain. However, this diagnosis should only be made after two negative x-rays 2 weeks apart.[1,2]

900. E. None of the above.

The treatment of choice for the patient discussed in question 899 is immobilization in a plaster cast that extends down the thumb to the level of the interphalangeal joint, and molded firmly around the first metacarpal bone. This immobilization should be undertaken in spite of the negative x-ray finding on first examination. Failure to properly immobilize the scaphoid may result in avascular necrosis of the bone.[1,2]

901. D. The history of trauma, the signs, and the symptoms suggest a fracture of the lateral malleolus. Although the physical findings of an ankle sprain are similar, the injury (being thrown from a motorcycle) is more suggestive of a more significant bony injury.[1,2]

902. E. The treatment of choice for the patient described in question 901 is a walking plaster boot for 6 weeks. In the absence of significant deformity and the confirmation on x-ray of a singular injury to the lateral malleolus, no other treatment is indicated. With this injury, there is unlikely to be significant displacement that would demand fixation.[1,2]

903. E. Acute compartment syndrome is caused by increasing tissue pressure in a closed fascial space. The fascial compartments of the leg and forearm are most commonly involved. The most common causes of acute compartment syndrome are a fracture with subsequent hemorrhage, and limb compression or a crushing injury. Intracompartmental fluid pressure is increased, leading to ischemia. Severe ischemia for 6–8 hours leads to muscle and nerve death, with resulting contracture.[1,2]

On physical examination, there is usually swelling and palpable tenseness over the muscle compartment. Paresis, pain with stretch of the involved muscle, and sensory deficit are also common findings.

The treatment of choice is fasciotomy.[1,2]

904. E. Before specific orthopedic injuries are assessed and treated, the patient's overall condition (ABCs) should be assessed. Shock should be treated as described in the chapter on trauma.

The trauma patient should be suspected of having multiple injuries. These should be assumed to be present until proven otherwise and searched for. Cervical spine injuries should be assumed to be present until excluded.

With any injured extremity, arterial injury should be suspected and the pulses assessed. Acute compartment syndrome should be ruled out.

Deformities should be corrected as soon as possible with regional or general anesthesia. Ideally, the injured area(s) should be splinted before the patient arrives in the emergency department. Open fractures should be cleaned and the area debrided as soon as possible. Tetanus prophylaxis should be given and antistaphylococcal antibiotics should be started. Orthopedic consultation should be immediately sought.

SUMMARY OF THE DIAGNOSIS AND TREATMENT OF FRACTURES AND OTHER ORTHOPEDIC INJURIES

1. Remember ABCs of resuscitation
2. Suspect and search for multiple injuries
3. Suspect and prevent potential spine injuries
4. Rule out arterial injury in affected limb
5. Rule out compartment syndrome
6. Recognize and treat open fractures and areas suspected of concealing open fractures by copious

irrigation, debridement, and the initiation of antibiotics. Obtain immediate orthopedic consultation

7. Correct deformities whenever possible
8. Splint each injured area

References

1. Day L et al. Orthopedics. In: May, LW, ed. Current surgical diagnosis and treatment. 8th Ed. Los Altos, CA: Lange Medical Publications, 1988; 919–1029.

2. Adams JC. Outline of fractures. 8th Ed. Edinburgh: Churchill and Livingstone, 1983.

PROBLEM 116. A 37-YEAR-OLD MALE WHO WAS FOUND DRUNK IN A SNOW-BANK

A 37-year-old male is brought into the emergency department after having been found drunk in a snowbank. He is unconscious and no history if available.

On physical examination his blood pressure is 90/60 mm Hg. His pulse is 50 and regular. His core temperature is 28° C. The ECG shows sinus bradycardia and a J wave after the QRS complex.

SELECT THE ONE BEST ANSWER TO THE FOLLOWING QUESTIONS:

905. Which of the following statements regarding the hypothermia in this patient is false?
    a) most hypothermic patients are intoxicated with ethanol or other drugs
    b) body temperatures from 32 to 35° C constitute mild hypothermia
    c) the Osborn "J" wave on the ECG is characteristic of hypothermia
    d) arrhythmias and dysrhythmias are common when the core body temperature drops below 30° C
    e) intravascular volume is usually maintained in hypothermia

906. The treatment of choice for the patient described above is:
    a) passive rewarming
    b) active external rewarming
    c) active core rewarming
    d) a and b
    e) none of the above

907. A 45-year-old is brought into the emergency department from his worksite with a numbness in both feet after working in -40° C weather for 6 hours.

    On examination, both feet are blanched. Sensation is decreased in both feet to the level of the ankles. Both feet are cold to touch and are bloodless. You suspect frostbite.

The most appropriate treatment of this injury at this time is:
    a) passive rewarming
    b) vigorous rubbing
    c) immersion in water at 42° C
    d) placement close to a radiant heater
    e) immersion in water at 30° C

908. A 4-year-old male is brought into the emergency department after having fallen through the ice into a lake. He was rescued 10 minutes later. Cardiopulmonary resuscitation was begun at the scene, and is being continued as the patient presents to the emergency department.

    On examination, there is no spontaneous breathing or cardiac activity. The child's core temperature is 28° C.

    At this time, the most appropriate action would be to:
    a) stop cardiopulmonary resuscitation
    b) continue CPR while rewarming the patient with active external rewarming
    c) continue CPR while rewarming the patient with inhalation rewarming
    d) continue CPR while rewarming the patient with peritoneal dialysis
    e) continue CPR while rewarming the patient with GI tract irrigation

ANSWER THE FOLLOWING QUESTIONS ACCORDING TO THE CODE:

A: 1, 2, and 3 are correct
B: 1 and 3 are correct
C: 2 and 4 are correct
D: Only 4 is correct
E: All of the above are correct

909. A 34-year-old male is brought to the emergency department by a friend after having worked outdoors all day in temperatures of 42° C. He complains of painful spasm of the skeletal muscles, most prominent in the lower extremities and the abdomen. He has had no other symptoms associated with these spasms.

On physical examination, the patient is alert and cooperative. His blood pressure is 120/80 mm Hg and his pulse 108/min. His temperature is 37° C. The rest of the physical examination is normal.

Which of the following statements regarding this patient's condition is(are) true?

1) this patient has heatstroke
2) this patient can be safely treated with outpatient therapy
3) this patient's temperature will likely go up in the next 3 hours
4) hyponatremia, hypokalemia, and respiratory alkalosis are commonly seen with this condition.

910. A 23-year-old female marathon runner presents to the emergency department after completing a marathon. During the last mile, she began to develop light-headedness, nausea, vomiting, severe headache, rapid heart rate, and rapid respiratory rate.

On examination, the patient's blood pressure is 90/70 mm Hg. Her pulse is 120/min and regular. The temperature is 37.5° C. The rest of the physical examination is normal.

Which of the following statements regarding this patient's condition is(are) true?

1) this patient has heatstroke
2) this patient can be safely treated as an outpatient
3) this patient's temperature will likely go up in the next few hours
4) this patient's syndrome is characterized by volume depletion

911. A 34-year-old male is brought into the emergency department by ambulance after having collapsed in a marathon. Apparently, at the 18 mile mark he fell to the ground unconscious.

On examination, his blood pressure is 110/75 mm Hg. His pulse is 128/min. The patient's temperature is 41° C. He is unconscious.

Which of the following statements regarding this patient's condition is(are) true?

1) this patient has heatstroke
2) the mortality rate of this condition may be as high as 40%
3) hepatic and renal abnormalities are common in this condition
4) treatment should be directed at lowering the core temperature as quickly as possible

ANSWERS

905. E. The majority of hypothermic patients are intoxicated with ethanol or other drugs. Ethanol is a vasodilator, and due to its anesthetic and CNS-depressant effects, intoxicated subjects do not feel the cold. Hypothermia may be associated with other drugs (including barbiturates, phenothiazines, and insulin), hypothyroidism, sepsis, and other acute illnesses.[1]

Hypothermia is defined as mild if the body temperature is between 32 and 35° C, and severe if it is below 32°. Below 30° C, shivering ceases.

Hypothermia causes characteristic ECG changes, and may induce certain life-threatening arrhythmias and dysrhythmias, including ventricular fibrillation and asystole. The Osborn (J) wave, a slow positive deflection at the end of the QRS complex, is characteristic, although not pathognomonic, of hypothermia.[1] The probability of dysrhythmias increases with decreasing body temperature.[1] Oxygen delivery to the tissues is impaired, and intravascular volume is lost due to a plasma shift to the extravascular space.[1]

Hypothermia produces a depression of central nervous system function. Confusion and lethargy may be followed by coma.[1]

906. C. Because of the severity of the hypothermia (core temperature of 28° C), active core rewarming is the method of choice for the correction of this patient's hypothermia.[1]

Core rewarming will warm the internal organs preferentially. This will decrease myocardial irritibility and improve cardiac function.[1]

The methods of active core rewarming include inhalation rewarming, heated IV fluids, GI tract irrigation, peritoneal dialysis, hemodialysis, and extracorporeal rewarming.[1]

Passive rewarming (removal from the cold environment and insulation techniques) allows patients to rewarm on their own. Core temperature, however, rises slowly with this method, and thus, it by itself is not appropriate for a patient with cardiovascular compromise.

Active external rewarming (water immersion, heated objects, radiant heat) may be successful in rapidly raising body temperature. The application of external heat, however, may cause peripheral vasodilation, and return cold blood to the core.[1]

The method of choice in rewarming a patient depends upon the duration, degree, and cause of the hypothermia. Cold water immersion, for example, produces little disturbance of volume, electrolyte, and acid-base status. Rapid external rewarming, therefore, is usually both safe and successful.

In patients who are in the early phase of hypothermia improvement usually occurs no matter what method is used. At temperatures above 30° C, the incidence of arrhythmias is low, and rapid rewarming is rarely necessary.

The most important consideration in the choice of method is the patient's cardiovascular status. Patients with a stable cardiac rhythm (including sinus bradycardia and atrial fibrillation) and stable vital signs do not need rapid rewarming.[1] These patients simply require passive rewarming and noninvasive internal modalities (e.g., moist warm oxygen and warm IV fluids).

Patients with cardiovascular compromise, including persistent hypotension and life-threatening dysrhythmias need to be rewarmed rapidly. At this time, the choice lies within the methods that have been described for active core rewarming.[1]

907. C. The initial clinical response to cold is known as "frostnip." Frostnip, a superficial and reversible injury, begins as a blanching and numbness of the involved area, followed by a sudden cessation of cold and discomfort.[2] The sudden loss of cold sensation at the injury site is a very reliable sign of impending frostbite. If treatment is initiated at this point, frostnip will not progress to frostbite.

The best initial treatment for frostnip and frostbite is rapid rewarming of the extremity in 42 degree water for at least 20 minutes. Slow rewarming is less effective and may actually increase tissue damage.[2]

The use of dry heat (such as with the use of a radiant heater) to treat frostnip and frostbite is dangerous due to a high probability of superficial burning and unnecessary tissue destruction.

Rubbing the affected part causes skin breakage, increases chance of infection, and does not produce adequate thawing of tissues.

Passive rewarming does not produce rapid enough rewarming and decreases the chance of preserving viable tissue.[2]

908. B. Cardiopulmonary resuscitation should not be stopped until the core temperature is at least 30–32° C.[1] Death in hypothermia is defined as a failure to revive after rewarming; CPR should be continued until the core temperature is at least 30–32° C.[1] Cold water immersion can be treated with rapid external rewarming.[1]

909. C. This patient has heat cramps.[3] Heat cramps are usually associated with strenuous physical activity. The painful spasm of skeletal muscles, including muscles of the extremities and abdomen occurs. Heat cramps occur because of the production of large amounts of sweat with associated sodium loss.

Hyperventilation may also play an etiologic role. Hyperventilation produces respiratory alkalosis, and may be associated with hypokalemia.

On physical examination, the body temperature is normal and there is no evidence of dehydration. Laboratory investigation may reveal hyponatremia, hypokalemia, hypomagnesemia, hypophosphatemia, and respiratory alkalosis.

Heat cramps are benign, and respond well to rest and oral electrolyte replacement.

Heatstroke is discussed in a subsequent question.

With heat cramps, there will not be an increase in body temperature.[3]

910. D. This patient has heat exhaustion. Heat exhaustion is characterized by volume depletion, and fluid and electrolyte losses due to sweating. Hypovolemia and tissue hypoperfusion occur.[3]

Heat exhaustion usually presents with fatigue, light-headedness, nausea and or vomiting, and sometimes headache. Significant hypovolemia with tachycardia, hyperventilation, and hypotension occur. The patient's body temperature is usually normal or only slightly elevated. Sweating may be profuse.[3]

The most common laboratory abnormality is hemoconcentration. If the patient has not taken fluids and/or has not yet been adequately rehydrated hypernatremia will likely be present. If partial rehydration has been achieved, relatively normal sodium and chloride levels may be seen.

The treatment of heat exhaustion is rest and volume replacement. Rapid administration of intravenous fluids. The choice of electrolyte solution depends on the patient's condition and the laboratory abnormalities identified.

With the significant laboratory abnormalities discussed, inpatient therapy is perferable to outpatient therapy until the laboratory parameters are normalized.

As in the syndrome of heat cramps, this patient's temperature will not go up.[3]

911. E. This patient has heatstroke. Heatstroke is defined as the combination of hyperpyrexia (often to 40° C or greater) and neurologic symptoms.[3] Although lack of sweating is common, it is not an absolute diagnostic criteria. Heatstroke is a medical emergency. The mortality of heatstroke may be as high as 40%.[3]

Risk factors for heatstroke include the extremes of age; cardiovascular disease; high environmental temperature and humidity; occupations such as athletes, laborers, and military recruits; pharmacologic agents including anticholinergic drugs, phenothiazines, tricyclic antidepressants, monoamine oxidase inhibitors, and inhalation anesthetics.[3]

Heatstroke usually presents abruptly, with the rapid onset of neurologic dysfunction.

The loss of the ability to sweat is one of the most important distinctions between heatstroke and the other heat syndromes. Although patients in early heatstroke usually demonstrate marked sweating, at some point the patient will lose the ability to sweat and demonstrate the characteristic hot dry skin.[3]

Hepatic, renal, and hematologic abnormalities are common in heatstroke. Hepatic failure, renal failure, and disseminated intravascular coagulation may occur.

Fluid and electrolyte abnormalities vary with the onset and duration of heatstroke, underlying disease, and the prior use of medications (especially diuretics).[3] In contradistinction to heat exhaustion, dehydration and volume depletion may not occur in heatstroke. Vigorous fluid replacement may result in pulmonary edema.[3]

Heatstroke is treated by removing all clothing, and by applying cool water to the entire skin prior to reaching the emergency department. Once in the emergency department, external, artificial cooling methods should be utilized. Hypothermia blankets, ice packs applied to the groin and axillae, ice water gastric lavage and enemas, and iced water peritoneal dialysis will lower temperature rapidly. The other system disorders associated with elevated core temperature usually improve as the temperature is lowered.[3]

SUMMARY OF THE DIAGNOSIS AND TREATMENT OF ENVIRONMENTAL INJURIES

I. **Cold injuries:**

Frostnip and Frostbite

Frostnip: superficial and reversible

Frostbite: superficial or deep (some tissue damage)

Treatment of frostnip and frostbite: immersion of extremity at 42° C for 20 minutes

Hypothermia

Hypothermia: mild (core temperature 32–35° C) or severe (less than 32° C)

Treatment of mild hypothermia: passive rewarming and active external rewarming

Treatment of severe hypothermia: active core rewarming

Remember: "No one is dead until warm and dead."[4]

Heat syndromes

Heat cramps: no disturbance of core body temperature; treatment with oral electrolyte replacement is adequate.

Heat exhaustion: characterized by volume depletion. No increase in core temperature is seen. Intravenous fluid to correct hypovolemia and electrolyte disturbances is the treatment of choice.

Heatstroke: hyperpyrexia and neurologic symptoms. Absence of sweating is characteristic. Rapid, aggressive, lowering of body temperature is the treatment of choice.

References

1. Bessen H. Hypothermia. In: Tintinalli J, Krome R, Ruiz E, eds. Emergency medicine: a comprehensive study guide. 2nd Ed. New York: McGraw-Hill, 1988; 745–747.

2. Heller B. Frostbite. In: Tintinalli J, Krome R, Ruiz E, eds. Emergency medicine: a comprehensive study guide. 2nd Ed. New York: McGraw-Hill, 1988; 748–752.

3. Vance M. Heat Emergencies. In: Tintinalli J, Krome R, Ruiz E, eds. Emergency medicine: a comprehensive study

guide. 2nd Ed. New York: McGraw-Hill, 1988; 753–756.

4. Southwick FS, Dalglish PH. Recovery after prolonged asystolic cardiac arrest in profound hypothermia. JAMA 1980; 243:1250–1253.

PROBLEM 117: A 48-YEAR-OLD FEMALE WITH A SWOLLEN ANKLE

A 48-year-old female is brought to the emergency department after having sustained an injury to her ankle. She was walking, slipped on a piece of ice on the sidewalk, and twisted her ankle. She has a significant amount of pain.

On examination, she has an acutely swollen right ankle. There is some discoloration on the lateral side of the ankle. There is limitation of plantar flexion and dorsiflexion. There is also limitation of inversion.

SELECT THE ONE BEST ANSWER TO THE FOLLOWING QUESTIONS:

912. The injury this patient most likely has is:
    a) a grade I sprain of the medial collateral ligament
    b) a grade II or III sprain of the medial collateral ligament
    c) a grade I sprain of the lateral collateral ligament
    d) a grade II or III sprain of the lateral collateral ligament
    e) a fracture of the distal fibula

913. The treatment of choice in this patient is:
    a) a plaster cast
    b) active range of motion exercises
    c) nonweight bearing, and a splint or halfcast
    d) a tensor bandage
    e) surgical repair of the ligaments

914. A 26-year-old professional football player is brought to the emergency department after being hit on the lateral side of the left knee. His knee buckled and he is now in significant pain.

    On examination, there is swelling over the medial side of the left knee. On physical examination, there is significant varus when pressure is applied to the lateral side of the left knee. The right knee is normal.

    The most likely injury in this patient is:
    a) a tear of the left lateral meniscus
    b) a tear of the left medial meniscus
    c) a tear of the left lateral collateral ligament
    d) a tear of the left medial collateral ligament
    e) a fracture of the intercondylar eminence of the left knee

915. The treatment of choice for the injury in the patient described in question 914 is:
    a) ice and elevation
    b) a halfcast
    c) a fullcast
    d) a tensor bandage
    e) surgical repair

916. A 22-year-old football player is brought into emergency after having his right leg twisted while carrying the football. As he was being tackled, he felt a sharp pain at the anteromedial aspect of the right knee joint. He was unable to straighten his knee fully, and was carried off the field by his teammates.

    On examination, there is significant swelling on the medial side of the right knee joint. As well, there is tenderness at the joint line on the medial side, limitation of the last few degrees of extension by a springy resistance, and sharp anteromedial pain when passive extension is forced.

    The most likely diagnosis in this patient is:
    a) torn right medial meniscus
    b) torn right lateral meniscus
    c) torn right medial collateral ligament
    d) torn right anterior cruciate ligament
    e) fractured patella

917. The treatment of choice for the injury to the patient described in question 916 is:
    a) nonweight bearing and a halfcast
    b) a full cast
    c) ice, elevation, and a tensor bandage
    d) arthroscopic surgery
    e) active physiotherapy

918. A 23-year-old female presents to the emergency department after being injured in a motor vehicle

accident. She complains of pain in the area of the quadriceps muscle on the right side.

On examination there is tenderness over the midportion of the right quadriceps. The area is discolored. An x-ray of the right femur is normal. There are no other injuries noted.

The correct diagnosis in this patient is:
a) right quadriceps strain
b) right quadriceps sprain
c) right quadriceps hemorrhage
d) right quadriceps avulsion
e) none of the above

919. The treatment of choice for the patient described in question 918 is:
a) surgical repair
b) a halfcast
c) a fullcast
d) ice, rest, elevation, compression
e) none of the above

ANSWERS

912. D. This patient most likely has a grade II or III sprain of the lateral collateral ligament of the right ankle.

A sprain is defined as a complete or partial tear of the ligaments occurring either within the ligaments themselves or as they are torn off at their attachement to bone. Swelling and tenderness over a ligament and pain when it is stretched suggest a sprain. Excessive motion of the joint when the ligament is stretched confirms the diagnosis. Sprains are graded according to the following criteria:

Grade I: A minor incomplete tear. The joint is tender and painful, but there is no laxity. Swelling and ecchymosis are usually minimal

Grade II: A significant incomplete tear. On physical examination, there is laxity. Swelling and ecchymosis may occur.

Grade III: Total disruption or tear of the ligament involved. No end point is felt when the joint is stressed. Swelling and ecchymosis are prominent.

The most common ankle injury is an inversion injury in which there is partial or complete disruption of the lateral collateral ligament complex.[1]

913. C. The treatment of choice in this patient is ice, elevation, nonweight bearing, and the application of a splint or halfcast. If a halfcast is applied, it should be molded into slight eversion.

This patient should be nonweight bearing for at least 3 weeks, and if there is a complete disruption of the ligament, it may take up to 6 weeks to properly heal.

A full cast is inappropriate because of the degree of swelling.

A tensor bandage does not provide enough support.

Surgical intervention is not indicated in most ankle sprains.

Active range of motion exercises at this time are inappropriate.

914. D. The most likely injury in this patient is a tear of the left medial collateral ligament. The mechanism of injury (blow to the lateral side of the left knee) plus the swelling on the medial side of the knee and the varus deformity on physical examination suggest a significant sprain of the left medial collateral ligament.[1]

915. E. The treatment of choice for a torn medial collateral ligament in a football player is surgical repair. Surgical repair is preferrable when the patient is an athlete who wishes to continue playing his sport of choice.

In other individuals, especially older individuals who are not involved in athletics, a more conservative approach may be indicated. This would include nonweight bearing, ice, a splint, and elevation of the injured extremity. Complete healing will take up to 3 months.[1]

916. A. This patient has a torn right medial meniscus.

The history of the injury is quite characteristic. Usually, a torn medial meniscus is the result of a twisting injury. The patient then falls (or is tackled) and has pain at the anteromedial aspect of the knee joint. He is unable to continue doing what he was doing, or only do it with difficulty. The knee becomes acutely swollen and there is only a sensation of "locking." This "locking" is really an inability to fully extend the knee.

On examination there is swelling on the medial side of the knee, wasting of the quadriceps (if the injury occurred some time ago), local tenderness at the joint line anteromedially, and limitation of the last few degrees of extension by a springy resistance, with sharp anterior-medial pain if passive extension is forced.

Knee sprains (grade II or III) can usually be distinguished from meniscal tears by two features: (1) varus or valgus deformity on stressing of the knee ligaments in ligamentous injuries; and (2) tenderness along the joint line in meniscal injuries.

Twisting injuries commonly also give rise to anterior cruciate ligament tears.[1]

917. D. The treatment of choice for the patient described in question 916 is arthroscopic surgery. With the arthroscope, the torn cartilage can easily be removed. Failure to remove a significant torn portion of cartilage will not only prohibit his future professional football career, but can also cause significant stress and wearing down of the articular surfaces of the knee joint.

918. A. This patient has a right quadriceps strain. A strain is an overstretching of some portion of musculature. As with sprains, every degree of strain, ranging from the overstretching of a few muscle fibers to the complete rupture of a muscle or muscle group can occur. It can occur at any site in the body.

919. D. The treatment of choice for the patient discussed in question 916 is ice, rest, elevation, and compression with a splint or tensor bandage. This should be followed by physiotherapy.

SUMMARY OF THE DIAGNOSIS AND TREATMENT OF SPRAINS AND STRAINS

1. **Sprain:**
   a) definition: a complete or partial tear of ligaments
   b) classification: grades I, II, and III
   c) most common sites: ankle (anterior fibulotalar ligament of lateral collateral ligament complex) and knee (medial, lateral, and cruciate ligaments)
   d) treatment: ankle—conservative: nonweight bearing, splint or halfcast;
   knee—surgical repair (especially if patient is young or involved in athletics

2. **Strain:**
   a) definition: overstretching of some portion of musculature. As with sprains, may range from tear of a few fibers to complete disruption.
   b) treatment:
   I: ice
   C: compression
   E: elevation
   followed by active physiotherapy

3. **Meniscal injuries of knee:** Diagnosed by swelling along injured side of knee and tenderness along joint line. Arthroscopic surgery is recommended as treatment.

Reference

1. Conolly J, Jardon O. Orthopedics in family practice. In: Rakel R (ed). Textbook of family practice. 3rd Ed. Philadelphia, PA: WB Saunders, 1984. 698–778.

PROBLEM 118: A 24-YEAR-OLD FEMALE BROUGHT INTO EMERGENCY WITH A SUSPECTED DRUG OVERDOSE

A 24-year-old female is brought into the emergency department of your local hospital with a suspected drug overdose. She was found by a friend, unconscious beside her bed, with a number of unmarked pill containers beside her. Her friend does not know any other details of her medical history.

You are called by the intern, who is on his first day on the emergency service. He asks you "what should I do now?"

SELECT THE ONE BEST ANSWER TO THE FOLLOWING QUESTIONS:

920. The first step in the management of the potential drug overdose victim is:
   a) administration of syrup of ipecac
   b) administration of naloxone
   c) administration of dextrose in water
   d) administration of activated charcoal
   e) none of the above

921. Which of the following conditions resulting in coma or altered level of consciousness can be treated quickly if recognized immediately?
   a) hypoxia
   b) hypoglycemia

c) opioid overdose
d) b and c
e) all of the above

ANSWER THE FOLLOWING QUESTIONS ACCORDING TO THE CODE:

A: 1, 2, and 3 are correct
B: 1 and 3 are correct
C: 2 and 4 are correct
D: Only 4 is correct
E: All of the above are correct

922. Which of the following is/are usually indicated in the initial assessment of the possible overdose patient?
1) history from anyone who has knowledge of the patient
2) physical examination with particular attention to vital signs and neurologic status
3) electrolytes
4) a "complete" toxicology screen

923. Which of the following is/are associated with an increased anion-gap metabolic acidosis?
1) salicylates
2) methanol
3) ethylene glycol
4) solvents

924. Which of the following statements regarding decontamination is/are true?
1) poison-specific management should be undertaken only after initial stabilization
2) syrup of ipecac is contraindicated in patients with ingestion of caustic substances or pure hydrocarbons
3) lavage is the preferred method of evacuating the stomach in patients who are unconscious
4) aspiration is not a significant problem in the decontamination of the poison victim

925. Which of the following statements regarding the use of activated charcoal for decontamination is/are true?
1) activated charcoal should follow syrup of ipecac or gastric lavage in most cases of poisoning
2) activated charcoal is usually mixed with a cathartic
3) activated charcoal may have to be delivered by lavage tube or nasogastric tube
4) the usual dose of activated charcoal is 5 g/kg

926. Which of the following statements regarding elimination of a poison is/are true?
1) pH-dependent diuresis can be useful in many situations
2) multidose activated charcoal has been abandoned as a method of effectively eliminating poisons from the body
3) hemodialysis or hemoperfusion may be useful in some cases
4) acid diuresis is a well-established form of therapy

927. Which of the following are recommended antidotes for the poisons listed?
1) acetaminophen: N-acetylcysteine
2) methanol: ethanol
3) opiates: naloxone
4) organophosphates: atropine

ANSWERS

920. E. None of the above. The first step in the management of the potential overdose victim is the assessement and support of the ABCs (airway, breathing, circulation) of life support. Before any medications are administered a secure airway should be established, respiratory and circulatory system function should be assessed and supported, and an intravenous line should be established.[1]

921. E. All of the above. The second step in the management of the potential overdose victim is the treatment of causes that can be treated effectively if recognized early. These causes include hypoxia, hypoglycemia, and opioid overdose. Therefore, all patients who present to the emergency department with altered level of consciousness should receive 2 mg of naloxone, 50 cc of 50% dextrose in water, and supplemental oxygen by Venturi mask or nasal specs. In addition, 50–100 mg of thiamine should be given to prevent Wernicke's encephalopathy in a patient who may be thiamine-depleted (an alcoholic).[1]

922. A. After you have stablized the patient, you should proceed to trying to establish the identity of the particular poison.

A physical examination with emphasis on vital signs, including temperature, and the neurologic examination should be performed as quickly as possible.

Although the patient will not be able to supply accurate (if any) information, as much information as possible should be obtained from the family, friends, the patient's physician or anyone else.

Laboratory testing should include serum electrolytes, arterial blood gases, a 12-lead electrocardiogram, an x-ray of the abdomen to look for certain radiopaque medications, and specific drug levels that may be indicated. The "routine toxicology screen" is generally inappropriate.[1]

923. E. The etiology of metabolic acidosis is dependent upon the determination of the presence or absence of a normal anion gap, which can be defined by the following formula:
Anion Gap: = Na+ - (Cl- + HCO3-)

The normal anion gap is 14 to 16. Patients who present with increased anion gap, and appear to be suffering from acute poisoning, usually have ingested toxic amounts of salicylates, methanol, ethylene glycol, iron, paraldehyde, phenformin, isoniazid, or certain solvents such as toluene.[1]

924. A. Poison-specific management should only be undertaken after initial stabilization. Syrup of ipecac (15 cc for children and 30 cc for adults) is a valuable treatment in many cases of poisoning, but should not be used in a patient in coma, a patient who has convulsions, or a patient who has ingested caustics or pure hydrocarbons.[1] Also, ipecac should be used in any situation in which the suspected substance may cause a decreased level of consciousness or seizures within the 30 to 40 minute delay period before ipecac results in vomiting.[1]

Lavage is the preferred method of ingestion decontamination in an unconscious patient. Aspiration is a complication and should be avoided by a head-down, left lateral decubitus position. The preferred solution for carrying out the lavage in adults is tepid tap water (warmed saline solution in children). The lavage should be continued until the fluid return is clear.[1]

925. A. Further decontamination with activated charcoal should usually follow emesis induced by syrup of ipecac or gastric lavage.[1]

The standard dose of activated charcoal is 1 g/kg. In the unconscious or uncompliant patient activated charcoal will have to be administered by the lavage or nasogastric tubes respectively. In the conscious patient, an aqueous suspension can be used.

Activated charcoal is usually given with a cathartic such as magnesium sulfate, magnesium

citrate, or sorbitol. to hasten bowel transit. This will hasten bowel-transit time and prevent the constipation.

Activated charcoal is as effective, if not more effective, than either gastric lavage or ipecac-induced emesis.[1]

926. B. Once a poison has been absorbed, techniques to promote its elimination from the body should be implemented. The techniques that have the greatest value are alkaline pH-dependent diuresis (alkalinization of the urine for the elimination of salicylates and phenobarbitol), multidose activated charcoal and hemodialysis and hemoprofusion.[1]

927. E. In some poison cases, specific antidote therapy is indicated. Some toxic substances and their antidotes include acetaminophen: N-acetylcysteine, methanol: ethanol, opiates: naloxone; and organophosphates: atropine.[1]

SUMMARY OF THE GENERAL MANAGMENT PRINCIPLES FOR THE OVERDOSED PATIENT

1. **Stabilization:** ABCs

2. **Drugs immediately given:** 50% dextrose, naloxone, thiamine, oxygen

3. **Assessment:** Physical examination (particular attention to vital signs and neurologic status), history (from whom ever available), and laboratory evaluation including electrolytes, arterial blood gases, 12-lead ECG, x-ray abdomen, and specific drug levels if indicated. Complete toxicology screen should only be used in select situations

4. **Decontamination:** Emesis with ipecac, gastric lavage, activated charcoal and cathartic

5. **Elimination:** pH-dependent diuresis, multidose activated charcoal, and extracorporeal removal

6. Specific antidote therapy

7. **Anticipate and treat complications:** Seizures, coma, hypotension, and hyperthermia

Reference

1. Vicas I. Management principles for the overdosed patient.
    Can Fam Physician 1988; 34: 2251–2255.

Index

Premenstrual tension syndrome, 142-145
Prostate hyperplasia, benign, 263-265
Prostate carcinoma, 263-265
Prostatitis, chronic, 276-281
Psychotherapy, 173-174
Pulmonary embolism, 19-22

R

Renal colic, 269-271
Renal failure, chronic, 102-104
Rheumatoid arthritis, 48-52
Rhinitis, allergic, 218-221
Roseola, 209-211
Rubella, 209-211
Rubeola, 209-211

S

Scarlet fever, 209-211
Screening, 304-305
Seborrheic dermatitis, infantile, 227-230
Seizures, 88-91
Sensitivity, 295-299
Short stature, child, 212-214
Sleep apnea, 189-191
Somatization disorder, 176-179
Somatoform pain disorder, 176-179
Somatoform disorders, 176-179
Specificity, 295-299
Spousal abuse, 168-170
Sprain, 324-326
Status epilepticus, 88-91
Stillbirth, 171-173
Strain, 324-326

Stroke, 22-26
Subarachnoid hemorrhage, 22-26
Suicide, 193-195
Supportive psychotherapy, 173-174

T

Teething, child, 238-240
Transient ischemia attacks, 22-26
Trauma, multiple, 314-317
Tibial torsion, child, 217-218
Tremor, benign essential, 291-294

U

Ulcer, 92-95
Ulceration, corneal, 265-269
Ulcerative colitis, 63-67
Urinary incontinence, elderly, 283-285
Urinary tract infection, elderly, 276-281
Uterine bleeding, dysfunctional, 133-136
Urticaria, 71-74

V

Vacuum extraction of fetus, 108-111
Vaginal birth after cesarian section, 115-117
Vaginismus, 186-189
Vaginitis, 151-154
Vestibular neuronitis, 258-261
Viral upper respiratory tract infection, child, 238-240

W

Warts, 261-263